Epilepsy - Update on Classification, Etiologies, Instrumental Diagnosis and Treatment

Edited by Sandro Misciagna

Published in London, United Kingdom

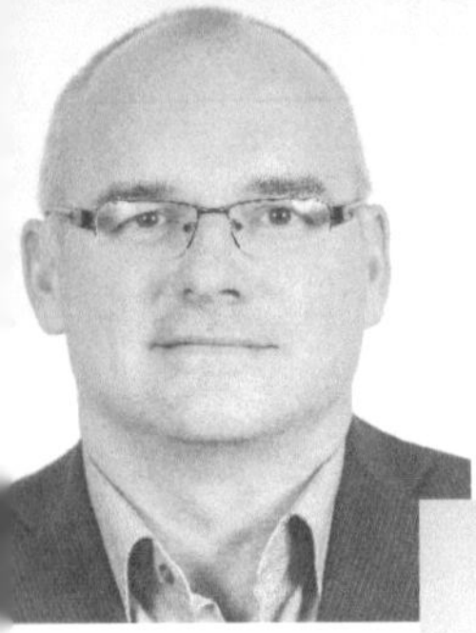
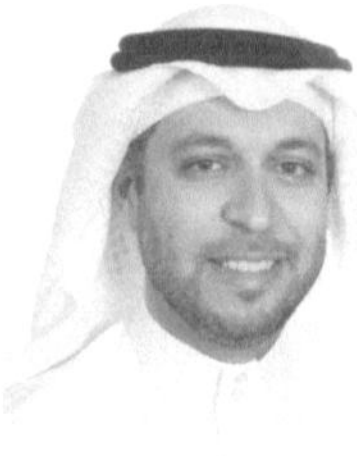
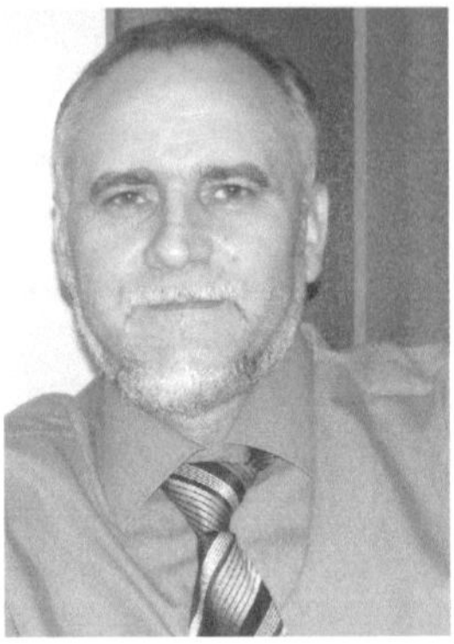
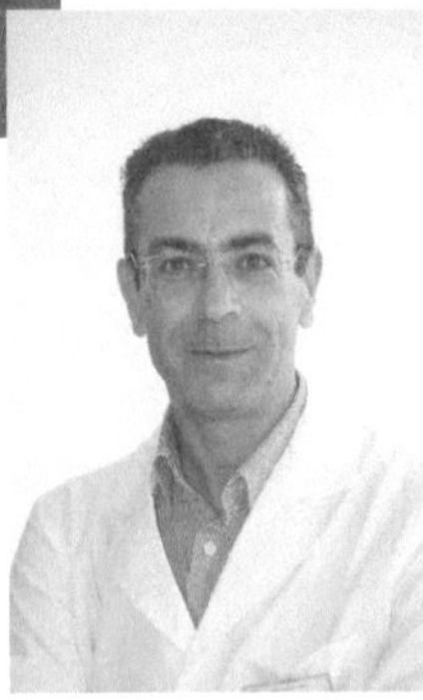
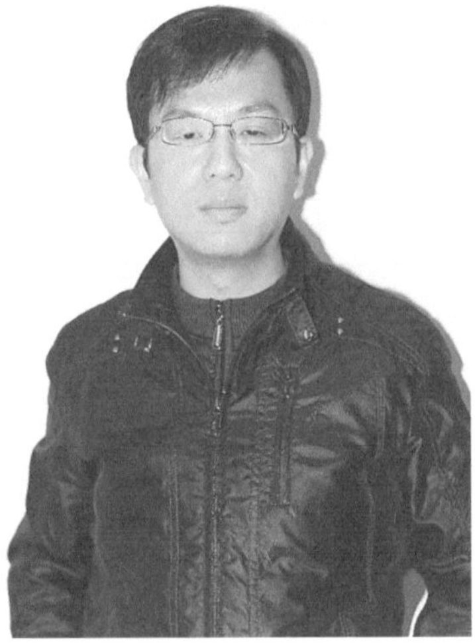
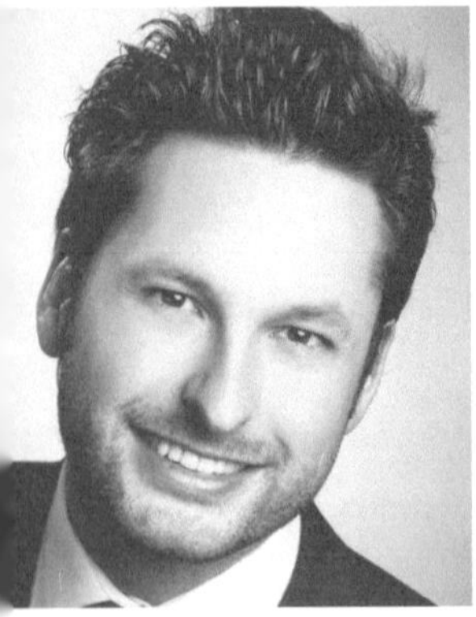
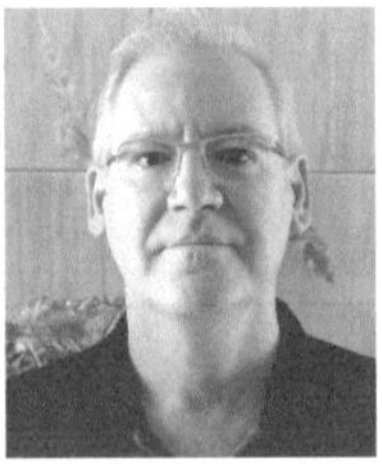

IntechOpen

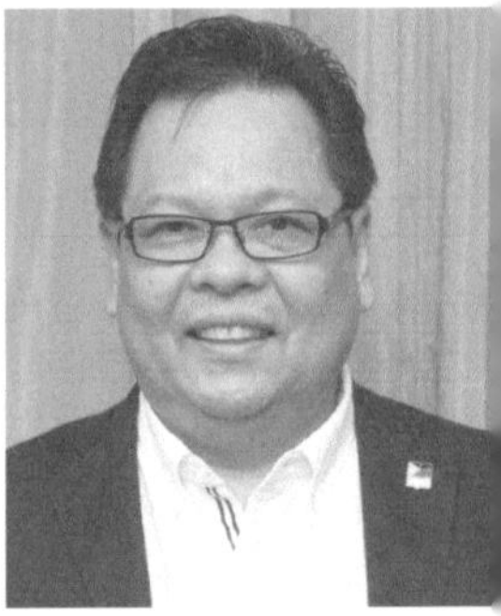
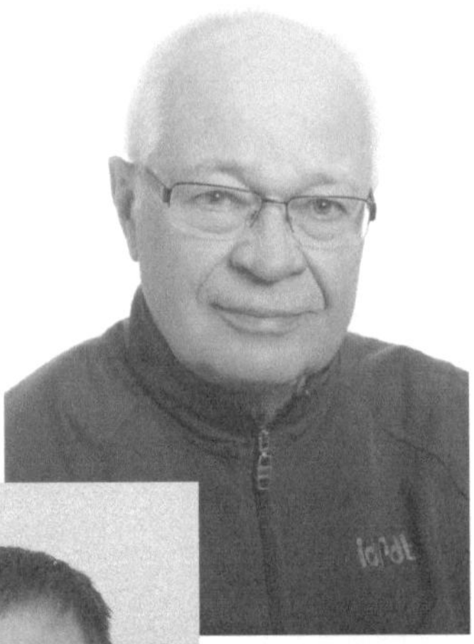
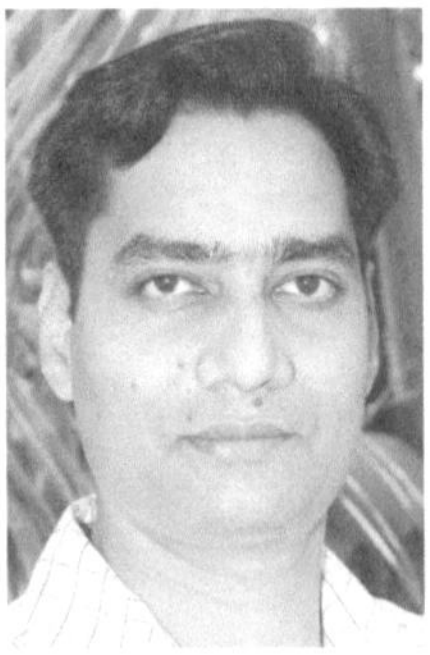
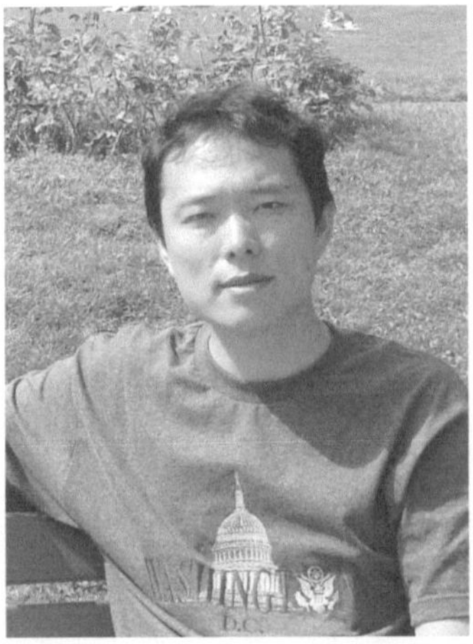
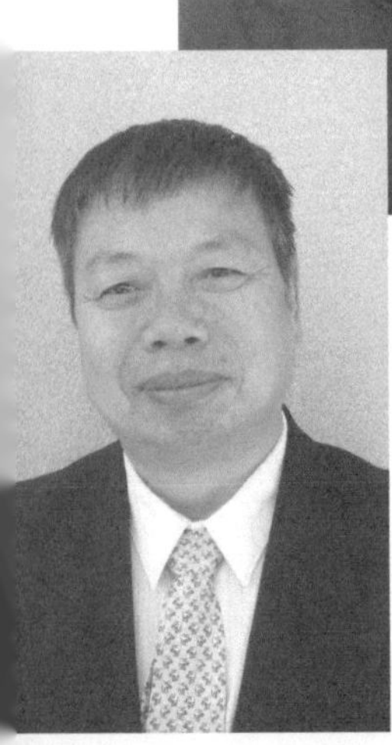
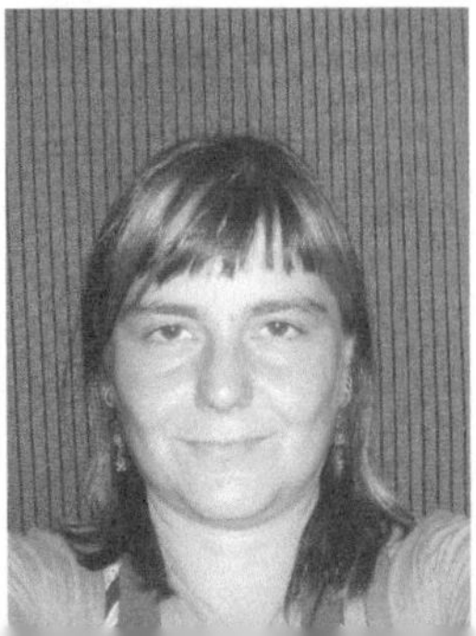

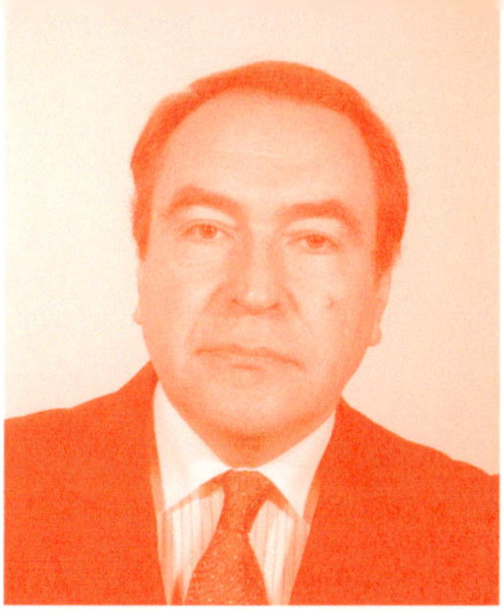
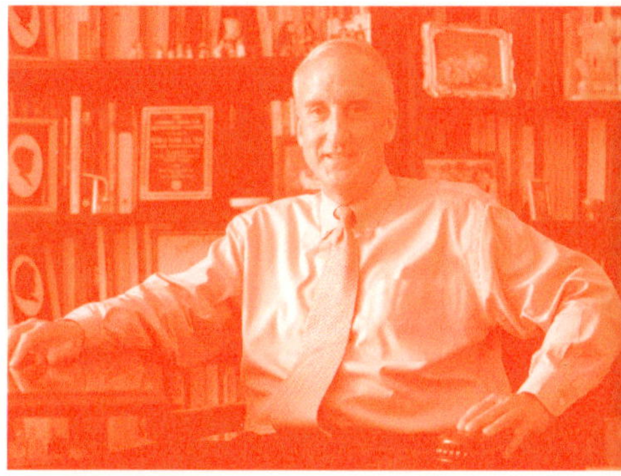
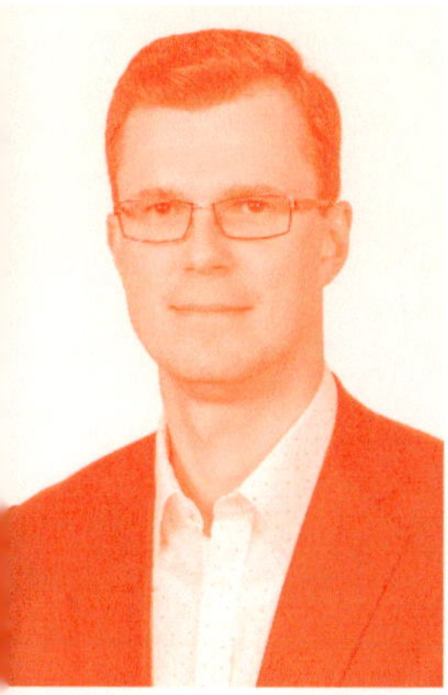
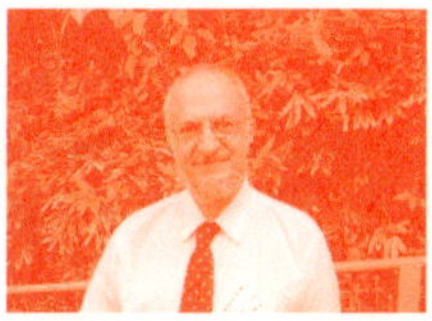
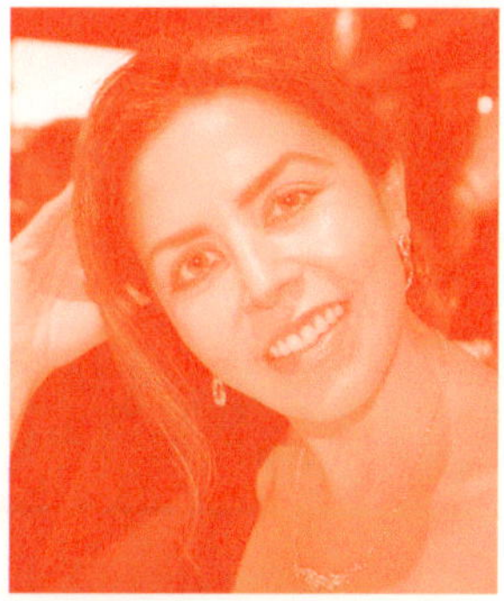

Supporting open minds since 2005

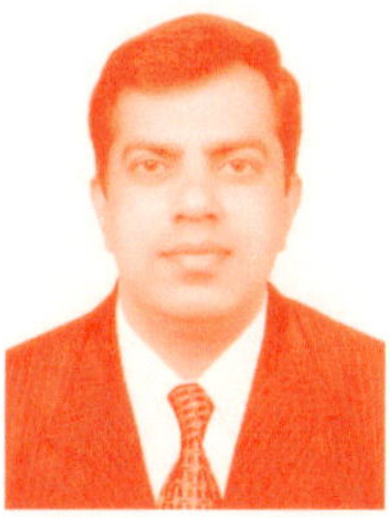
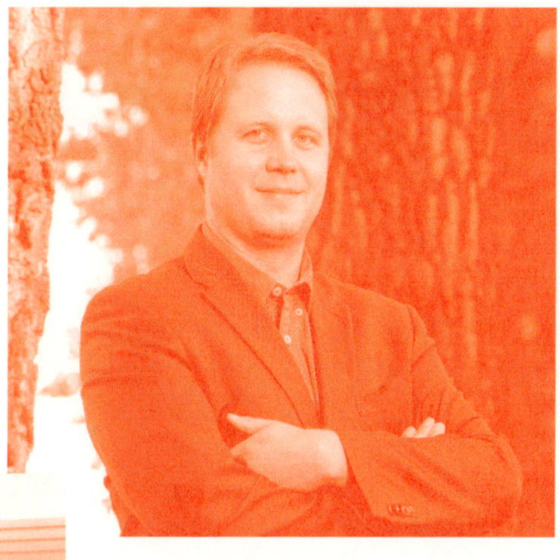
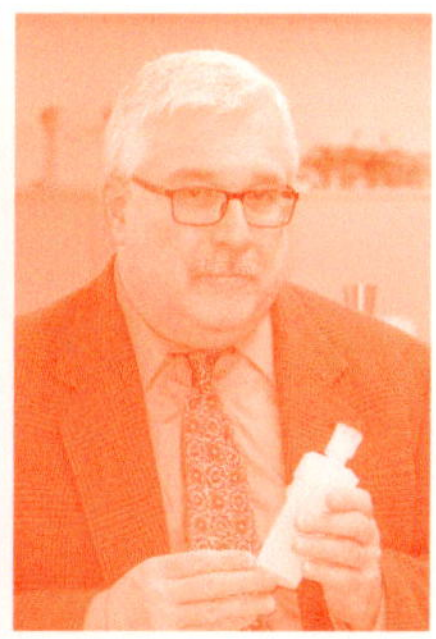
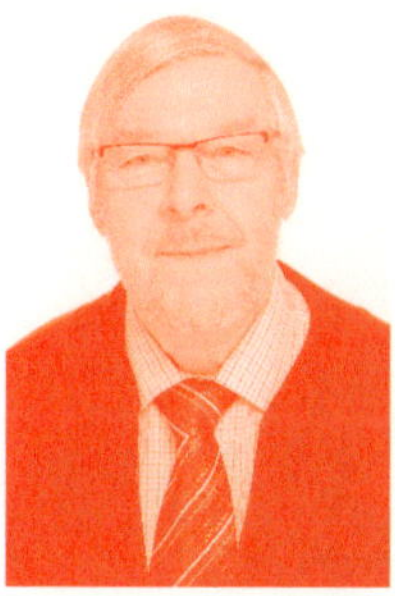
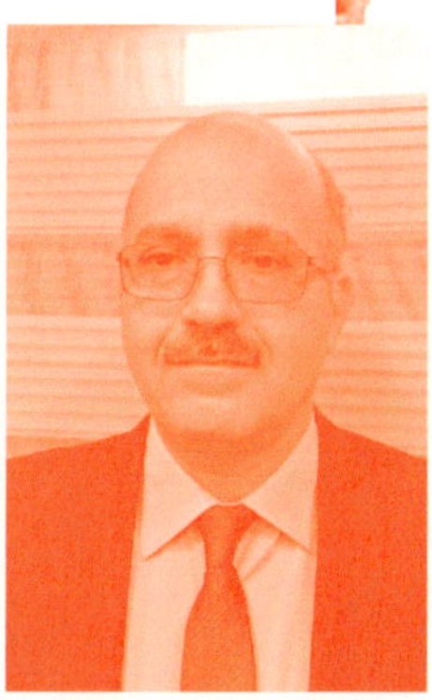
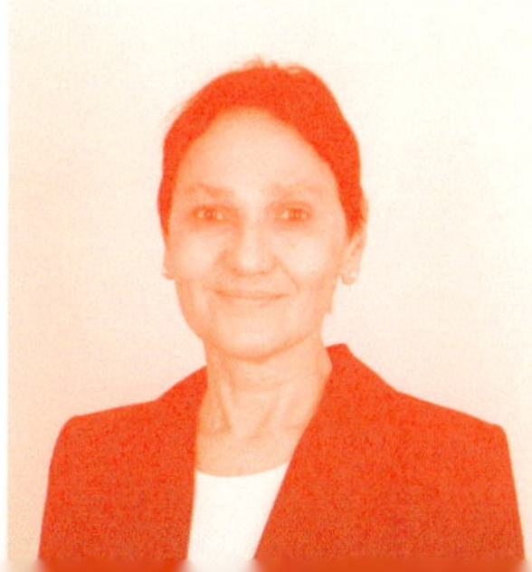
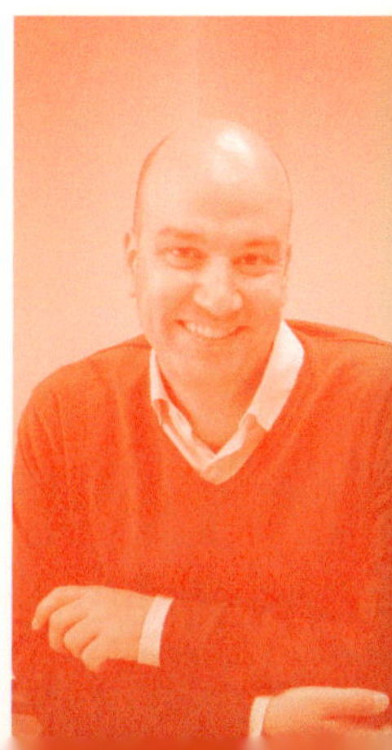

Epilepsy - Update on Classification, Etiologies, Instrumental Diagnosis and Treatment
http://dx.doi.org/10.5772/intechopen.87314
Edited by Sandro Misciagna

Contributors
Sasikumar Gurumoorthy, Naresh Babu Muppalaneni, G. Sandhya Kumari, Shaik Jakeer Hussain, Gurajapu Raja Sumant, Aydin Akan, Ozlem Karabiber Cura, Tak Lap Poon, Joseph Nelson Siewe Fodjo, Richard M. Millis, Vasavi R. Gorantla, Sabyasachi Maity, Ulviyya Guliyeva, Nana Tatishvili, Rauan Kaiyrzhanov, Katja Brückner, Kaoru Obata, Masako Kinoshita, Kazuaki Sato, Hiroya Ohara, Zhiyuan Li, Huifang Zhao, Hideki Azuma, Irma Khachidze, Mashael Omar AlKhateeb, Hesham AlDhalaan, Sandro Misciagna

First published in London, United Kingdom, 2021 by IntechOpen
IntechOpen is the global imprint of INTECHOPEN LIMITED, registered in England and Wales, registration number: 11086078, 5 Princes Gate Court, London, SW7 2QJ, United Kingdom
Printed in Croatia

British Library Cataloguing-in-Publication Data
A catalogue record for this book is available from the British Library

Additional hard and PDF copies can be obtained from orders@intechopen.com

Epilepsy - Update on Classification, Etiologies, Instrumental Diagnosis and Treatment
Edited by Sandro Misciagna
p. cm.
Print ISBN 978-1-83962-288-5
Online ISBN 978-1-83962-289-2
eBook (PDF) ISBN 978-1-83962-290-8

Meet the editor

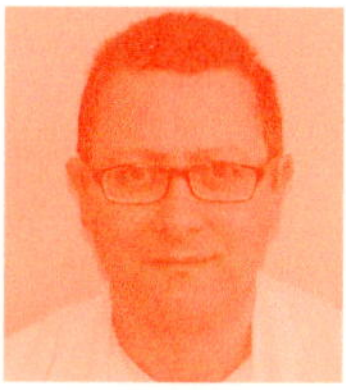

Dr. Sandro Misciagna was born in Italy in 1969. He received a degree in medicine in 1995 and another in neurology in 1999 from The Catholic University, Rome. From 1993 to 1995, he was involved in research of cerebellar functions. From 1994 to 2003, he attended the Neuropsychological department involved in research in cognitive and behavioural disorders. From 2001 to 2003, he taught neuropsychology, neurology, and cognitive rehabilitation. In 2003, he obtained a Ph.D. in Neuroscience with a thesis on the behavioural and cognitive profile of frontotemporal dementia. Dr. Misciagna has worked in various neurology departments, Alzheimer's clinics, neuropsychiatric clinics, and neuro-rehabilitative departments. In November 2016, he began working as a neurologist at Belcolle Hospital, Viterbo, where he has run the epilepsy centre since February 2019.

Contents

Preface XI

Section 1
General Definition and Classification of Epilepsy 1

Chapter 1 3
Definition, Classification, and Burden of Epilepsy
by Joseph Nelson Siewe Fodjo

Chapter 2 17
Epileptic EEG Classification by Using Advanced Signal Decomposition Methods
by Ozlem Karabiber Cura and Aydin Akan

Section 2
Etiologies of Epilepsy and Epileptic Syndromes 37

Chapter 3 39
Rolandic Epilepsy: Self-Limited Epilepsy with Centrotemporal Spikes
by Ulviyya Guliyeva, Nana Nino Tatishvili and Rauan Kaiyrzhanov

Chapter 4 61
Review in Autism and Epilepsy
by Mashael AlKhateeb and Hesham AlDhalaan

Chapter 5 69
Cerebrovascular Disease; A Leading Cause of Epilepsy
by Kaoru Obata, Kazuaki Sato, Hiroya Ohara and Masako Kinoshita

Section 3
Neurophysiological Techniques to Study Epilepsy and Epileptic Seizures 93

Chapter 6 95
Clinical Applications of Brain Mapping in Epilepsy
by Sandro Misciagna

Chapter 7 109
Is EEG a Useful Examination Tool for Diagnosis of Epilepsy and Comorbid Psychiatric Disorders?
by Hideki Azuma

Chapter 8 127
EEG Signal Denoising Using Haar Transform and Maximal Overlap Discrete Wavelet Transform (MODWT) for the Finding of Epilepsy
by Sasikumar Gurumoorthy, Naresh Babu Muppalaneni and G. Sandhya Kumari

Chapter 9 135
Epileptic Seizure Prediction
by Shaik Jakeer Hussain and Gurajapu Raja Sumant

Chapter 10 151
The Dynamic of EEG Characteristics in Epileptic Children during the Treatment with Valproic Acid
by Irma Khachidze

Section 4
Pharmacological, Surgical and Experimental Therapies for Epilepsy 161

Chapter 11 163
Cognitive and Psychological Side Effects of Antiepileptic Drugs
by Katja Eva Brückner

Chapter 12 175
Challenges Related to Epilepsy Management in Sudan, an Example of Low-Middle Income Country
by Ismat Babiker, Awab Saad, Basil Ibrahim and Mohamed Abdelsadig

Chapter 13 187
Presurgical Evaluation of Epilepsy Surgery
by Tak Lap Poon

Chapter 14 205
Pyramid Exploration Intervention, Environmental Enrichment, Aerobic Swimming Exercise and Brain Neuroplasticity in the Kainate Rat Model of Temporal Lobe Epilepsy
by Vasavi R. Gorantla, Sabyasachi Maity and Richard M. Millis

Chapter 15 219
Current Status and Potential Challenges of Cell-Based Therapy for Treating Status Epilepticus and Chronic Epilepsy
by Huifang Zhao and Zhiyuan Li

Preface

A seizure is the manifestation of an abnormal, hypersynchronous discharge of a population of cortical neurons that may produce subjective symptoms or objective signs, in which case it is a clinical seizure.

Clinical seizures are usually classified according to the International Classification of Epileptic Seizures proposed by the International League Against Epilepsy (ILAE), which is the best one currently available. This classification introduces different levels of classification with respect to the semiological mode of onset (focal, generalized, or unknown), physical manifestations (motor, non-motor, or unknown), etiologies (structural, genetic, infectious, metabolic, immune, unknown), state of consciousness, and possible evolution to a bilateral tonic-clonic seizure.

The incidence of new-onset seizures in the general population is approximately 80 per 100,000 per year; approximately 60 percent of these patients will have epilepsy.

The diagnosis of a particular seizure type, and of a specific type of epileptic syndrome, directs the clinical diagnosis of these patients and their initial therapy.

Some types of epilepsy are more common in children, such as Self-limited Epilepsy with Centro Temporal Spikes (SECTS) also known as Rolandic epilepsy. SECTS is quite common in children: 15%–25% of all epileptic syndromes are diagnosed between the ages of 5 and 15 years, with a peak around 6 years. In children, it is common to find an association between epilepsy and neurodevelopmental disorders such as autism. Autistic disorders are common in children with genetic anomalies including Rett syndrome, fragile X syndrome, tuberous sclerosis, Potocki-Lupski syndrome, Smith-Lemli-Opitz syndrome, and cortical dysplasia. About 30 percent of autistic patients have epileptic anomalies in electroencephalography (EEG) registrations. The relation between autism and epilepsy can probably be explained by the existence of common neural networks characterized with alterations in subcortical systems or basal ganglia-substantia nigra connectivity. Other studies show evidence of dysfunction in cerebral neuroreceptors such as glutamate receptors, serotonin receptor 2A, and GABA-A receptors; for example, excessive glutamatergic activity is associated with epileptiform activity.

In adults, secondary forms of epilepsy are frequent after cerebrovascular insults such as cerebral infarction, intracerebral hemorrhage, and subarachnoid hemorrhage. In this case it is especially important to distinguish between early seizures and late seizures, since the former are more indicative of symptomatic seizures, while the latter could be a signal of post-stroke epilepsy and thus should be treated with specific antiepileptic drugs.

In the last two decades, enormous advances have occurred in the understanding of epilepsy. Techniques such as EEG, neuroimaging, neurosurgery, and neuropsychology are giving us a better understanding of the mechanisms of the pathogenesis of epilepsy.

EEG is the gold standard for diagnosis of epilepsy and a useful examination, especially when epileptic abnormalities emerge as paroxysmal activities or typical epileptic grapho-elements. EEG is an instrument for monitoring the course of the disease and the efficacy of treatment. EEG is useful for investigating epilepsy especially in combination with rating scales and clinical examination.

Recent EEG techniques have allowed automatic detection of epileptic seizures, classification of EEG signals, and distinguishing seizures and pre-seizures. Techniques consisting of quantitative analysis of EEG have been potentially used in spike detection, localization of epileptic focus, and determination of the type of epilepsy. EEG evaluation can determine antiepileptic drug efficacy in the management of epileptic children.

Additionally, major developments are taking place in the laboratories of scientists studying genetics, embryogenesis, neuropathology, neurochemistry, and pharmacology. These advances provide a much better understanding of why patients develop epilepsy, improving the way in which epileptic patients are cared for.

This book discusses the pharmacological treatment of epilepsy with older antiepileptic drugs (e.g., phenobarbital, carbamazepine, phenytoin, valproate) as well as newer drugs (e.g., topiramate, zonisamide, levetiracetam, lamotrigine, lacosamide, perampanel), neurosurgical treatments, and treatments based on the use of stem cells. Pharmacological approaches sometimes cause side effects such as dizziness, nausea, headache, and diplopia. Antiepileptic drugs (AEDs) can potentially interfere with other drugs in the treatment of special groups of patients such as children or women (increased risk of teratogenicity). One of the most common side effects of AEDs are cognitive disorders that adversely affect information processing, reaction times, and levels of concentration. Cognitive side effects are more common with older drugs and can be identified via neuropsychological examinations by experienced neuropsychologists. Strategies to reduce cognitive side effects include using monotherapies, slowly increasing medication dose, and considering the quality of life and performances of patients.

The surgical approach to epilepsy can be proposed in patients with drug-resistant epilepsy, a condition that affects about 30 percent of patients. When treating these patients, it is important to consider the potential cause of drug resistance as an inappropriate choice of AEDs or problems of poor compliance, often considered as "pseudoresistence." Surgical candidates must be evaluated by neurophysiology techniques (interictal EEG, video EEG), structural imaging (MRI protocols, diffusion tensor imaging, PET, SPECT, fMRI, MEG), neuropsychological assessment (eventually associated with WADA test of fMRI), psychiatric assessment, and invasive studies (invasive EEG monitoring, use of subdural electrodes, intracerebral electrodes, epidural electrodes, foramen ovale electrodes). A neurosurgical approach may involve curative surgery (e.g., callosotomy, hemispherectomy) or modulatory surgery (deep brain stimulation, vague nerve stimulation, gamma knife radiosurgery). Stem cell therapies are promising for epilepsy. Mesenchymal stem cell (MSC) therapy was discovered for the first time in 1966, but only in 2007 was it suggested for use in epilepsy, after evidence that cytokines and other factors secreted by MSCs could stimulate endogenous protection and recovery response. Approaches based on stem cell transplantation can use different sites of administration (endovenous, intraperitoneally, intra-hippocampal transplantation) and with different measures of investigation (electrophysiological, behavioral task, the study of GABA levels, histopathological investigations, immunohistochemically essay).

Neural stem cells or neural progenitor cells have the potential for use in temporal lobe epilepsy, which accounts for approximately 40 percent of all epilepsy cases. Models of stem cell transplantation using different sites of administration (intravenous, intraperitoneal) seem to show positive effects such as anticonvulsant effects, changes in the anatomy of the epileptic hippocampus, and micro-changes in neural circuitry.

Sandro Misciagna
Neurology Department,
Belcolle Hospital,
Viterbo, Italy

Section 1

General Definition and Classification of Epilepsy

Chapter 1

Definition, Classification, and Burden of Epilepsy

Joseph Nelson Siewe Fodjo

Abstract

Epilepsy is one of the most common neurological diseases in the world, and is characterized by recurrent unprovoked seizures (fits) that can occur at all ages. The causes of epilepsy are multiple, ranging from perinatal problems, traumatic brain insults, metabolic abnormalities, to infections of the central nervous system; sometimes, the causes are not known. Consensual international norms have been established for the proper diagnosis and management of epilepsy, including specificities for vulnerable populations such as children and pregnant women. Specific emphasis must be laid on low and middle income countries, where about 80% of all persons with epilepsy reside. In such resource-limited settings, epilepsy patients are often confronted with sub-optimal care, reduced access to treatment, and frequent epilepsy complications. Early epilepsy diagnosis and proper anti-epileptic treatment usually result in satisfactory seizure control, and enable persons with epilepsy to lead a normal life. Besides the usual medications, psychosocial support and stigma reducing interventions are crucial to improve the quality of life of affected persons and their families.

Keywords: epilepsy, seizure, epidemiology, etiology, management

1. Introduction

Epilepsy is a chronic disease of the brain estimated to affect 50 million people worldwide according to World Health Organization (WHO) [1]. It is characterized by repetitive, unprovoked epileptic seizures which vary widely in their clinical presentations. Although a meticulous patient history complemented by sound clinical/paraclinical investigations often unveil the underlying cause of epilepsy, the exact etiology remains unknown in about half of cases [2]. Proper diagnosis and treatment of epilepsy are paramount to achieve seizure control and ensure an optimal quality of life for affected individuals.

1.1 Definition of epilepsy

In 2005, the International League Against Epilepsy (ILAE) defined epilepsy as "a disorder of the brain characterized by an enduring predisposition to generate epileptic seizures, and by the neurobiologic, cognitive, psychological, and social consequences of this condition" [3]. An epileptic seizure, on the other hand, refers to "a transient occurrence of signs and/or symptoms due to abnormal excessive or synchronous neuronal activity in the brain" [3]. While these definitions remain very conceptual, they are difficult to apply in a real-life clinical setting. Therefore, a Task Force was commissioned to formulate an operational definition of epilepsy; the definition of epilepsy was thus broadened to accommodate three practical circumstances (**Box 1**) [4].

Epilepsy is a disease of the brain defined by any of the following conditions:

- At least two unprovoked (or reflex) seizures occurring >24 h apart
- One unprovoked (or reflex) seizure and a probability of further seizures similar to the general recurrence risk (at least 60%) after two unprovoked seizures, occurring over the next 10 years
- Diagnosis of an epilepsy syndrome

Epilepsy is considered to be resolved for individuals who had an age-dependent epilepsy syndrome but are now past the applicable age or those who have remained seizure-free for the last 10 years, with no seizure medicines for the last 5 years.

Box 1.
Operational (practical) clinical definition of epilepsy [4].

Emphasis must be laid on some points in this operational definition. Firstly, the seizures must be unprovoked, and not as a result of an acute, punctual event such as head trauma, substance abuse/withdrawal, metabolic imbalance, infection of the central nervous system or fever. As concerns the minimal risk of recurrence fixed at 60%, it is merely approximative of the likelihood of future seizure (mostly based on paraclinical findings on the electroencephalogram (EEG) or brain imaging [5]) and should not be interpreted as an absolute cut-off [4]. Another point to note is the minimal time difference of 24 hours between the seizures, but without a maximum time interval; in practice, the ILAE maintains the lifetime occurrence of two unprovoked seizures as a diagnostic criterion for epilepsy. Finally, epilepsy syndromes have been elaborately documented by the ILAE; each syndrome is characterized by specific electroclinical and/or genetic features [6].

1.2 Diagnosis of epilepsy

The diagnosis of epilepsy is essentially clinical. Based on the criteria listed in **Box 1**, the epilepsy diagnosis can be made if an individual fulfills the ILAE criteria. In a hospital setting, the following paraclinical workups can be performed to further investigate the epilepsy diagnosis: EEG, brain imaging (by scan or magnetic resonance), and blood tests (to investigate metabolic or genetic epilepsies).

In field research settings, the ILAE recommends epilepsy assessment using a door-to-door approach [7]. Several tools have been developed for epilepsy screening during epilepsy studies [8–11]; for studies conducted in the sub-Saharan setting in particular, the Institute of Neurological Epidemiology and Tropical Neurology of Limoges (France) developed a questionnaire with the support of the Pan-African Association of Neurological Sciences and the ILAE (Commission on Tropical Diseases, 1993–1997) [11]. This questionnaire was validated in Mauritania (sensitivity: 95.1%; specificity: 65.6%) and has since then been widely used for epilepsy surveys in Africa [11]. It has the advantages of being brief, usable by non-physicians, and diagnosing seizure types other than generalized tonic-clonic episodes (for instance, absences and focal seizures). To ensure accurate outcomes, it is important that a neurologist or physician trained in epilepsy confirms all suspected epilepsy cases clinically, following the ILAE diagnostic criteria.

1.3 Epidemiology and burden of epilepsy

Although epilepsy occurs in a ubiquitous manner, its burden is unevenly spread in different regions of the world depending on the local distribution of risk factors, access to treatment, and population demography. A recent meta-analysis found an overall lifetime prevalence of epilepsy of 7.60 per 1000 population (95% CI 6.17–9.38); this was higher in low and middle income countries (LMICs) (8.75 per 1000; 95% CI 7.23–10.59) than in high income countries (5.18 per 1000; 95% CI 3.75–7.15) [12]. A similar pattern was observed regarding epilepsy incidence: it was higher in LMICs compared to high-income countries, 139.0 per 100,000 person years (95% CI 69.4–278.2) vs. 48.9 per 100,000 person years (95% CI 39.0–61.1) [12].

These numbers clearly demonstrate that epilepsy poses a greater problem among populations living in LMICs compared to those in industrialized countries [2]. Indeed, nearly 80% of the global burden of epilepsy occurs in the people living in LMICs [1]. In sub-Saharan Africa specifically, a median epilepsy prevalence of 14.2 per 1000 (IQR 8·0–33·2) was documented, with over 90% of cases being younger than 20 years [13]. Annual epilepsy incidence was also high, reaching 81.7 per 100,000. Mortality was greatest in the 18–24 years age group, suggesting a relatively low life expectancy among persons with epilepsy (PWE) in Africa [13]. Suggested explanations for this pattern include the epilepsy risk factors that are often reported in resource-poor settings such as perinatal brain insults, traumatic head injury and infections of the central nervous system [13]. A variable genetic predisposition to manifest seizures in different populations may also explain the regional disparities observed in the occurrence of epilepsy worldwide, as people of different ethnic origins within a given population were found to have different incidence rates for epilepsy [14].

According to the 2016 Global Burden of Disease Collaborators, epilepsy accounted for >13 million Disability Adjusted Life Years (DALYs – a measure of the number of years of healthy life lost to epilepsy within a given population), and was responsible for 0.5% of the total disease burden in 2016 [15]. Again, important geographical differences were noted with epilepsy ranking among the top five neurological diseases in low-income regions. That study also found significant reductions in mortality and DALY among PWE between 1990 and 2016, reflecting some improvement in epilepsy healthcare and treatment.

2. Seizure/epilepsy classification and etiologies

International standards and norms have been adopted to classify seizures and epilepsies.

2.1 Classification of seizures

In 2017, the ILAE released the most recent guidelines for classifying seizures and epilepsies [5, 6, 16, 17]. Seizure classification begins with the mode of onset, whether focal or generalized [16]; the onset may also be unknown if the patient/caregiver does not recall the details of the initial seizure manifestations. Focal-onset seizures are further categorized into two depending on the state of consciousness during any part of the seizure: retained awareness versus impaired awareness (**Figure 1**) [16]. Irrespective of whether the onset is focal or generalized, seizures are grouped based on their physical manifestations as being motor (visible external movements) or non-motor (**Figure 1**). There is also a special group for focal

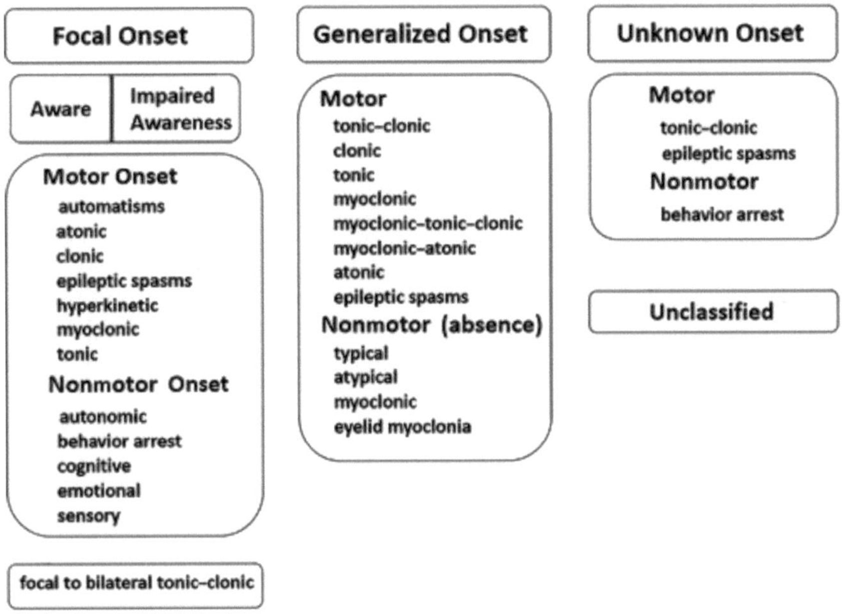

Figure 1.
ILAE 2017 classification of seizure types (extended version) [16] (used with permission).

onset seizures which evolve to generalized seizures, known as focal to bilateral tonic-clonic seizures [16]. Of note, absence seizures are considered as generalized non-motor seizures [16]. However, in case some seizure descriptions do not appropriately fit into any of these categories, they can be considered as "unclassified".

2.2 Classification of epilepsies

For epilepsies, the classification starts with the seizure type [6], and the certainty that the nature of the seizure(s) justifies the diagnosis of epilepsy [4]. Patients who do not meet criteria for epilepsy (for example, a single seizure or repeated provoked seizures) should be classified as to a seizure type, but classification should stop there [5]. Once the epilepsy diagnosis is confirmed, the epilepsy type can be deduced as focal, generalized, combined generalized & focal, or unknown (**Figure 2**) [6]. The epilepsy type is decided mainly on clinical grounds, and the diagnosis may be supported by EEG findings [6]. The final (facultative) level in epilepsy classification is the epilepsy syndrome diagnosis; an epilepsy syndrome refers to a cluster of features incorporating seizure types, EEG results, and brain imaging features that tend to occur together [6]. Each epilepsy syndrome often has specific features such as age at onset and remission (where applicable), seizure triggers, diurnal variation, and sometimes prognosis. Distinctive co-morbidities such as intellectual and psychiatric abnormalities may also be associated with specific epilepsy syndromes, as has been observed with the nodding syndrome [18]. Other common epilepsy syndromes include: Childhood Absence Epilepsy, Juvenile Absence Epilepsy, Juvenile Myoclonic Epilepsy, and Generalized Tonic-Clonic Seizures Alone; these are all forms of idiopathic generalized epilepsies [6]. Classification of epilepsy into syndromes often has etiologic, prognostic, and treatment implications [6].

A new feature in the 2017 epilepsy classification is that it integrates an etiology component as well as co-morbidities in epilepsy (**Figure 2**). Six etiological axes were enumerated by the ILAE task force: structural, genetic, infectious, metabolic,

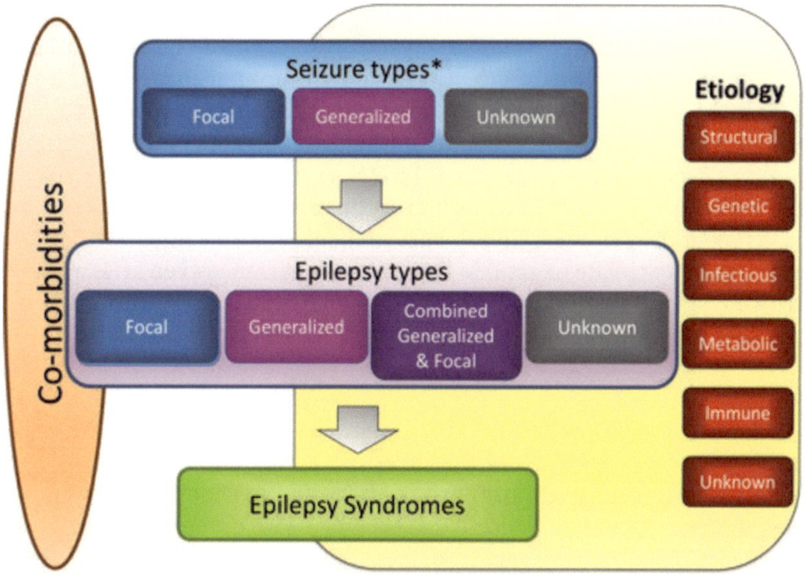

Figure 2.
ILAE framework for the classification of epilepsies [6] (used with permission).

immune, and unknown etiologies. Co-morbidities which should be considered on a case-by-case basis when diagnosing/classifying epilepsy include: intellectual decline, psychiatric and behavioral abnormalities, psychosocial problems, sleep disorders, and motor deficits [6].

2.3 Epilepsy etiologies

2.3.1 Structural etiologies

These are caused by structural brain abnormalities which have been shown to substantially increase the risk of developing epilepsy. These abnormalities are usually detectable by neuroimaging and in association with electroclinical assessments, lead to a reasonable inference that they are responsible for the enduring predisposition to unprovoked seizures [3, 6]. Structural etiologies could be primitive (for instance congenital malformations), or acquired (from a stroke, head trauma, infection, hypoxic-ischemic encephalopathy) [6].

2.3.2 Genetic etiologies

Epilepsy etiology is considered as genetic if there exists a specific disease-causing variant in a gene or copy number variant, believed to be the explanation for the observed epileptogenicity [5]. Of note, genetic mutations are not always inherited, as several epileptogenic de novo mutations have been identified [6]. The genetic alteration often causes a very heterogeneous phenotypic spectrum. A few genetic epilepsies identified to date include: the syndrome of Benign Familial Neonatal Epilepsy (KCNQ2 or KCNQ3 mutations) [19] and the Dravet syndrome (SCN1A mutations) [20].

2.3.3 Infectious etiologies

These are the most common preventable causes of epilepsy, particularly in sub-Saharan Africa [13, 21]. The concept of an infectious etiology is that the epilepsy directly results from a known infection in which seizures are a core symptom [6]; it is the persistence of these seizures even after resolution of the acute infection that is referred to as epilepsy of infectious origin. Common examples of infectious etiologies include neurocysticercosis, tuberculosis, HIV, cerebral malaria, subacute sclerosing panencephalitis, cerebral toxoplasmosis, and congenital infections such as Zika virus and cytomegalovirus [6, 22]. A recent cohort study supports the addition of onchocerciasis to this list, as the more infected participants had an increased risk of developing epilepsy later in life [23]. These infections sometimes have a structural correlate to explain the seizure recurrence even after anti-infectious treatment; this results in a substantial overlap with the acquired structural causes of epilepsy [5].

2.3.4 Metabolic etiologies

In some cases, the core cause of the epilepsy results from a metabolic derangement. Clinical entities such as porphyria, uremia, aminoacidopathies, or pyridoxine-dependent seizures all fall within this category. These conditions may also be associated with a pre-existing genetic defect, although a few can be acquired such as cerebral folate deficiency [6].

2.3.5 Immune etiologies

There are a rising number of persons in whom the epilepsy is caused by an autoimmune condition, as evidenced by an autoimmune-mediated central nervous system inflammation [6]. Examples include anti-NMDA (N-methyl-D-aspartate) receptor encephalitis and anti-LGI1 encephalitis [24]. The anti-leimodin antibodies hypothesis for central nervous system damage would equally place Nodding syndrome in this category [25].

2.3.6 Unknown etiology

For many PWE, the exact etiology may not be known. In such cases, diagnosis and management are solely based on electroclinical findings [6]. Nevertheless in some settings, epidemiological observations may provide clues as to a possible epilepsy etiology within a given vicinity. For instance, a pooled analysis of 37 studies showed that the etiologic fraction of epilepsy was estimated to be 63.0% (95% CI: 61.4 ± 64.5) in persons exposed to cysticercosis [26]. Therefore, in cysticercosis-endemic settings, it would be reasonable to assume that a considerable number of epilepsy cases are due to neurological complications of *Taenia solium* infection even without laboratory confirmation. Similarly, in onchocerciasis-endemic villages of Cameroon, the contribution of infection with *O. volvulus* to epilepsy was very high (population-attributable fraction: 91.7%, 95% CI 56.7–98.4; p = 0.0021) [23]. Hence in communities with proven high ongoing transmission of *O. volvulus*, many epilepsies of "unknown" etiology could as well be caused by onchocerciasis.

3. Epilepsy management in specific settings

About four fifth of PWE currently reside in LMICs where epilepsy care is often sub-optimal, resulting in a 75% treatment gap (proportion of PWE needing treatment who do not receive the necessary anti-epileptic drugs) [1]. It is therefore important to discuss epilepsy in these contexts, and propose ways to improve PWE management in such settings. Another special population worth looking into is the women of reproductive age suffering from epilepsy. The risk with these women is the teratogenic effects of anti-epileptic drugs, which renders their management before, during, and after pregnancy quite delicate.

3.1 Managing epilepsy in resource-limited settings

Improved management of PWE in resource-limited settings may be achieved by decentralizing epilepsy care. Approaches to diagnose and manage epilepsy and related complications can be simplified and taught to non-physicians, who will be in charge of running local epilepsy clinics under the supervision of physicians or specialists [27, 28]. Setting up a community-based epilepsy surveillance system will enable early diagnosis and treatment of PWE thereby preventing complications. To reduce the treatment gap, a regular supply of subsidized anti-epileptic drugs (AEDs) appropriate for different seizure types should be instituted. Daily intake of the adequate AEDs would eventually achieve seizure control in at least 70% of PWE [1]. The first-line AEDs that are routinely used in sub-Saharan Africa include phenobarbital, carbamazepine, phenytoin, and valproate [29]. Their indications and prescribed dosages as recommended by the WHO are detailed in **Table 1** [30]. AED treatment must be initiated as monotherapy with progressive dose increase based on the response to the treatment and seizure control. Phenobarbital, the most available and affordable AED (annual cost per PWE: 5 US dollars [29]), is used as first-line treatment for most seizure types but is not recommended for absences. It is usually initiated at 2–3 mg/kg/day and could be increased every 2–3 weeks by 15 mg if seizures continue, without going above the maximal recommended dose. When switching to another AED, phenobarbital should be tapered progressively (15 mg reduction every 2 weeks) while starting the newly prescribed AED as soon as the tapering begins. This approach minimizes the risk of rebound seizures upon stopping phenobarbital [31].

Besides the AEDs in **Table 1** which are commonly used in resource-limited settings, newer AEDs have been developed and are widely used in high-income countries; these include: gabapentin (GBP), topiramate (TPM), lamotrigine (LTG), levetiracetam (LEV), rufinamide (RFN), vigabatrin (VGB), oxcarbazepine (OXC), perampanel (PER), lacosamide (LCM) and eslicarbazepine acetate [36]. Although these are more expensive and less available in LMICs compared to the routine first-line AEDs, they are superior in achieving seizure control with relatively less side effects and fewer drug interactions.

Another essential component of epilepsy care in resource-limited settings is stigma reduction. In rural communities of Africa, PWE and their families are often stigmatized as a result of misconceptions regarding the origin and transmissibility of epilepsy [37]. Therefore, it is important that community awareness programs on epilepsy, as well as other interventions should be implemented to reduce stigma and facilitate the social rehabilitation of PWE [38].

3.2 Epilepsy in women of child-bearing age

In addition to seizures and related complications experienced by all PWE, women with epilepsy (WWE) require a more comprehensive management strategy that takes into account reproductive health needs [39]. Indeed, optimal seizure control is recommended to ensure positive health and gestational outcomes for these women. However, most of the first-line AED routinely used in Africa (**Table 1**) may reduce the efficacy of hormonal contraceptives [40] or increase the risk for foetal malformations if taken during pregnancy [41]. Therefore, a tailored management approach is recommended for WWE and should include

Drug	Indication and frequency of use	Required dosage		Remark
		Children	Adults	
Phenobarbital	Recommended by WHO as first line AED for most seizure types, except absences; cheap and readily available [30, 32]. Used by 74.6% of PWE [33].	Given once or twice daily Starting dose: 2–3 mg/kg/day Maintenance: 3–6 mg/kg/day	Given once daily Starting dose: 60 mg/day Maintenance: 60–180 mg/day	Steady state reached after 14–21 days. Possible side effects: Drowsiness, skin rash, lethargy and hyperactivity in children, hepatic failure, Stevens Johnson syndrome
Carbamazepine	Indicated for focal seizures, and could be used in generalized convulsive seizures [31]. Used by 27.4% of PWE [33]	Given twice daily Starting dose: 5 mg/kg/day Maintenance: 10–30 mg/kg/day	Given twice daily Starting dose: 100–200 mg/day Maintenance: 400–1400 mg/day	Steady state reached in 8 days. Possible side effects: allergic skin reactions, bone marrow suppression with long-term use, blurred vision, diplopia, ataxia, nausea. Contraindicated in absences and myoclonus [31]
Phenytoin	Indicated for treating some generalized seizures and status epilepticus [34]. Used by 22.2% of PWE [33]	Given once/twice daily Starting dose: 3–4 mg/kg/day Maintenance: 3–8 mg/kg/day (max 300 mg daily)	Given once or twice daily Starting dose: 150–200 mg/day Maintenance: 200–400 mg/day	Possible side effects: drowsiness, ataxia, slurred speech, motor twitching and mental confusion, coarsening of facial features, hepatitis, gum hyperplasia, hirsutism, skin reaction including Stevens Johnson syndrome
Valproate	Broad spectrum anticonvulsant that can be used for both focal and generalized onset seizures. Specifically indicated for absence, atonic and myoclonic seizures [34]. Preferred drug for nodding seizures [35]. Used by 14.7% of PWE [33]	Given twice daily Starting dose: 5–10 mg/kg/day Maintenance: 15–30 mg/kg/day	Given twice daily Starting dose: 400 mg/day Maintenance: 400–2000 mg/day	Possible side effects: sedation, tremor, transient hair loss, increase in body weight, impaired hepatic function. Use in women of childbearing age is discouraged

Table 1.
Description of common first-line AEDs in resource-limited settings.

the following components: regular evaluation of the treatment regimen/dose and adjustments if needed; contraception and pre-conceptual counseling; psychosocial support and stigma-reducing interventions to improve their self-esteem and quality of life [42].

4. Public health interventions for epilepsy

The high epilepsy burden, unequaled treatment gap, and low quality of life of PWE in low-income settings have been a global health concern during the pass decades. Following the launching of the Global Campaign Against Epilepsy in the early 2000s by the International League Against Epilepsy (ILAE) and International Bureau for Epilepsy (IBE), a number of epilepsy demonstration projects which used a primary healthcare approach were launched in five developing countries: China, Senegal, Zimbabwe, Brazil, and Argentina [43, 44]. In 2015, epilepsy was acknowledged as a major public health problem during the 68th World Health Assembly, and participating countries engaged to step care up epilepsy care [45]. Eventually, the Mental Health Gap Action Programme (mhGAP) enabled the development of evidence-based guidelines for managing neurological conditions including epilepsy in resource-limited settings [30].

Outcomes from the various demonstration projects [46] as well as more recent studies in Guinea [28] and South Africa [47] are in favor of a community-based approach whereby local non-specialized staff and community health workers cater for the PWE. Phenobarbital, a cheap and available first-line AED, is the WHO's recommended molecule of choice for large scale epilepsy treatment [48]. Another important public health component in epilepsy is education and information campaigns, aimed at reducing the epilepsy-related stigma and its consequences on the quality of life of the PWE [32, 46].

5. Conclusion

Epilepsy remains a common neurological disorder with a wide clinical spectrum and a panoply of etiologies. Consensual diagnostic and therapeutic approaches have been established for epilepsy and they constantly evolve as more aspects of this condition are being uncovered by science. LMICs are the most affected by epilepsy, and should therefore be prioritized for interventions aimed at reducing the epilepsy burden.

Acknowledgements

I will like to thank the Global Health Institute of the University of Antwerp and the Brain Research Africa Initiative (BRAIN) Cameroon for their mentorship and support during my PhD project on epilepsy in Africa.

Conflict of interest

The author declares he has no conflict of interest.

Author details

Joseph Nelson Siewe Fodjo
Global Health Institute, University of Antwerp, Antwerp, Belgium

*Address all correspondence to: josephnelson.siewefodjo@uantwerpen.be

References

[1] World Health Organization. Epilepsy fact sheet [Internet]. 2019. Available from: https://www.who.int/news-room/fact-sheets/detail/epilepsy [Accessed: 12 March 2019]

[2] Beghi E. The epidemiology of epilepsy. Neuroepidemiology. 2020;**54**:185-191

[3] Fisher RS, Boas W van E, Blume W, Elger C, Genton P, Lee P, et al. Epileptic seizures and epilepsy: Definitions proposed by the international league against epilepsy (ILAE) and the International Bureau for Epilepsy (IBE). Epilepsia. 2005;**46**:470-472

[4] Fisher RS, Acevedo C, Arzimanoglou A, Bogacz A, Cross JH, Elger CE, et al. ILAE official report: A practical clinical definition of epilepsy. Epilepsia. 2014;**55**:475-482

[5] Falco-Walter JJ, Scheffer IE, Fisher RS. The new definition and classification of seizures and epilepsy. Epilepsy Research. 2018;**139**:73-79

[6] Scheffer IE, Berkovic S, Capovilla G, Connolly MB, French J, Guilhoto L, et al. ILAE classification of the epilepsies: Position paper of the ILAE Commission for Classification and Terminology. Epilepsia. 2017;**58**:512-521

[7] Thurman DJ, Beghi E, Begley CE, Berg AT, Buchhalter JR, Ding D, et al. Standards for epidemiologic studies and surveillance of epilepsy: Standards for epidemiologic studies and surveillance of epilepsy. Epilepsia. 2011;**52**:2-26

[8] Konanki R, Mishra D, Gulati S, Aneja S, Deshmukh V, Silberberg D, et al. INCLEN diagnostic tool for epilepsy (INDT-EPI) for primary care physicians: Development and validation. Indian Pediatrics. 2014;**51**:539-543

[9] Ngugi AK, Bottomley C, Chengo E, Kombe MZ, Kazungu M, Bauni E, et al. The validation of a three-stage screening methodology for detecting active convulsive epilepsy in population-based studies in health and demographic surveillance systems. Emerging Themes in Epidemiology. 2012;**9**:8

[10] Giuliano L, Cicero CE, Crespo Gómez EB, Padilla S, Bruno E, Camargo M, et al. A screening questionnaire for convulsive seizures: A three-stage field-validation in rural Bolivia. Romigi A, editor. PLoS One. 2017;**12**:e0173945

[11] Diagana M, Preux PM, Tuillas M, Ould Hamady A, Druet-Cabanac M. Dépistage de l'épilepsie en zones tropicales: validation d'un questionnaire en Mauritanie. Bulletin de la Société de Pathologie Exotique. 2006;**99**:103-107

[12] Fiest KM, Sauro KM, Wiebe S, Patten SB, Kwon C-S, Dykeman J, et al. Prevalence and incidence of epilepsy: A systematic review and meta-analysis of international studies. Neurology. 2017;**88**:296-303

[13] Ba-Diop A, Marin B, Druet-Cabanac M, Ngoungou EB, Newton CR, Preux P-M. Epidemiology, causes, and treatment of epilepsy in sub-Saharan Africa. The Lancet Neurology. 2014;**13**:1029-1044

[14] Beghi E, Hesdorffer D. Prevalence of epilepsy-an unknown quantity. Epilepsia. 2014;**55**:963-967

[15] Feigin VL, Nichols E, Alam T, Bannick MS, Beghi E, Blake N, et al. Global, regional, and national burden of neurological disorders, 1990-2016: A systematic analysis for the global burden of disease study 2016. The Lancet Neurology. 2019;**18**:459-480

[16] Fisher RS, Cross JH, French JA, Higurashi N, Hirsch E, Jansen FE, et al. Operational classification of

seizure types by the international league against epilepsy: Position paper of the ILAE Commission for Classification and Terminology. Epilepsia. 2017;**58**:522-530

[17] Fisher RS, Cross JH, D'Souza C, French JA, Haut SR, Higurashi N, et al. Instruction manual for the ILAE 2017 operational classification of seizure types. Epilepsia. 2017;**58**:531-542

[18] Dowell SF, Sejvar JJ, Riek L, Vandemaele KAH, Lamunu M, Kuesel AC, et al. Nodding Syndrome. Emerging Infectious Diseases. 2013;**19**:1374-1383

[19] Grinton BE, Heron SE, Pelekanos JT, Zuberi SM, Kivity S, Afawi Z, et al. Familial neonatal seizures in 36 families: Clinical and genetic features correlate with outcome. Epilepsia. 2015;**56**:1071-1080

[20] Brunklaus A, Dorris L, Ellis R, Reavey E, Lee E, Forbes G, et al. The clinical utility of an SCN1A genetic diagnosis in infantile-onset epilepsy: Clinical utility of SCN1A testing. Developmental Medicine and Child Neurology. 2013;**55**:154-161

[21] Carrizosa Moog J, Kakooza-Mwesige A, Tan CT. Epilepsy in the tropics: Emerging etiologies. Seizure. 2017;**44**:108-112

[22] Baraff LJ, Lee SI, Schriger DL. Outcomes of bacterial meningitis in children: A meta-analysis. The Pediatric Infectious Disease Journal. 1993;**12**:389-394

[23] Chesnais CB, Nana-Djeunga HC, Njamnshi AK, Lenou-Nanga CG, Boullé C, Bissek A-CZ-K, et al. The temporal relationship between onchocerciasis and epilepsy: A population-based cohort study. The Lancet Infectious Diseases. 2018;**18**: 1278-1286

[24] Lancaster E, Dalmau J. Neuronal autoantigens—Pathogenesis, associated disorders and antibody testing. Nature Reviews. Neurology. 2012;**8**:380-390

[25] Johnson TP, Tyagi R, Lee PR, Lee M-H, Johnson KR, Kowalak J, et al. Nodding syndrome may be an autoimmune reaction to the parasitic worm Onchocerca volvulus. Science Translational Medicine. 2017;**9**:eaaf6953

[26] Debacq G, Moyano LM, Garcia HH, Boumediene F, Marin B, Ngoungou EB, et al. Systematic review and meta-analysis estimating association of cysticercosis and neurocysticercosis with epilepsy. Flisser A, editor. PLoS Neglected Tropical Diseases. 2017;**11**:e0005153

[27] Siewe Fodjo JN, Dekker MCJ, Idro R, Mandro MN, Preux P-M, Njamnshi AK, et al. Comprehensive management of epilepsy in onchocerciasis-endemic areas: Lessons learnt from community-based surveys. Infectious Diseases of Poverty. 2019;**8**(11). Available from: https://doi.org/10.1186/s40249-019-0523-y

[28] van Diessen E, van der Maas F, Cabral V, Otte WM. Community-based rehabilitation offers cost-effective epilepsy treatment in rural Guinea-Bissau. Epilepsy & Behavior. 2018;**79**:23-25

[29] Caraballo R, Fejerman N. Management of epilepsy in resource-limited settings. Epileptic Disorders. 2015;**17**:13-18

[30] World Health Organization, editor. World Health Organization, Editors. mhGAP Intervention Guide for Mental, Neurological and Substance Use Disorders in Non-specialized Health Settings: Version 1.0. Geneva: World Health Organization; 2010

[31] Howlett W. Neurology in Africa: clinical skills and neurological disorders [Internet]. Tanzania; 2012. Available from: http://www.uib.no/filearchive/

neurologyinafrica_bora-complete-book.pdf

[32] World Health Organisation. Epilepsy in the WHO African Region: Bridging the Gap. Geneva: WHO; 2004

[33] Ibinda F, Odermatt P, Kariuki SM, Kakooza-Mwesige A, Wagner RG, Owusu-Agyei S, et al. Magnitude and factors associated with nonadherence to antiepileptic drug treatment in Africa: A cross-sectional multisite study. Epilepsia Open. 2017;**2**:226-235

[34] NICE. Epilepsies: Diagnosis and management [Internet]. National Institute for Health and Care Excellence; 2012. Available from: www.nice.org.uk/guidance/cg137 [Accessed: 03 December 2017]

[35] Idro R, Namusoke H, Abbo C, Mutamba BB, Kakooza-Mwesige A, Opoka RO, et al. Patients with nodding syndrome in Uganda improve with symptomatic treatment: A cross-sectional study. BMJ Open. 2014;**4**: e006476

[36] Hanaya R, Arita K. The new antiepileptic drugs: Their neuropharmacology and clinical indications. Neurologia Medico-Chirurgica (Tokyo). 2016;**56**:205-220

[37] O'Neill S, Irani J, Siewe Fodjo JN, Nono D, Abbo C, Sato Y, et al. Stigma and epilepsy in onchocerciasis-endemic regions in Africa: A review and recommendations from the onchocerciasis-associated epilepsy working group. Infectious Diseases of Poverty. 2019;**8**:34

[38] Kaddumukasa M, Kaddumukasa MN, Buwembo W, Munabi IG, Blixen C, Lhatoo S, et al. Epilepsy misconceptions and stigma reduction interventions in sub-Saharan Africa, a systematic review. Epilepsy & Behavior. 2018;**85**:21-27

[39] Stephen LJ, Harden C, Tomson T, Brodie MJ. Management of epilepsy in women. The Lancet Neurology. 2019;**18**:481-491

[40] Brodie MJ, Mintzer S, Pack AM, Gidal BE, Vecht CJ, Schmidt D. Enzyme induction with antiepileptic drugs: Cause for concern?: Enzyme induction with AEDs. Epilepsia. 2013;**54**:11-27

[41] Tomson T, Battino D, Bonizzoni E, Craig J, Lindhout D, Perucca E, et al. Comparative risk of major congenital malformations with eight different antiepileptic drugs: A prospective cohort study of the EURAP registry. The Lancet Neurology. 2018;**17**:530-538

[42] Menon S, Siewe Fodjo JN, Weckhuysen S, Bhwana D, Njamnshi AK, Dekker M, et al. Women with epilepsy in sub–Saharan Africa: A review of the reproductive health challenges and perspectives for management. Seizure. 2019;**71**:312-317

[43] ILAE/IBE/WHO. Global Campaign against Epilepsy [Internet]. 2003. Available from: https://www.who.int/mental_health/management/en/GcaeBroEn.pdf?ua=1

[44] Pal DK. China begins long march to epilepsy control. The Lancet Neurology. 2003;**2**:525

[45] WHO. Sixty-eighth World Health Assembly adopts resolution on epilepsy [Internet]. WHO. Available from: https://www.who.int/mental_health/neurology/epilepsy/resolution_68_20/en/ [Accessed: 21 July 2019]

[46] Wolf P, Reynolds E. International League Against Epilepsy – commissions, task forces and the Global Campaign Against Epilepsy. International League Against Epilepsy 1909-2009 A Centenary History [Internet]. Available from: https://www.ilae.org/7A4746E0-7C57-11E7-B3A0141877632E8F

[47] Wagner RG. The Burden of Epilepsy: using population-based

data to define the burden and model a cost-effective intervention for the treatment of epilepsy in rural South Africa [PhD thesis]. Umea, Sweden: Umea University; 2016. Available from: http://umu.diva-portal.org/smash/get/diva2:926968/FULLTEXT03.pdf

[48] Scott RA, Lhatoo SD, Sander JWAS. The treatment of epilepsy in developing countries: Where do we go from here? Bulletin of the World Health Organization. 2001;**79**:344-351

Chapter 2

Epileptic EEG Classification by Using Advanced Signal Decomposition Methods

Ozlem Karabiber Cura and Aydin Akan

Abstract

Electroencephalography (EEG) signals are frequently used for the detection of epileptic seizures. In this chapter, advanced signal analysis methods such as Empirical Mode Decomposition (EMD), Ensembe (EMD), Dynamic mode decomposition (DMD), and Synchrosqueezing Transform (SST) are utilized to classify epileptic EEG signals. EMD and its derivative, EEMD are recently developed methods used to decompose nonstationary and nonlinear signals such as EEG into a finite number of oscillations called intrinsic mode functions (IMFs). In this study multichannel EEG signals collected from epilepsy patients are decomposed into IMFs, and then essential IMFs are selected. Finally, time- and spectral-domain, and nonlinear features are extracted from selected IMFs and classified. DMD is a new matrix decomposition method proposed as an iterative solution to problems in fluid flow analysis. We present single-channel, and multi-channel EEG based DMD approaches for the analysis of epileptic EEG signals. As a third method, we use the SST representations of seizure and pre-seizure EEG data. Various features are calculated and classified by Support Vector Machine (SVM), k-Nearest Neighbor (kNN), Naive Bayes (NB), Logistic Regression (LR), Boosted Trees (BT), and Subspace kNN (S-kNN) to detect pre-seizure and seizure signals. Simulation results demonstrate that the proposed approaches achieve outstanding validation accuracy rates.

Keywords: epileptic EEG classification, empirical mode decomposition (EMD), dynamic mode decomposition (DMD), synchrosqueezing transform (SST), machine learning

1. Introduction

Epilepsy, affecting approximately 4 and 10 per 1000 people of the world's population, is one of the most common acute neurological diseases. EEG is the most frequently used technique for the diagnosis of epilepsy, prediction, detection, and classification of epileptic seizures owing to cost, safety, and easy applicability [1, 2]. In order to detect or monitor epilepsy patients, long-term electroencephalogram (EEG) signals, which are records of the electrical activity generated by the brain, should be inspected visually by expert neurologists. However, this examination method is very time-consuming, bothersome, not efficient, and subjective process. Therefore, utilizing signal processing, machine learning, and artificial intelligence methods for automatic seizure prediction and detection from epileptic EEG signals has become an active research field [2–5].

In the literature, seizure prediction and detection studies have been carried out using successful signal processing approaches in which many spectral, temporal, nonlinear, and statistical properties are calculated.

Automatic seizure detection and prediction studies have been conducted based on time-domain features such as energy, mean value, skewness, and kurtosis values [6–8], exponential energy [6] and, and frequency domain features such as Power spectral density features [9].

Also, entropy-based features such as fuzzy entropy (FuzzyEn), and sample entropy (SampEn) [10], sigmoid entropy [11], approximate entropy (ApEn) [12], weighted Permutation Entropy (WPE) [13], have also been commonly utilized to detect and predict epileptic seizures.

Additionally, in several epileptic seizure detections and prediction study, non-linear features such as cross-bispectrum [4], fractal dimension, detrended fluctuation analysis (DFA), Hurst's exponent [3, 12] have been utilized and promising results have been provided.

On the other hand, various Time-Frequency (FT) analysis approaches have been also performed for epileptic seizure distinguish. The wavelet transform and its derivative [5, 14], Discrete WT (DWT) and Wavelet Packed Decomposition (WPD) [7] based approaches were successfully utilized in the seizure classification studies. Another TF analysis approaches such as The Hilbert Vibration Decomposition (HVD) [15], Variational Mode Decomposition (VMD), Hilbert transforms (HT) [16], the smoothed pseudo-Wigner-Ville distribution (SPWVD) [17], Hilbert–Huang transform (HHT) [18], short-time Fourier transform (STFT) [14, 19], the analytic time-frequency flexible wavelet transform (ATFFWT) [20], The Wigner–Ville distribution (WVD) [21] have been frequently used in seizure detection and prediction studies.

EMD [7, 8, 22] and its derivative approaches such as bivariate empirical mode decomposition (BEMD) [23], multivariate empirical Mode Decomposition (MEMD) [24], ensemble Empirical Mode Decomposition (EEMD) [25] that decompose a given signal into a limited number of zero-mean oscillations called Intrinsic Mode Functions (IMFs) have been developed for the analysis of nonlinear and non-stationary signals and have been successfully used in many seizure detection or prediction studies.

Generally, traditional Fourier-based methods such as CWT or STFT are not very effective in the TF analysis of non-stationary biosignals like EEG [26–28]. Successful seizure classification studies have been carried out using the Synchrosqueezing Transform (SST) method [28], which has been developed based on CWT and STFT [26–29], in order to achieve better TF representations (TFRs) in recent years.

The dynamic mode decomposition (DMD) and derivative approaches, a new matrix decomposition method, that introduced as a solution to problems encountered in fluid flow analysis by Schmidt [30], has recently been used to analyze epileptic EEG signals [31, 32].

In this chapter, three different advanced signal analysis methods are utilized for the classification of seizure and seizure-free EEG signals. The pre-seizure and seizure EEG segments were investigated using *(i)* EMD and its derivative EEMD methods, *(ii)* DMD method, and finally, *(iii)* SST and traditional STFT methods to achieve high classification performances. The rest of this chapter is organized as follows. In Section 2, EEG data set used in this study and employed signal analysis methods are described. Computer simulation results and discussion on the results of three different approaches are presented in Section 3. Conclusions of the study are drawn in Section 4.

2. Classification of epileptic EEG signals

In this study, three different approaches are presented to distinguish seizure and seizure-free EEG segments. In the first method, various temporal, spectral, and non-linear features are extracted from the IMFs obtained using EMD and EEMD approaches. In the second method we present, epileptic EEG segments are analyzed using a simple matrix decomposition method, namely the DMD approach. Finally, in the third approach the SST method with high TF resolution is utilized to extract features and achieve high classification performance in distinguishing seizure and seizure-free EEG segments. The results of these three approaches are compared in line with the classification performances of various machine learning algorithms used in our study.

2.1 Data set (IKCU EEG data set)

In our study, EEG data recorded using the Neurofax EEG device from 16 different epilepsy patients (5 Female; 11 Male, the average age is 37.3∓7) in the Department of Neurology, Faculty of Medicine, İzmir Katip Celebi University are used. These EEG recordings are collected with a sampling frequency of 100 Hz using surface electrodes from 18 different EEG channels (Fp1-F7, F7-T1, T1-T3, T3-T5, T5-O1, Fp1-F3, F3-C3, C3-P3, P3-O1, Fp2-F8, F8-T2, T2-T4, T4-T6, T6-O2, Fp2-F4 F4-C4, C4-P4, P4-O2). It was informed by expert neurologists that the attacks in the used EEG data set are Frontal and Temporal lobes focused. Hence, 10 EEG channels (Fp1-F7, F7-T1, T1-T3, T3-T5, Fp1-F3, Fp2-F8, F8-T2, T2-T4, T4-T6, Fp2-F4) with a predominance of temporal and frontal lobes are used in our study. These EEG data are used in our study by obtaining the Ethical Approval of İzmir Katip Çelebi University Non-Invasive Clinical Research Ethics Committee dated 08.08.2019 and numbered 296.

2.2 Empirical mode decomposition and its variant

EMD approach in which signals decomposed into Intrinsic Mode Functions (IMF) with zero-mean oscillations, is the adaptive time-frequency analysis method for the non-linear and non-stationary processes. The sum of these obtained IMFs must be equal to the original signal [22, 24].

$$x[n] = \left(\sum_{l=1}^{L} IMF_l[n] \right) + R_L[n] \tag{1}$$

where $x[n]$ is the original analyzed signal, L denotes the number of IMFs and $R_L[n]$ indicates the residue.

Despite the successful results of the traditional EMD approach to analyze the non-stationary process, the problem named "mode mixing" is encountered where similar oscillations occur in different modes or different oscillations are observed in the same mode. In the EEMD method, by adding Gaussian white noise to the analyzed signal, the continuity of the signal in different frequency regions is ensured, and the mode mixing problem has been tried to be overcome. Then, the noisy signals obtained by adding white noises with different statistical properties were decomposed into IMFs by the EMD method. As a result of the EEMD method, the average IMFs value is obtained by taking the average of the IMFs group obtained as much as the number of white noise added [25].

$$x^i[n] = x[n] + g^i[n], \qquad i = 1, 2, \ldots, K. \tag{2}$$

Here, ensemble number is denoted by K value, $g^i[n]$ is indicates the added Gaussian noise at i^{th} iteration.

By using EMD approach, IMFs ($IMF^i_j[n], j = 1, \ldots, J^i$) of noisy signal $x^i[n]$ is obtained for the ith iteration. IMFs are calculated for the EEMD approach by taking the average of the IMFs obtained after the number of ensembles (K) iterations.

$$\overline{IMF_j[n]} = \frac{1}{K}\sum_{i=1}^{K} IMF^i_j[n] \tag{3}$$

The first 3 IMFs obtained for an example pre-seizure and seizure EEG segments using EMD and EEMD methods are shown in **Figure 1**.

In our proposed EMD and EEMD based approach, IMFs of pre-seizure and seizure EEG segments are obtained. Following, the IMF selection process is performed using energy-based, correlation-based, power spectral density-distance based and statistical p-value based metrics, as described in [8]. Time (Energy, Mean value, Skewness, and Kurtosis values) [6, 7], spectral (Total power, Spectral Entropy, 1st, 2nd, and 3rd spectral moments) [9], and non-linear (Hurst Exponent and Higuchi Fractal Dimension) [3, 12] features are calculated using 3 highly voted

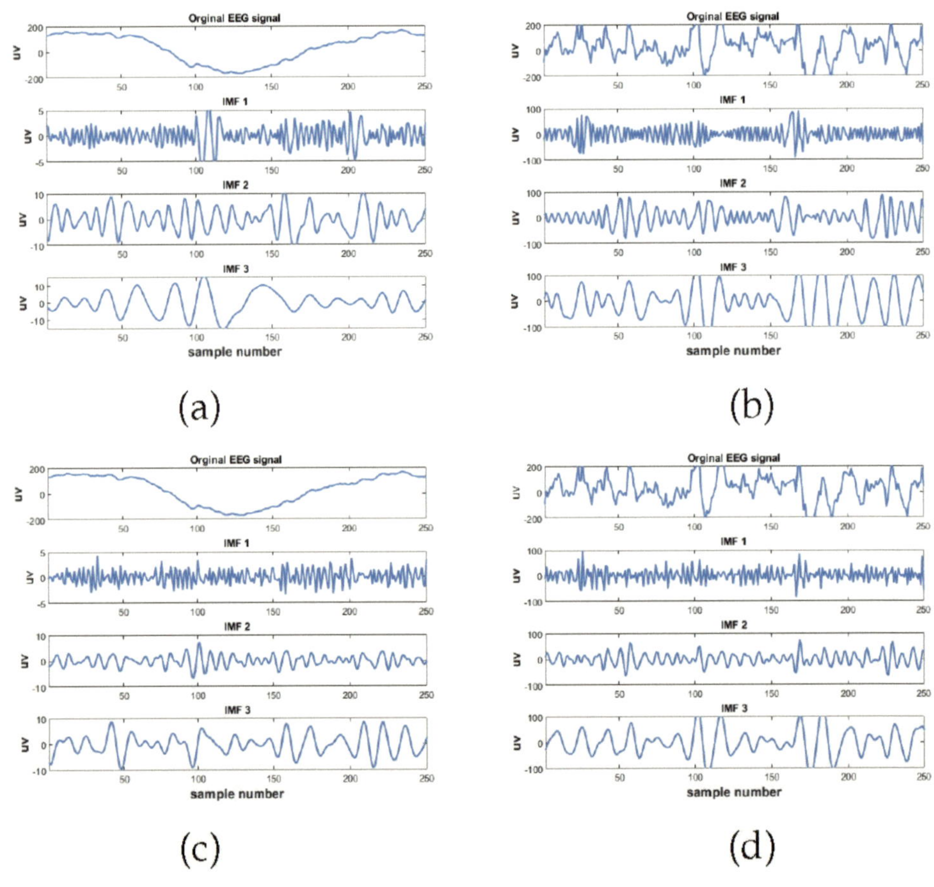

Figure 1.
Pre-seizure EEG signal and it's first three IMF obtained using (a) EMD, and (c) EEMD approaches; seizure EEG signal and it's first three IMF obtained using (b) EMD and (d) EEMD approaches.

IMFs (IMF1, IMF3, and IMF2) determined in the IMF selection process [8]. Thus, 4 time domain, 5 spectral, and 2 non-linear features are calculated for each pre-seizure and seizure EEG segment. For comparison, the same features are calculated from the EEG segment itself, without using the EMD or EEMD method. In addition, the same features are calculated from the sub-bands of the DWT approach, which is a conventional analysis method and compared with the results of the EMD and EEMD approach. In our experiments, Daubechies4 (db4) mother wavelet and 3 level subband decomposition are used [7, 33].

2.3 Dynamic mode decomposition

In fluid flow analysis studies, generally, computationally expensive Global stability analysis method where classical approaches are used, is performed. Proper Orthogonal Decomposition (POD) method based on snapshots of flow and achieving the most active modes is used in these methods. DMD approach based on matrix decomposition has been proffered as a solution to computationally cost of these previous approaches. Systems are analyzed in space using the DMD method in which temporal orthogonality is used. However, using the POD method utilizing spatial orthogonality, systems could be analyzed in time [30]. The behavior of non-linear and dynamic systems such as biological signals cannot be completely revealed by classical time-frequency analysis methods. By evaluating the measurements collected over a certain period of time with the DMD method, both the system can be expressed with a function, and information about the future behavior of the system can be predicted. The basic idea of the DMD method is to obtain the dynamic modes that best represent the system by achieving the eigenvalues and eigenvectors of the system that linearized with the Least-Squares Approximation (LSA) method [31, 34].

In literature, previously, $K \times T-$ sized multi-channel EEG signals are evaluated using the DMD approach. Here, T is the sample size of a single EEG channel, and N is the number of channels. Using this data matrix, $K \times L-$ sized X data matrices in which L denotes the time samples named "snapshot" is obtained, and the DMD algorithm is applied to this obtained data matrices [31]. In our study, both the multi-channel DMD approach used in the literature is performed and the single-channel DMD approach is proposed, unlike the literature, and $K \times L-$ sized X data matrices are constructed using this two different approaches.

In the **single-channel DMD approach (SC-DMD)**, the single-channel EEG signals with $T-$ samples long are divided into non-overlapping, L samples long EEG segments. The $(K \times L)$ EEG data matrices are constructed using K of these obtained segments. For our epileptic seizure classification experiment, $L = 140$ and $K = 5$ are chosen.

Additionally, in the **multi-channel DMD approach (MC-DMD)**, $(K \times L)$ EEG data matrices with no overlap are generated using $L = 140$ samples of $K = 5$ different EEG channels. In our experiment, these data matrices are obtained using the $K = 5-$EEG channel in the left hemisphere (Fp1-F7, F7-T1, T1-T3, T3-T5, Fp1-F3) and the $K = 5-$EEG channel in the right hemisphere (Fp2-F8, F8-T2, T2-T4, T4-T6, Fp2-F4). Also (10×120) EEG data matrices are constructed using the $K = 10-$EEG channel with $L = 120$ sample long in both hemispheres.

In order to achieve a sufficient number of modes to demonstrate the dynamics of neurological activity efficiently, the number of (K) measurements must be at least twice the number of L time points named snapshots [16]. Therefore, the data augmentation process is applied to the data matrix X based on the Hankel matrix creation principle as detailed in [34] and the $N \times M, (N \geq 2M)$ dimensional augmented data matrix X_a is obtained.

$$X_a = \begin{bmatrix} \vdots & \vdots & \cdots & \vdots \\ x_1 & x_2 & \cdots & x_{M-1} \\ \vdots & \vdots & \cdots & \vdots \end{bmatrix} \qquad X'_a = \begin{bmatrix} \vdots & \vdots & \cdots & \vdots \\ x_2 & x_3 & \cdots & x_M \\ \vdots & \vdots & \cdots & \vdots \end{bmatrix} \tag{4}$$

$$X'_a = AX_a \tag{5}$$

Transition matrix A that denoted in Eq. (5) should be obtained to achieve relation based on the high-dimensional linear regression between Xa matrix and its time-shifted version X'_a matrix (given in Eq. (4)). This transition matrix can be calculated using the pseudo-inverse of the X_a matrix $\left(A = X'_a X_a^+\right)$, but for higher-dimensional data such as biosignal, this can cause computational complexity. Using the DMD algorithm;

Singular value decomposition (SVD) of augmented data matrix $X_a = U\Sigma V^*$ is calculated, and formulation of transition matrix rewrite again using the Left singular vectors U, the inverse of the singular values Σ^{-1}, and the Right singular vectors V $A = X'_a X_a^+ = X'_a V \Sigma^{-1} U^*$. The low-rank approximation value $\tilde{A}$ of the transition matrix A can be obtained using Eq. (6)

$$\tilde{A} = U^* X'_a V \Sigma^{-1} \tag{6}$$

The Eigen decomposition of $\tilde{A}$ matrix is calculated ($\tilde{A}W = W\Omega$) and the matrix of eigenvectors W, the diagonal matrix Ω of eigenvalues are achieved. Finally, DMD modes of augmented data matrix X_a are calculated using Eq. (7) where each column of ϕ includes the DMD mode ϕ_m related to eigenvalues λ_m [31, 34].

$$\phi = X'_a V \Sigma^{-1} W \tag{7}$$

In our DMD based epileptic seizure classification experiment, using the DMD spectrum, various features based on DMD subband powers and Higher-order DMD spectral moments (DMD-HOS) are calculated and classification performances of approaches are compared.

The real part, of DMD modes associated with the complex eigenvalues λ_m, indicates the decay frequency of the dynamic modes, while the imaginary part of these modes shows the oscillation frequencies of the dynamic modes. To obtain the DMD spectrum of pre-seizure and seizure EEG segments, oscillation frequencies, and powers, of the dynamic modes, should be calculated. The oscillation frequencies f_m (Hz) are calculated using $\Delta t = 0.01s$ time difference between sequential snapshots, and the complex eigenvalues λ_m of DMD modes; $f_m = |imag\left(\frac{\omega_m}{2\pi}\right)|$, $\omega_m = \frac{log\,(\lambda_m)}{\Delta t}$ (the imaginary part of a complex number is calculated using $imag(.)$ operation). The frequency set $F_{DMD} = \{f_m\}$ is obtained by aligning the oscillation frequencies containing different mode frequencies. Additionally, power $P_m = \|\phi_m\|^2$ of these modes are calculated using the Euclidian norm [34]. The total DMD mode power $\{f_m\} \in F_{DMD}$ (given in Eq. (8)) for the f_m frequency is calculated by summing the power value of L_k DMD modes at the f_m frequency. This process is repeated for all frequencies in the F_{DMD} set and a single DMD power corresponding to each frequency is calculated. In order to obtain the **DMD spectrum**, the obtained DMD power set P_{DMD}, $\forall\{P_{DMD}(f_m)\} \in P_{DMD}$ is plotted according to the oscillation frequency set F_{DMD}.

$$P_{DMD}(f_m) = \sum_{i=1}^{L_k} P_m^i(f_m) \qquad \forall\{f_m\} \in F_{DMD}. \tag{8}$$

To reveal the advantages of the DMD approach, the traditional Power Spectral Density is estimated using the Welch method [5, 35] where the Hamming window and 50% overlapping are chosen, for each seizure, and pre-seizure EEG segments (140 samples long = 1.4 sec). Examples of the proposed Single-Channel EEG based DMD spectra and traditional Welch PSD estimates for pre-seizure and seizure epileptic EEG data are demonstrated in **Figure 2**. The similarity between the average PSD values of the 5 EEG segments (shown with bold black lines in **Figure 2(c)** and **(f)**) whose PSDs are calculated separately by the Welch method and the DMD spectrum, given in **Figure 2(b)** and **(e)**, is remarkable.

In DMD based epileptic seizure detection approach, sub-band powers based and DMD-HOS moments based features are introduced using the DMD spectrum. In computer-aided epileptic seizure detection and prediction studies, EEG subband powers of different frequency bands like delta (0–4 Hz), theta (4–8 Hz), alpha (8–12 Hz), beta (12–30 Hz), and gamma (30–60 Hz), and DMD-HOS moments are calculated using conventional Power Spectral Density [17, 40]. Using the estimated DMD spectrum, similar to the classical PSD approach, Delta (P_δ), Theta (P_θ), Alpha (P_α), Beta (P_β), and Gamma (P_γ)) **subband powers** are calculated as

$$P_{sb} = \sum_{f_m \in f_{sb}} P_{DMD}(f_m), \quad sb = \{\delta, \theta, \alpha, \beta, \gamma\} \qquad P_T = \sum_{f_m} P_{DMD}(f_m) \tag{9}$$

We propose another set of features called **DMD-HOS moments** $M^j_{DMD}, j = 1, 2, 3, \cdots$ defined by

$$M^j_{DMD} = \sum_{f_m \in F_{DMD}} (f_m)^j P_{DMD}(f_m), \qquad j = 1, 2, 3, \cdots \tag{10}$$

In Eqs. (9) and (10), f_{sb} is a subset of oscillation frequencies in $F_{DMD} = \{f_m\}$ of extracted DMD modes corresponding to sub-band frequencies $\{f_\delta, f_\theta, f_\alpha, f_\beta, f_\gamma\}$

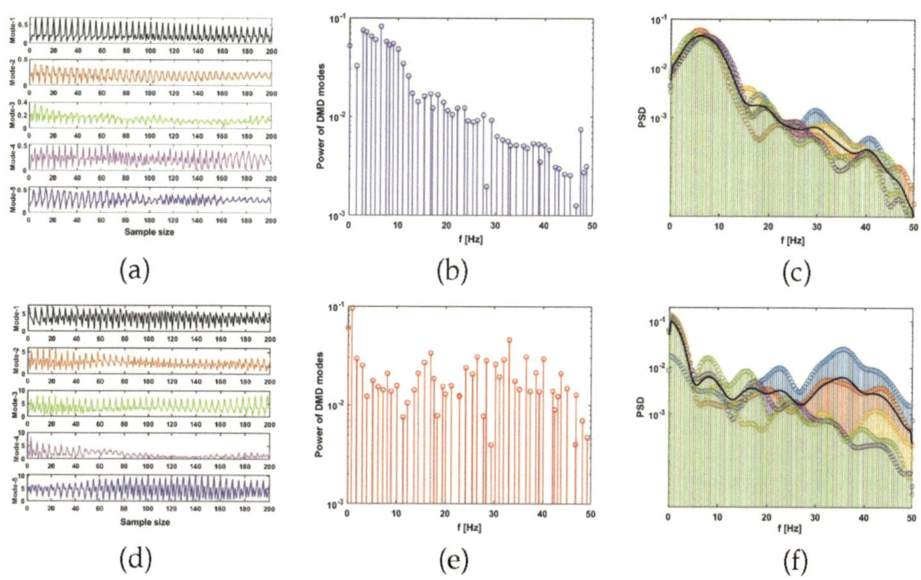

Figure 2.
First 5 DMD modes of 5 pre-seizure EEG segments (a) and its DMD spectrum (b) obtained using Single Channel EEG based dynamic mode decomposition, PSD of these 5 pre-seizure EEG segments together (c); first 5 DMD modes of 5 seizure EEG segments (d) and its DMD spectrum (e) obtained using Single Channel EEG based dynamic mode decomposition, PSD of these 5 seizure EEG segments together (f). Bold black lines denote the average of 5 PSD in (c) and (f).

of EEG, P_T denotes the total power of DMD spectrum, and M^j_{DMD} indicates the jth order DMD spectral moment. In our computations, we extract 6 DMD subband power-based features, and 3 DMD-HOS moments features for each seizure and pre-seizure EEG segment.

2.4 Synchrosqueezing transform

Synchrosqueezing Transform is a member of TF reassignment methods (RM) family which developed to improve the localization properties of TFRs. In RM methods, using the reassignment process, TF coefficients $X(t,\omega)$ that computed utilizing classical TF analysis method, are reassigned into the instantaneous frequency (IF) trajectory close to the ideal TFR which have high frequency and time resolution $(t,\omega) \mapsto (\tau_0(t,\omega), \omega_0(t,\omega))$. On the other hand, using the squeezing process, this TF coefficients $X(t,\omega)$ are squeezed into the IF trajectory close to the ideal TFR which have high-resolution in only frequency $(t,\omega) \mapsto (t, \omega_0(t,\omega))$. Although lower TF resolution is achieved using the SST method, signal reconstruction may be performed [29, 36].

SST method based on STFT or CWT can be performed to obtain high-resolution TFRs of signals. Hence, the TF coefficients of the studied signals are obtained by STFT or CWT, and by using these coefficients with the SST approach, high-resolution TFR is obtained.

In the STFT method, the signal is divided into short-time, and usually overlapping segments and the Fourier transforms of these short-term segments are calculated. In our computations, STFT of 1-second EEG segment $x(t)$, are calculated as, $X(t,\omega) = \int_{-\infty}^{\infty} x(\tau) w(\tau - t) e^{-j\omega\tau} d\tau$ where $w(t)$ denotes the used window function. Using the Fourier transforms of analyzed segment $X(\omega)$ and used window function $W(\omega)$, STFT may be rewritten again as given in Eq. (11).

$$X(t,\omega) = \frac{1}{2\pi} \int_{-\infty}^{\infty} X(\xi) W(\omega - \xi) e^{j\xi t} d\xi. \tag{11}$$

In the SST approach, computing the derivative of STFT $X(t,\omega)$ according to time, the instantaneous frequency $\omega_0(t,\omega) = -j \frac{\partial_t X(t,\omega)}{X(t,\omega)}$ is obtained. By using synchrosqueezing operator $\int_{-\infty}^{\infty} \delta(\eta - \omega_0(t - \omega)) d\omega$ of SST and IF $\omega_0(\mathrm{t}, \omega)$, SST $T(t,\eta)$ with high-resolution is obtained by collecting the STFT coefficients which have the same frequency where they should appear.

$$T(t,\eta) = \int_{-\infty}^{\infty} X(t,\omega) \delta(\eta - \omega_0(t - \omega)) d\omega \tag{12}$$

An example TF representations of 1-sec pre-seizure and seizure EEG segments achieved utilizing SST and STFT approaches are shown in **Figure 3**. We observe in **Figures 3(b)**, **(c)**, **(e)** and **(f)** that the SST approach is able to represent pre-seizure and seizure EEG segments better in the TF plane than the STFT method. Although the window size, which is the most important parameter of STFT [19], is chosen to give the best time and frequency resolution, the SST approach provided better TF resolution.

In our SST based epileptic seizure detection study, high-resolution joint TF distributions of pre-seizure and seizure EEG segments are calculated. Two different feature extraction approaches are presented to achieve efficient features from the magnitude square of the SST matrix $S(n, \omega_k)$:

a. Log-normalized **higher-order joint TF (HOJ-TF) moments,** $\overline{<n^i\,\omega_k^j>}; i,j = 1, 2, \ldots$ [37],

$$\overline{<n^i\,\omega_k^j>} = \log\left(\frac{\sum_{n=0}^{N-1}\sum_{k=0}^{N-1} n^i \omega_k^j S(n,\omega_k)}{i!j!}\right), \qquad i,j = 1, \ldots \tag{13}$$

where N is the length of the EEG segments, and $\omega_k = \frac{2\pi}{N}k, k = 0, \ldots, N-1$.

b. TFR obtained by SST is used as image and **Gray Level Co-occurrence Matrix (GLCM)** texture descriptors are obtained from this TFR image.

GLCM is a prediction of the joint probability distribution of two neighboring gray-level image pixel pairs with a certain position that consists of distance (d) and direction (θ) information. The GLCM of this image can be expressed as given in Eq. (14) using image pixel pair position information ($\Delta = (\theta, d)$).

$$G_\Delta(i,j) \qquad (i,j = 0, 1, \ldots, N_g - 1) \tag{14}$$

where, i and j indicate the intensity values of two pixels, and N_g is the number of gray levels in the image [28, 38]. Second-order statistical features such as contrast, correlation, energy, and homogeneity [39] are calculated as features from the GLCM matrix of TF images corresponding to pre-seizure and seizure EEG segments. In order to evaluate the performance of the SST approach, same features are calculated using the magnitude square of STFT, i.e., the spectrogram $|X(t,\omega)|^2$, which is a classical TF approach and is also used in the SST algorithm [19]. In our experiments, 3 HOJ-TF moments based features, and 4 GLCM based features are calculated for each pre-seizure and seizure EEG segment using both SST and STFT approaches.

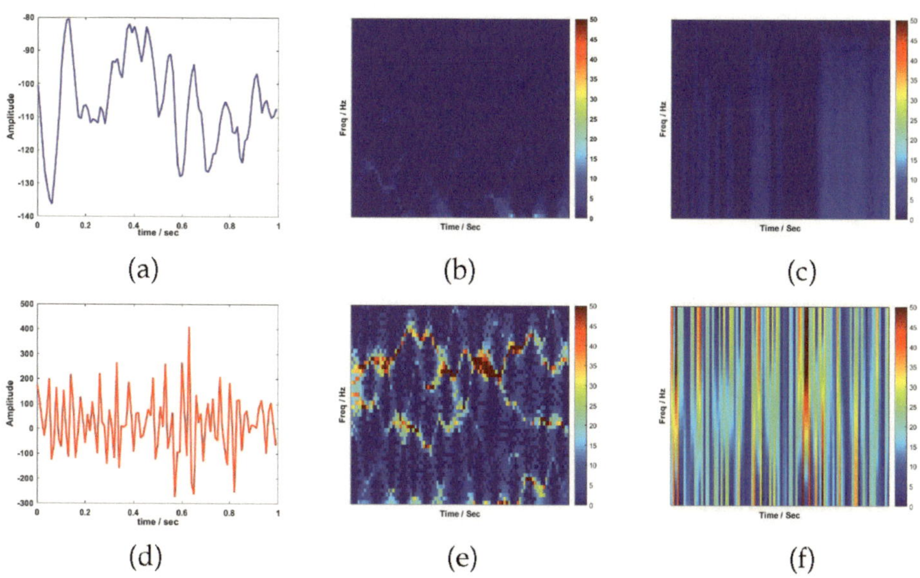

Figure 3.
(a) 1-sec pre-seizure EEG segment, its (b) magnitude SST, and (c) magnitude STFT; (d) 1-sec seizure EEG segment, its (e) magnitude SST, and (f) magnitude STFT.

2.4.1. Classification and performance evaluation

In the proposed study, features extracted utilizing the three different approaches are classified using six different classifiers such as SVM, kNN, NB to distinguish seizure and pre-seizure EEG segments.

In SVM, one of the well-known supervised learning algorithms, decision boundaries, called hyper-planes', is determined to categorize data. While there are many possible hyper-planes that may be constructed, it is essential to determine the hyper-plane where the best classification performance is obtained. The optimal hyper-plane is achieved by maximizing the margin, which is the distance between different classes' support vectors. Once the optimum hyper-plane is determined, the data falling on different sides of the hyper-plane are assigned as elements of different classes. While this process used for the only linearly separable datasets, using the kernel functions SVM is performed to distinguish linearly non-separable datasets. In our proposed study, linear kernel function is performed [10, 13].

The basic and efficient machine learning method kNN is one of the most widely used supervised learning approaches. The distance between each sample x_0 to be classified in the test data and the training data is calculated for all data set which is randomly divided into tests and trains. By determining the k neighbors that have the minimum distance, the most common class among these k neighbors is assigned as the class of this sample. Although there are various distance calculation metrics such as Euclidean, Manhattan, Minkowski, and Hamming, the Euclidean distance metric, which is the most commonly used in the literature, is used in our study. In addition, the value of k is chosen as 10 for the proposed study [39, 40].

The NB classifier is one of the probabilistic classifiers in which the classification is performed according to Bayes' theorem. Membership probabilities $P(M_i/x_0)$ (M_i indicates the class, c denotes the number of class) to "c" classes of sample x_0 to be classified are calculated, separately. This sample is assigned as a member of the class in which the highest probability of membership among the "c" class is calculated [39, 40].

To achieve a stable classification accuracy, 10–fold cross-validation is employed in our experiment. Using Accuracy (ACC), and $F1$-score metrics, performance evaluation of proposed methods and utilized classifiers are investigated.

$$ACC = \frac{TP + TN}{TP + FN + FP + TN}, \quad F_{Score} = 2 * \frac{PRE * REC}{PRE + REC} \tag{15}$$

where true-positive (TP) is the number of samples of *class*_1 classified in the same class, and true-negative (TN) denotes the number of samples of *class*_0 classified in *class*_0. While false-positive (FP) is the number of samples not in *class*_1 but classified in *class*_1, false-negative (FN) indicates the number of samples in *class*_1 but classified in *class*_0. Recall and Precision metrics are formulated respectively as, $REC = \frac{TP}{TP+FN}$, and $PRE = \frac{TN}{FP+TN}$ [18].

3. Experiments and results

In the following, we give the performance evaluation of seizure and pre-seizure EEG classification by using three different advanced signal representation methods presented in Section 2. The classification process is performed using SVM, kNN, and NB classifiers and compared the performance of each approach and classifier. In the **Tables 1–5**, highest classification performances are indicated with boldface numbers for each approach and component.

		SVM		kNN		NB	
Approach	**Components**	**ACC**	**F-Score**	**ACC**	**F-Score**	**ACC**	**F-Score**
EMD	IMF1	94.31	94.16	94.38	94.31	94.31	94.03
	IMF2	94.12	93.85	92.62	92.48	93.13	92.79
	IMF3	93.38	93.36	94.63	94.45	95.63	95.48
	IMF1-IMF2	**94.56**	**94.40**	93.81	93.70	94.56	94.33
	IMF1-IMF3	92.06	92.38	**95.63**	**95.53**	**96.88**	**96.77**
	IMF2-IMF3	94.50	94.35	94.81	94.66	95.88	95.74
	IMF1-3	90	90.99	94.88	94.81	96.19	96.07
EEMD	IMF1	**96.06**	**96.04**	94.44	94.43	93.75	93.60
	IMF2	92.44	92.19	91.81	91.69	93.50	93.12
	IMF3	94.50	94.42	94.06	94.02	95.44	95.27
	IMF1-IMF2	94.94	94.86	94.81	94.76	94.12	93.91
	IMF1-IMF3	81.69	80.29	95.94	95.90	**97**	**96.91**
	IMF2-IMF3	94.44	94.32	94.25	94.21	95.38	95.18
	IMF1-3	94.19	94.39	**97**	**96.97**	95.75	95.62
DWT	AC + DC1-3	80.81	76.83	93.44	93.38	**94.56**	**94.43**
EEG	all EEG	59.75	66.33	**93.25**	**93.35**	78.94	74.41

Table 1.
Performance results (%) of EMD and EEMD based seizure detection approach.

		SVM		kNN		NB	
Approach	**Components**	**ACC**	**F-Score**	**ACC**	**F-Score**	**ACC**	**F-Score**
SC-DMD	Right Hems.	90.3	91.9	90.8	92.9	89.4	91.2
	Left Hems.	93.7	95.1	**94.1**	**95.5**	93.4	94.6
	Two Hems.	91.7	93.4	92.3	93.9	91.3	92.8
MC-DMD	Right Hems.	90.6	91.9	89.3	90.9	89.5	91.7
	Left Hems.	92.9	94.8	**93.9**	**95.5**	92.7	93.8
	Two Hems.	94.7	95.9	94.5	95.9	93.5	94.4
PSD	Right Hems.	86.1	88.7	87.2	89.9	86.7	86.2
	Left Hems.	92.1	93.4	**92.2**	**93.9**	91.3	93.4
	Two Hems.	89.1	91.3	89.5	91.5	88.3	90.7

Table 2.
Performance results (%) for seizure detection using the subband power based feature set of DMD based approach.

3.1 Results of EMD methods

In EMD and EEMD based seizure detection approaches, various features in the time-domain, spectral-domain, and non-linear are calculated to separate the seizure and pre-seizure EEG segments. To compare the performances of EMD based approaches, DWT approach is implemented to the pre-seizure and seizure EEG

		SVM		kNN		NB	
Approach	**Components**	**ACC**	**F-Score**	**ACC**	**F-Score**	**ACC**	**F-Score**
SC-DMD	Right Hems.	87.3	89.4	88.4	90.5	83.1	85.8
	Left Hems.	**92.2**	**93.9**	91.2	93.9	90.1	92.9
	Two Hems.	89.7	92.4	90.2	92.5	87	89.3
MC-DMD	Right Hems.	88.9	90.9	85.9	89.4	81.2	84.4
	Left Hems.	**92.9**	**93.4**	92	93.9	87.6	89.7
	Two Hems.	92.8	94.4	92.2	93.5	88.8	90.4
PSD	Right Hems.	85.6	87.6	88.1	90.9	86.8	88.2
	Left Hems.	**92.5**	**93.9**	91.6	93.5	92.5	93.9
	Two Hems.	88.6	90.3	89.4	91.5	89.2	91.3

Table 3.
Performance results (%) for seizure detection using the DMD-HOS moment based feature set of DMD based approach.

		SVM		kNN		NB	
Approach	**Components**	**ACC**	**F-Score**	**ACC**	**F-Score**	**ACC**	**F-Score**
SST	Right Hems.	88.4	91.1	**88.5**	**91.1**	83.6	86.2
	Left Hems.	**93.1**	**94.6**	92.5	94.2	92.1	93.7
	Two Hems.	**90.5**	**92.6**	90.1	92.3	88	90.2
STFT	Right Hems.	**87.2**	**90.1**	86.6	89.5	79.1	81.7
	Left Hems.	**92.1**	**93.8**	91.6	93.5	85.3	87.7
	Two Hems.	**89.5**	**91.7**	89.1	91.4	82.2	84.8

Table 4.
Performance results (%) for seizure detection using the HOJ-TF moment based feature set of SST and STFT based approaches.

		SVM		kNN		NB	
Approach	**Components**	**ACC**	**F-Score**	**ACC**	**F-Score**	**ACC**	**F-Score**
SST	Right Hems.	**88.6**	**91.2**	88.4	91	88.1	90.6
	Left Hems.	92.5	94.1	**92.6**	**94.2**	92.2	93.9
	Two Hems.	**90.4**	**92.4**	90	92.2	90.1	92.2
STFT	Right Hems.	**85.4**	**88.6**	85	88.2	83.8	87.3
	Left Hems.	90.3	92.4	**90.4**	**92.4**	88.7	91.1
	Two Hems.	**87.5**	**90.2**	87.4	90	86.2	89.1

Table 5.
Performance results (%) for seizure detection using the GLCM based feature set of SST and STFT based approaches.

segments, and same features are calculated from the Approximation Coefficient (AC) and 3 Detail Coefficients (DC) of DWT. Additionally, without using any signal processing approach the same features are extracted from the EEG signals itself.

The performance evaluation results for different IMF combinations are demonstrated in **Table 1**. In all tables, we indicate the highest classification performance with boldface numbers for each case. In **Table 1**, the components column shows that the features for classifications are calculated by using the corresponding component. For example, the classification results of the features calculated using IMF1 are given in the first row, and the classification results of the features calculated from the EEG signal itself are given in the last row. NB classifier provides the highest classification successes for both EMD (96.88% ACC, 96.77% *F*1-score) and EEMD (97% ACC, 96.91% *F*1-score) approaches by using features calculated from IMF1-IMF3 (the first two IMFs decided by the IMF selection process) of the corresponding approach. While, the maximum (94.56% ACC, 94.43% *F*1-score) classification successes are achieved using the NB classifier for the DWT approach; using the kNN classifier and EEG signals itself, maximum (93.25% ACC, 93.35% *F*1-score) values are obtained.

3.2 Results of DMD methods

Performance evaluation results of SC-DMD and MC-DMD based and PSD based epileptic seizure detection approaches are summarized in **Tables 2–3**. For the SC-DMD and PSD approaches, the classification results of the feature set created by combining the features obtained from the Left Hemisphere (Fp1-F7, F7-T1, T1-T3, T3-T5, Fp1-F3), Right hemisphere (Fp2-F8, F8-T2, T2-T4, T4-T6, Fp2-F4), and both hemisphere (Fp1-F7, F7-T1, T1-T3, T3-T5, Fp1-F3, Fp2-F8, F8-T2, T2-T4, T4-T6, Fp2-F4) channels separately are denoted with "Left Hems", "Right Hems "and "Two Hems", while the same components show the classification results of DMD features obtained from the EEG data matrix created using the respective hemisphere channels in the MC-DMD approach.

For all three approaches, the highest classification performance for both the subband based feature set and the moment based feature set is obtained from the Left Hems. While the kNN classifier is yield to highest classification accuracy 94.1% and *F*1-score 95.5% for subband power-based feature set obtained from the Left Hems of SC-DMD approach, the maximum 92.2% ACC and 93.9% *F*1-score values are achieved with the SVM classifier using the moment-based feature set of the SC-DMD approach. On the other hand, in the MC-DMD approach, the classification performances of subband power-based (kNN: 93.9% ACC, 95.5% *F*1-score) and moment-based (SVM: 92.9% ACC, 93.4% *F*1-score) feature sets are close to each other for Left Hems and Two Hems. Additionally, using the PSD approach, a maximum of 92.2%, and 92.5% classification accuracies are achieved using the kNN and SVM classifiers for the subband power-based and moment-based feature sets of Left Hems, respectively. The results show that both SC-DMD and MC-DMD approaches are more successful than the classical PSD approach.

3.3 Results of SST and STFT methods

Performance evaluation results of the SST based approach are given in **Tables 4** and **5**. Analyzes for SST and STFT approaches are carried out separately for each channel. The classification result of the feature set created by combining the features obtained from the left hemisphere channels is given with the "Left Hems" component. Similarly, while the classification result of the feature set obtained for the right hemisphere is given with "Right Hems", the classification result of the feature set created by combining the features obtained from all channels is given with the "Two Hems" component.

Classification performance of HOJ-TF based feature set is higher than that of GLCM based feature set for each component of SST and STFT approaches. In both approaches, the classification success of both the HOJ-TF moment based feature set and the GLCM based feature set is higher in Left Hems than in Right Hems. While the highest 93.1% ACC and 94.6% $F1$-score are provided with SVM classifier by using the HOJ-TF moment-based feature set for Left Hems of SST, the maximum 92.6% ACC and 94.2% $F1$-score are obtained with the kNN classifier using the GLCM based feature set. On the other hand, in the STFT approach, 92.1% ACC and 93.8% $F1$-score values are achieved with the SVM using the HOJ-TF moment-based feature set, while the classification performance of GLCM based feature set is 90.4% ACC, and 92.4% $F1$-score for kNN classifier.

$F1$-scores obtained by the proposed methods, and by the classical approaches are calculated for comparison and given in **Figure 4**. The $F1$-scores of the proposed EMD and EEMD-based approaches, in **Figure 4a**, are higher than those of DWT and EEG-based approaches, except for the kNN classifier. In the DMD-based seizure detection approach, higher $F1$-score values are obtained in all classifiers than that of the traditional PSD approach for the subband power-based feature set, while the DMD approach provided higher $F1$-score values in the moment-based feature set, except for the NB classifier, shown in **Figure 4b**. Finally, in the SST-based epileptic seizure detection approach, higher $F1$-score values are obtained for each feature set and classifier compared to the STFT approach as shown in **Figure 4c**.

Channel-based classification performances of the proposed SC-DMD, SST, EMD, and EEMD approaches are given with a topographic maps in **Figure 5**. The topographic map is created by averaging the ACC values obtained with all classifiers for each method. It was stated by the expert neurologists that epileptic attacks in the used data set are left hemisphere-focused. It is noteworthy that the channel-based classification success of the EEG-based seizure detection approach (shown in **Figure 5a**) is very low, while is very high for the EEMD-based seizure detection approach (given in **Figure 5c**). It is also remarkable that in all proposed methods, the channels in the left hemisphere yielded successful results of seizure detection (given in **Figure 5b–5e**).

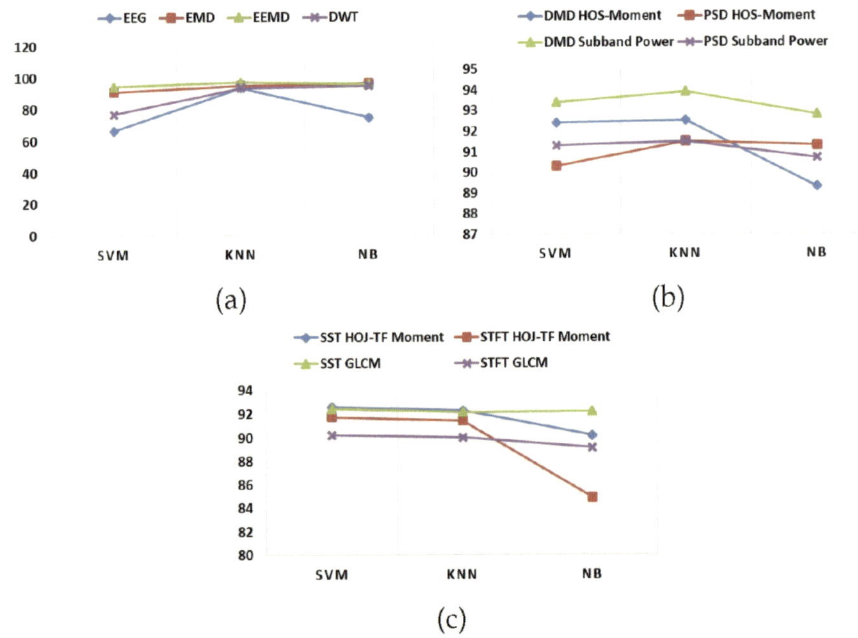

Figure 4.
Changing of F1-score values of (a) EMD and EEMD based, (b) DMD based, and (c) SST and STFT based epileptic seizure detection approaches.

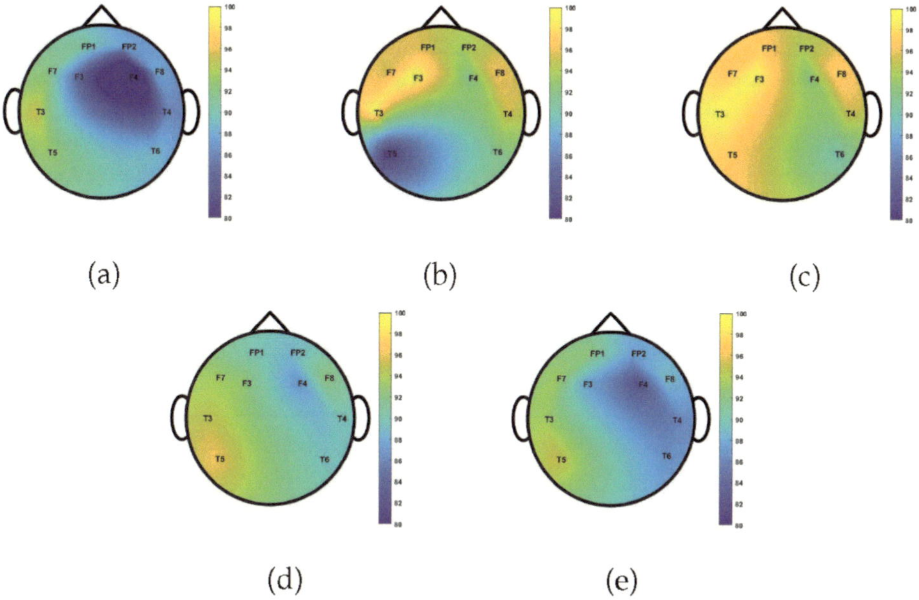

Figure 5.
Topographic map of channel based classification accuracies of (a) EEG based (b) EMD based (c) EEMD based (d) SC-DMD based, and (e) SST based approaches.

4. Conclusions

In our study, epileptic seizure detection is performed using EMD and derivative approaches, the DMD approach, which is a matrix decomposition method, and the SST approach, a new TF method. Pre-seizure and seizure EEG segments are decomposed into IMFs using the EMD and EEMD method, and time, spectral and non-linear features are calculated using the first 3 IMFs (IMF1, IMF3, IMF2) after the IMF selection process which detailed in our previous study [18]. In order to compare the success of EMD and EEMD methods, the same features are obtained using the approximation and detail coefficient of the DWT approach and directly from the EEG signal itself. While the EEMD method gives more successful results than the EMD approach for all conditions and classifiers, the most unsuccessful classification results are obtained by using features calculated from the EEG signal itself.

DMD spectra are obtained for pre-seizure and seizure EEG segments using the DMD approach, which is a simple matrix decomposition method. Although the DMD spectrum has been defined in the literature [31, 34], different features other than DMD powers have not been calculated using this spectrum. In our study, it is proposed to calculate DMD subband powers and DMD-HOS moments as features. In addition, although the multi-channel DMD approach has been used in the literature, the single-channel DMD approach has been proposed in our study. The success of the DMD approach is compared with the classical PSD obtained using the Welch method. The classification performance of both MC-DMD and SC-DMD approaches is higher than that of the PSD approach. In addition, the proposed SC-DMD based approach has been at least as successful as the MC-DMD based approach.

Another seizure detection study is carried out using the high TF resolution SST approach which proposed to overcome the disadvantages of classical TF approaches. HOJ-TF moment-based and GLCM-based features are calculated as features using the magnitude square of SST. The same features are computed using the STFT method that is the classical TF analysis method to compare the success of SST. The SST approach provided higher classification accuracy than STFT for each condition and classifier.

EMD and EEMD approaches with high computational complexity [18], yielded more successful results than the other two approaches. As a result of these evaluations, it may be concluded that the suggested DMD and SST-based approaches that have lower computational complexity [28, 41] can successfully be used in the detection of epileptic EEG signals.

Acknowledgements

This paper was supported by Izmir Katip Celebi University Scientific Research Projects Coordination Unit: Project numbers: 2019-GAP-MÜMF-0003 and 2019-TDR-FEBE-0005.

Conflict of interest

The authors declare no conflicts of interest directly related to this study.

Thanks

We would like to thank Asst. Prof. Dr. Hatice Sabiha TÃ¼re and Asst.Prof.Dr. Sibel Kocaaslan Atli for their support in providing epileptic EEG recordings.

Abbreviations

EMD	empirical mode decomposition
EEMD	ensembe empirical mode decomposition
IMFs	intrinsic mode functions
DMD	dynamic mode decomposition
SST	synchrosqueezing transform
SC-DMD	single-channel DMD approach
MC-DMD	multi-channel DMD approach
DMD-HOS	higher-order DMD spectra
HOJ-TF	higher-order joint TF
GLCM	gray level co-occurrence matrix

DOI: http://dx.doi.org/10.5772/intechopen.93810

Author details

Ozlem Karabiber Cura[1†] and Aydin Akan[2*†]

1 Department of Biomedical Engineering, Izmir Katip Celebi University, Cigli, Izmir, Turkey

2 Department of Electrical and Electronics Engineering, Izmir University of Economics, Balcova, Izmir, Turkey

*Address all correspondence to: akan.aydin@ieu.edu.tr

† These authors contributed equally.

References

[1] S Raghu, Natarajan Sriraam, Shyam Vasudeva Rao, Alangar Sathyaranjan Hegde, and Pieter L Kubben. Automated detection of epileptic seizures using successive decomposition index and support vector machine classifier in long-term eeg. *Neural Computing and Applications*, pages 1–20, 2019

[2] J. Song, Q. Li, B. Zhang, M. B. Westover, and R. Zhang. A new neural mass model driven method and its application in early epileptic seizure detection. *IEEE Transactions on Biomedical Engineering*, 67(8):2194–2205, 2020

[3] Manish Sharma, Ram Bilas Pachori, and U Rajendra Acharya. A new approach to characterize epileptic seizures using analytic time-frequency flexible wavelet transform and fractal dimension. *Pattern Recognition Letters*, 94:172–179, 2017

[4] Naghmeh Mahmoodian, Axel Boese, Michael Friebe, and Javad Haddadnia. Epileptic seizure detection using cross-bispectrum of electroencephalogram signal. *Seizure*, 66:4–11, 2019

[5] Qi Yuan, Weidong Zhou, Liren Zhang, Fan Zhang, Fangzhou Xu, Yan Leng, Dongmei Wei, and Meina Chen. Epileptic seizure detection based on imbalanced classification and wavelet packet transform. *Seizure*, 50:99–108, 2017

[6] OK Fasil and R Rajesh. Time-domain exponential energy for epileptic EEG signal classification. *Neuroscience Letters*, 694:1–8, 2019

[7] Emina Alickovic, Jasmin Kevric, and Abdulhamit Subasi. Performance evaluation of empirical mode decomposition, discrete wavelet transform, and wavelet packed decomposition for automated epileptic seizure detection and prediction. *Biomedical signal processing and control*, 39:94–102, 2018

[8] Ozlem Karabiber Cura, Sibel Kocaaslan Atli, Hatice Sabiha Türe, and Aydin Akan. Epileptic seizure classifications using empirical mode decomposition and its derivative. *BioMedical Engineering OnLine*, 19(1):1–22, 2020

[9] Zafer Iscan, Zümray Dokur, and Tamer Demiralp. Classification of electroencephalogram signals with combined time and frequency features. *Expert Systems with Applications*, 38(8): 10499–10505, 2011

[10] Jie Xiang, Conggai Li, Haifang Li, Rui Cao, Bin Wang, Xiaohong Han, and Junjie Chen. The detection of epileptic seizure signals based on fuzzy entropy. *Journal of neuroscience methods*, 243:18–25, 2015

[11] S Raghu, Natarajan Sriraam, Yasin Temel, Shyam Vasudeva Rao, Alangar Satyaranjandas Hegde, and Pieter L Kubben. Performance evaluation of dwt based sigmoid entropy in time and frequency domains for automated detection of epileptic seizures using svm classifier. *Computers in biology and medicine*, 110:127–143, 2019

[12] Qi Yuan, Weidong Zhou, Shufang Li, and Dongmei Cai. Epileptic EEG classification based on extreme learning machine and nonlinear features. *Epilepsy research*, 96(1-2):29–38, 2011

[13] Noha S Tawfik, Sherin M Youssef, and Mohamed Kholief. A hybrid automated detection of epileptic seizures in EEG records. *Computers & Electrical Engineering*, 53:177–190, 2016

[14] M Kemal Kıymık, İnan Güler, Alper Dizibüyük, and Mehmet Akın. Comparison of STFT and wavelet transform methods in determining

epileptic seizure activity in EEG signals for real-time application. *Computers in biology and medicine*, 35(7):603–616, 2005

[15] Barkın Büyükçakır, Furkan Elmaz, and Ali Yener Mutlu. Hilbert vibration decomposition-based epileptic seizure prediction with neural network. Computers in Biology and Medicine, 119:103665, 2020

[16] Susanta Kumar Rout and Pradyut Kumar Biswal. An efficient error-minimized random vector functional link network for epileptic seizure classification using VMD. *Biomedical Signal Processing and Control*, 57:101787, 2020

[17] Alexandros T Tzallas, Markos G Tsipouras, and Dimitrios I Fotiadis. Automatic seizure detection based on time-frequency analysis and artificial neural networks. *Computational Intelligence and Neuroscience*, 2007, 2007

[18] Kai Fu, Jianfeng Qu, Yi Chai, and Yong Dong. Classification of seizure based on the time-frequency image of EEG signals using HHT and SVM. *Biomedical Signal Processing and Control*, 13:15–22, 2014

[19] Ricardo Ramos-Aguilar, J. Arturo Olvera-López, Ivan Olmos-Pineda, and Susana Sánchez-Urrieta. Feature extraction from EEG spectrograms for epileptic seizure detection. *Pattern Recognition Letters*, 133:202–209, 2020

[20] Manish Sharma, Ram Bilas Pachori, and U. [Rajendra Acharya]. A new approach to characterize epileptic seizures using analytic time-frequency flexible wavelet transform and fractal dimension. *Pattern Recognition Letters*, 94:172–179, 2017

[21] M Deriche, S Arafat, S Al-Insaif, and M Siddiqui. Eigenspace time frequency based features for accurate seizure detection from EEG data. *IRBM*, 40(2): 122–132, 2019

[22] Shufang Li, Weidong Zhou, Qi Yuan, Shujuan Geng, and Dongmei Cai. Feature extraction and recognition of ictal EEG using EMD and SVM. *Computers in biology and medicine*, 43(7): 807–816, 2013

[23] Yang Zheng, Gang Wang, Kuo Li, Gang Bao, and Jue Wang. Epileptic seizure prediction using phase synchronization based on bivariate empirical mode decomposition. *Clinical Neurophysiology*, 125(6):1104–1111, 2014

[24] Asmat Zahra, Nadia Kanwal, Naveed ur Rehman, Shoaib Ehsan, and Klaus D. McDonald-Maier. Seizure detection from EEG signals using multivariate empirical mode decomposition. *Computers in Biology and Medicine*, 88:132–141, 2017

[25] Paschalis A Bizopoulos, Dimitrios G Tsalikakis, Alexandros T Tzallas, Dimitrios D Koutsouris, and Dimitrios I Fotiadis. EEG epileptic seizure detection using k-means clustering and marginal spectrum based on ensemble empirical mode decomposition. In *13th IEEE International Conference on BioInformatics and BioEngineering*, pages 1–4. IEEE, 2013

[26] S Ali, Mst Jannatul Ferdous, E Hamid, and KI Molla. Time-frequency coherence of multichannel EEG signals: Synchrosqueezing transform based analysis. *International Journal of Computer Science Trends and Technology*, 4(3):40–48, 2016

[27] Alireza Ahrabian, David Looney, Ljubiša Stanković, and Danilo P Mandic. Synchrosqueezing-based time-frequency analysis of multivariate data. *Signal Processing*, 106:331–341, 2015

[28] Shamzin Mamli and Hashem Kalbkhani. Gray-level co-occurrence matrix of fourier synchro-squeezed transform for epileptic seizure detection. *Biocybernetics and Biomedical Engineering*, 39(1):87–99, 2019

[29] Gaurav Thakur and Hau-Tieng Wu. Synchrosqueezing-based recovery of instantaneous frequency from nonuniform samples. *SIAM Journal on Mathematical Analysis*, 43(5):2078–2095, 2011

[30] Peter J Schmid. Dynamic mode decomposition of numerical and experimental data. *Journal of fluid mechanics*, 656:5–28, 2010

[31] Muhammad Sohaib J Solaija, Sajid Saleem, Khawar Khurshid, Syed Ali Hassan, and Awais Mehmood Kamboh. Dynamic mode decomposition based epileptic seizure detection from scalp EEG. *IEEE Access*, 6:38683–38692, 2018

[32] Muhammad Bilal, Muhammad Rizwan, Sajid Saleem, Muhammad Murtaza Khan, Mohammed Saeed Alkatheir, and Mohammed Alqarni. Automatic seizure detection using multi-resolution dynamic mode decomposition. *IEEE Access*, 7:61180–61194, 2019

[33] A Sharmila and P Geethanjali. DWT based detection of epileptic seizure from EEG signals using naïve bayes and k-NN classifiers. *Ieee Access*, 4:7716–7727, 2016

[34] Bingni W Brunton, Lise A Johnson, Jeffrey G Ojemann, and J Nathan Kutz. Extracting spatial–temporal coherent patterns in large-scale neural recordings using dynamic mode decomposition. *Journal of neuroscience methods*, 258:1–15, 2016

[35] Agustina Garcés Correa, Lorena Orosco, Pablo Diez, and Eric Laciar. Automatic detection of epileptic seizures in long-term EEG records. *Computers in biology and medicine*, 57: 66–73, 2015

[36] Chuan Li and Ming Liang. A generalized synchrosqueezing transform for enhancing signal time–frequency representation. *Signal Processing*, 92(9):2264–2274, 2012

[37] Aydin Akan and R. Başar Ünsal. Time–frequency analysis and classification of temporomandibular joint sounds. *Journal of the Franklin Institute*, 337(4):437–451, 2000

[38] Mryka Hall-Beyer. GLCM texture: A tutorial. *National Council on Geographic Information and Analysis Remote Sensing Core Curriculum*, 3, 2000

[39] Kaveh Samiee, Serkan Kiranyaz, Moncef Gabbouj, and Tapio Saramäki. Long-term epileptic EEG classification via 2d mapping and textural features. *Expert Systems with Applications*, 42(20): 7175–7185, 2015

[40] Siuly Siuly and Yan Li. Designing a robust feature extraction method based on optimum allocation and principal component analysis for epileptic eeg signal classification. *Computer Methods and Programs in Biomedicine*, 119(1): 29–42, 2015

[41] N Benjamin Erichson, Steven L Brunton, and J Nathan Kutz. Compressed dynamic mode decomposition for background modeling. *Journal of Real-Time Image Processing*, 16(5):1479–1492, 2019

Section 2

Etiologies of Epilepsy and Epileptic Syndromes

Chapter 3

Rolandic Epilepsy: Self-Limited Epilepsy with Centrotemporal Spikes

Ulviyya Guliyeva, Nana Nino Tatishvili and Rauan Kaiyrzhanov

Abstract

Childhood epilepsy with centrotemporal spikes, had been previously considered as benign childhood epilepsy. According to the new classification proposed by Sheffer I. and colleagues the term "benign" has been changed to "self-limited". Many studies reported that BECTS may cause transient or long lasting cognitive and behavioral disturbances. Rolandic epilepsy is the most frequent among the childhood focal epilepsy and may account for about 15–25% of all epileptic syndromes diagnosed between the ages of 5 to 15 years. The incidence range changes between 7.1–21 per 100000 in population younger than 15 years with male predominance. The age of onset in 90% of cases between 1 and 10 years with peak around 6–7 years. Seizures mainly occur during a night sleep, whereas the probability of awake seizures are less than 10%. The characteristic clinical features are: (1) focal motor seizure with unilateral orofacial tonic or clonic contractions; (2) speech arrest; (3) hypersalivation; (4) sensory symptoms represented by unilateral numbness or paresthesia of tongue, lips, gum and inner part of the check; (5) unilateral clonic jerk in leg and arm with postictal paresis; (6) generalized seizures. The EEG picture is distinctive in Rolandic epilepsy. The background activity is almost always preserved in awake state and during a sleep. The typical interictal EEG pattern is high voltage, diphasic spikes or sharp waves frequently with slow activity on central-midtemporal region. The centrotemporal spikes or rolandic spikes come from the lower rolandic region created a horizontal dipole with maximal electronegativity in the centrotemporal region and electropositivity in the frontal region usually seen unilateral or bilateral. In most cases children with RE have a good prognosis regarding both seizures and neurodevelopment. The remission of seizures usually occurs before the age of 18 years. The cognitive and behavior problem may happen in active period of disease which are reversable in most of patients.

Keywords: rolandic epilepsy, EEG, BECTS, epilepsy, atypical rolandic epilepsy, centrotemporal spikes, seizures, cognitive outcome

1. Introduction

Self-limited epilepsy with centrotemporal spikes (SECTS), well-known as Rolandic epilepsy is the most frequent among the childhood focal epilepsies and may account for about 15–25% of all epileptic syndromes diagnosed between the

IntechOpen

ages of 5 to 15 years [1]. It is termed 'rolandic' epilepsy because the focal seizures are originated from the region around the lower part of the central gyrus of Rolando. The incidence range changes between 7.1–21 per 100000 in a population younger than 15 years with male predominance [2]. The age of onset in 90% of cases between 1 and 10 years with a peak around 6–7 years and recovery occurs before the age of 15–16 years [2–4].

Self-limited epilepsy with centrotemporal spikes is a syndrome of brief hemifacial motor seizures, frequently having associated somatosensory symptoms, usually without impairment of consciousness which tend to evolve into GTCS [3–6]. Seizures are often related to sleep [7]. Genetic predisposition is frequent, and there is male predominance [3, 5, 8, 9]. An interictal EEG has normal background activity with biphasic high-voltage centrotemporal spikes, often followed by slow waves that are activated by sleep and tend to spread or shift from side to side [10]. Neurological and mental status before the debut of epilepsy is normal. There are no specific abnormalities on brain MRI or CT. Many studies reported that RE may cause transient or long-lasting cognitive and behavioral disturbances [4, 5, 11–40].

2. Terminology and classification

Panayiotopoulos described a concept of benign childhood susceptibility syndrome (BCSSS) to unify RE, Panayiotopoulos syndrome (PS) and childhood occipital epilepsy of Gastaut (ICOE-G) outlined the common features, course of diseases, prognosis, and the possible genetic predisposition in this group of associated syndromes [5].

1989 ILAE classification recognized three "age-related and localization-related epilepsies and syndromes": (1) benign childhood epilepsy with centrotemporal spikes (BCECTS); (2) childhood epilepsy with occipital paroxysms; (3) primary reading epilepsy [10].

ILAE Commission on Classification and Terminology lists three childhood idiopathic focal epilepsy syndromes: (1) benign childhood epilepsy with centrotemporal spikes (BCECTS); (2) Panayiotopoulos syndrome, and (3) late-onset childhood occipital epilepsy (Gastaut type) [13].

Rolandic epilepsy had undergone significant terminological and classification changes. RE had been previously considered as benign childhood epilepsy. Frequently reported cognitive and language impairments and behavioral disturbances in children with RE led to the replacement of the terms "benign" and "idiopathic" by the "self-limited" in the new classification proposed by Sheffer I. and colleagues [41].

3. Etiology

The role of genetic factors in RE has been presumed since the first high incidence of centrotemporal spikes in family members of patients with RE was reported in 1964 [42]. RE and related syndromes with atypical features do not follow a Mendelian inheritance mode [43]. The clinical and genetic studies have shown complex inheritance [43–51].

The genetics of CTS is not the same as the clinical genetics of RE [52]. Although CTS is the primary EEG characteristics of RE or ARE, they are also observed in healthy children [53] or the children with autistic spectrum disorders without seizures [54]. Only 10% of EEG trait carriers had seizures [55, 56]. An autosomal dominant mode of inheritance of CTS on EEG has been reported by several authors [42, 55, 56] but it is still debated [52]. The linkage of CTS to ELP4-PAX6 region on 11p13 and chromosome 15q13 [57], 16p12–11.2 [58], and 15q14 [59] have been identified.

Doose et al. investigated the broad spectrum clinical and EEG manifestation of 147 children with RE and their 1266 family members revealed a high incidence of febrile convulsion and afebrile GTCS in patients and their relatives suggested multifactorial inheritance. EEG recordings of probands and their siblings showed a high rate of generalized EEG traits [43].

A multicentral twin study of eighteen twin pairs (10 MZ, 8 DZ) based on a twin database done by Vadlamudi and colleagues demonstrated that the etiology of RE and its inheritance mode is much more complicated than considered before [44]. No twin pairs were concordant for RE. Only one monozygotic twin pair has shown centrotemporal spikes on EEG without seizures. Another intriguing finding from this twin data was that all twin pairs with atypical features RE, had a co-twin with seizures although discordant for RE, which emphasized that genetic factors may be more important in atypical cases of RE.

Mutations	Protein function	Special features	Reports
KCNQ2/KCNQ3	Voltage-gated potassium channel	BFNS plus RE	Maihara et al. [62]
		BFNS CTS trait	Coppola et al. [63]
		BFNS plus RE, RE, CTS trait	Neubauer et al. [64]
SRPX2	E2A/HLF fusion	RS, oral and speech dyspraxia, MR	Roll et al. [65]
ELP4	Elongator subunit	CTS trait, speech disorder, behavior disturbances, ADHD	Strug et al. [57]
GRIN2A	NMDAR subunit	Atypical RE (LKS/CSWS), intellectual disability, various dysmorphic features	Lemke et al. [66]
RBFXO1/3	ATAXIN 2-BINDING PROTEIN 1/ HEXARIBONUCLEOTIDE-BINDING PROTEIN 3	RE, atypical RE, CTS trait	Lal et al. [67]
DEPDC5	GATOR complex	RE, atypical RE	Lal et al. [50]
GABRG2	GABA receptors	RE, atypical RE	Reinthaler et al. [68]
CAMK2A	Subunit of calcium/ calmodulin-dependent protein kinase II	Atypical RE, intellectual disability and autism	Rudolf et al. [45]
GRIN2B	NMDAR subunit	Atypical RE, epileptic encephalopathy, intellectual disability	Rudolf et al. [45]
CHRNA4	Neuronal nicotinic acetylcholine receptor α4 subunits	RE (familial case)	Neng et al. [69]

Table 1.
Genetic mutations associated with RE/ARE spectrum.

The genetic basis of RE/ARE is polygenic and complex, the interaction of environmental factors or other genes should be considered in etiology of RE spectrum epilepsy syndromes [60, 61]. A number of genes were found to follow the Mendelian inheritance and be associated with RE/ARE (**Table 1**).

Lemke et al., have identified GRIN2A mutations in 20% of patients with ARE associated with neurocognitive disturbances [66].

Although mutations in PRRT2, KCNQ2, KCNQ3, RBFOX1, and DEPDC5 genes with an autosomal dominant transmission reported in patients with RE spectrum epilepsy syndromes, they have not been confirmed by the studies based on large case series [70].

With the exception of GRIN2A and ELP4, many genes currently associated with RE/ARE, including KCNQ2, KCNQ3, CHRNA4, DEPDC5, RBFOX1/3, BDNF, and GABAA-R, were initially linked to other neurogenetic conditions, and later their phenotypes were expanded to RE/ARE.

4. Clinical features

The main seizure type in RE according to the ILAE 2017 seizure classification is focal aware seizure consisting of motor-hemifacial tonic or clonic contractions, oro-pharyngo-laryngeal symptoms, sensory symptoms represented by unilateral numbness or paresthesia of tongue, lips, gum, and inner part of the check, and associated with speech arrest, hypersalivation, and focal to bilateral seizures [2–4, 41, 71]. Hemiconvulsions and bilateral tonic–clonic seizures are less frequently observed ictal features, mainly seen in younger children due to rapid distribution of focal onset seizures [2–4, 6]. Hemiconvulsions may be followed by post-ictal Todd's hemiparesis in 10% of cases [8, 72].

Seizures are brief, usually last from 30 sec to 2–3 minutes or longer if turn into bilateral tonic–clonic seizures [6, 18, 72]. Seizures mainly occur during night sleep or drowsiness, whereas the probability of awake seizures is less than 10% [73, 74]. Seizure frequency is low, most patients have less than 10 seizures, 10%–20% of patients have a single seizure [75]. Consciousness is completely preserved in around 60% of patients with RE [5].

Focal motor seizures in approximately one-third of cases manifest as unilateral oral-facial tonic or clonic contractions. These are brief (few seconds –1 min), a sudden burst of clonic contractions of the face, which may be entirely localized in the lower lip or spread to the ipsilateral upper and very rare to the lower extremities [1–5, 71, 76].

Tonic deviation of the mouth is frequently observed ictal motor manifestation [5].

Oro-pharyngo-laryngeal symptoms are mostly motor ictal phenomena with the involvement of the (epi-) glottis and pharynx (> 50%) produce guttural bizarre sounds, resembling gargling, grunting, wheezing [72]. These may be accompanied by contractions of the respiratory and abdominal muscles (vomiting like contractions) which appear in more than half of seizures [77]. They consist of unilateral sensory and motor manifestations inside the mouth, tongue, inner cheek, gums, teeth, and pharyngolaryngeal regions [3].

Speech arrest occurs in >40% of seizures with dys - or anarthria [3, 72]. The child usually is aware, with preserved receptive language, attempts to communicate with gestures, but unable to produce a single intelligible word [3, 5]. Speech arrest is considered more as a motor ictal manifestation associated with the loss of the power and coordination for the articulation of words [3]. There is no impairment of the cortical language mechanisms [4, 5].

Focal non-motor seizures commonly observed in RE.

Sensory symptoms may manifest as unilateral numbness or paraesthesias like tingling, prickling, freezing and their variations in the parts (rarely involve the whole area) of oral-facial-pharyngeal area, usually tongue, inner cheek, gum, teeth, lips [3, 4, 6]. Sensory seizures often occur in combination with motor seizures and hypersalivation [3, 5, 72].

Hypersalivation is one of the most characteristic autonomic ictal symptoms of RE, occurs in one-third of cases [2–5, 71]. It is frequently associated with hemifacial motor symptoms. As well as the awareness is not disturbed in most of the cases, children usually are able to describe their sensations as sudden filling of the mouth with saliva and air, difficulty in pronouncing words, a lot of saliva flowing from the mouth [5].

Other autonomic ictal manifestations as *ictal emesis* and *ictal syncope* may observe rarely in RE. Although autonomic seizures are the cardinal symptom of Panayiotopoulos syndrome, they are reported in RE [74, 78–82]. The overlap of the clinical and EEG features of PS and RE has been widely investigated by several authors [5, 74, 79, 80]. The cases where two different types of childhood focal seizures presented at the same time or one form of epilepsy progressed to another have been thoroughly reported by different investigators [74, 79–85].

Focal to bilateral tonic–clonic seizures are a frequent seizure type present in one to two-thirds of children with RE. FBTCSs mostly appear during night sleep [86].

Status epilepticus is seen rarely and usually associated with an atypical course of the disease [87].

Focal motor SE occurs more often than generalized convulsive SE [3]. This state consists of unilateral or bilateral hemifacial contraction, subtle perioral myoclonus, speech arrest, dysarthria, excessive drooling, swallowing difficulties [88–93].

5. EEG patterns

5.1 Interictal EEG

The EEG picture is distinctive in Rolandic epilepsy. The background activity is almost always preserved in an awake state and during sleep [91]. The characteristic interictal EEG pattern- centrotemporal spikes (CTS) or rolandic spikes are regarded as the neurobiological markers of RE. CTS is high-amplitude (usually > than 150 mkV) biphasic spikes or sharp waves of ~ 70–80 milliseconds duration frequently followed by a slow activity on the central-mid temporal region (C3/C4, T3/T4) [2–4]. More posterior localization of CTS is often observed in the youngest patients [94]. The spikes may occur isolated or in clusters, in one or both hemispheres [95, 96] (**Figure 1A** and **B**). A focal rhythmic slow activity over the centrotemporal region is occasionally observed [2]. The most typical finding of the rolandic spikes is their significant increase in frequency during NREM sleep [74] (**Figure 1C–E**). The spikes appear only in sleep in about a third of children [97].

EEG and magnetoencephalography (MEG) studies show a stable horizontal dipole coming from the lower rolandic region with maximal electronegativity in the centrotemporal region and electropositivity in the frontal region, usually seen unilateral or bilateral [98–100]. Spikes may often appear in the central, parietal, midline, or even occipital regions which do not exclude a diagnosis of RE [98].

Somatosensory stimulation by the tapping of hands or feet or electrical stimulation of fingers at 1 Hz may activate CTS and somatosensory evoked potentials (SEPs) on the contralateral hemisphere [101].

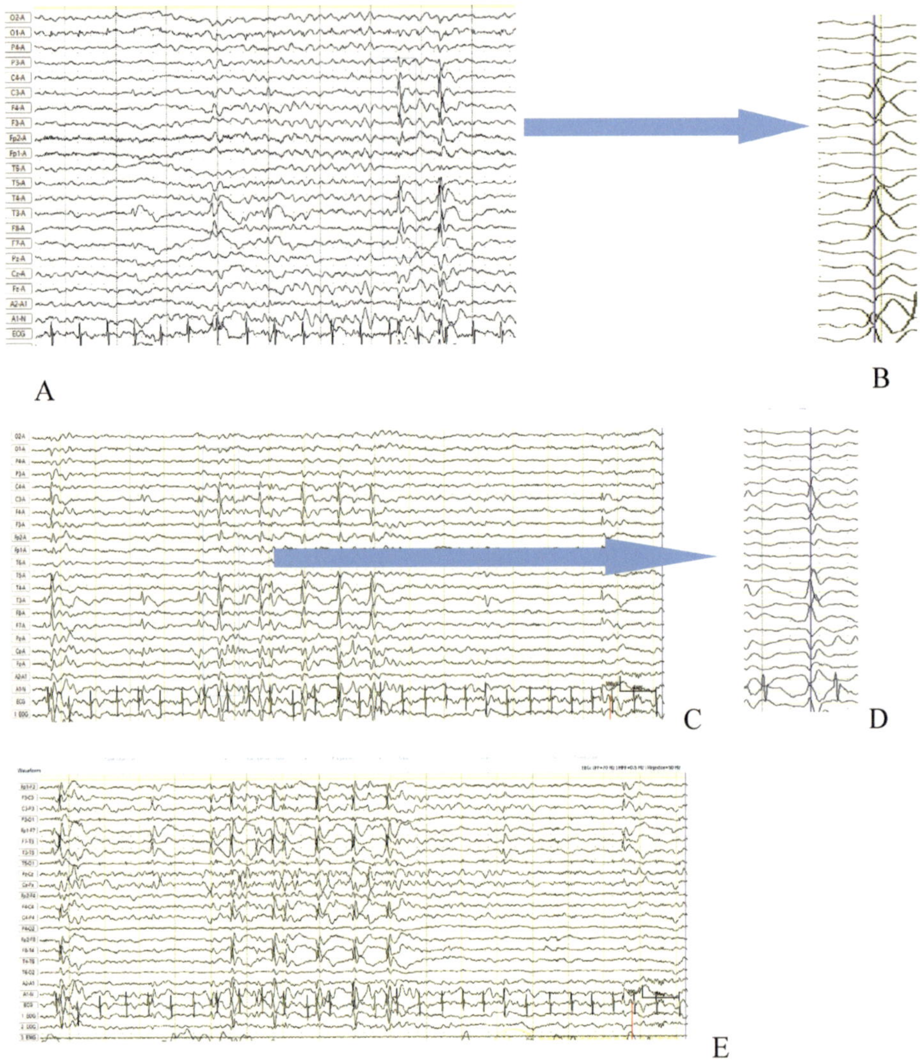

Figure 1.

7y.old boy with rolandic epilepsy. (A) Interictal awake EEG. Left centrotemporal spikes with rapid spreading to the right frontal-anterior temporal region. with maximum negativity over the C3T3,F7 and maximum positivity on the right-midline frontal-parietal region F4Fp2FzPzCz(AV montage, sensitivity 20Mkv/mm, paper speed 30mm/sec, LFF 70 Hz, HFF 0.5 Hz, Rejector 50 Hz). (B) Increased paper speed clearly demonstrates propagation of left centrotemporal spikes to the right frontal-anterior temporal region (AV montage, sensitivity 20 Mkv/mm, paper speed 120 mm/sec, LFF 70 Hz, HFF 0.5 Hz, Rejector 50 Hz). (C and D) Interictal 1NREM sleep EEG. The frequency of CTS of the same distribution is increased. (E) The same EEG sample in bipolar longitudinal montage demonstrates phase reversal on both right and left centrotemporal region (C3C4T3T4).

Brief interictal generalized bursts of 3–5 Hz slow waves with intermixed small spikes distinctive than a pattern 3 Hz spike–wave seen in CAE may observe in about 4% of patients with RE [85, 102].

Many studies have tried to identify the source of rolandic discharges using topographic analysis, source modeling techniques, dipole tracing method, magnetoencephalography (MEG), and functional MRI (fMRI) investigations [99–101, 103–106]. The functional MRI (fMRI) triggered by EEG of the rolandic spikes as well as MEG showed activation of the sensorimotor area [104], mainly in the orofacial division of the primary sensorimotor cortex [105]. However, it is challenging to distinguish the precentral or postcentral origin of CTS [103]. Ishitobi et al., suggested the precentral origin of rolandic spikes explained this theory by the continuity of cortical surface polarity from negative gyral cortex to the surface positive interhemispheric fissure based on the combination of scalp EEG and MEG [103]. Gregory and Wong analyzed 12 independent foci in 10 patients with RE assumed that the generator of a dipole discharge was located halfway between the maximum negative and positive poles, and was most likely situated at the depth of the lower rolandic fissure or Sylvian fissure [107]. The propagation pattern of rolandic spikes first studied by Jung et al., suggests that spike propagation was caused by intracortical spreading a single dipole across the central sulcus [108].

CTS are diagnostic markers of RE only in a suggestive clinical presentation [74]. It has been widely reported that 1.2 to 3.5% of normal healthy children population between 5 and 12 years old [109, 110], 6–34% of siblings and relatives of patients affected by RE [9, 111, 112], children with migraine, behavior disturbances, ADHD, variety of organic brain diseases with or without seizures, such as cerebral tumors, Rett syndrome, fragile X syndrome and focal cortical dysplasia [84, 113] also show CTS in routine EEG recording.

5.2 Ictal EEG

The first described ictal patterns are characterized by a quite monomorphic sequence of rhythmic sharp waves or spikes without significant post-ictal slowing [91, 114]. In 1990, Gutierrez et al. described an ictal event with speech arrest only characterized by a short train of ictal alpha activity, and then two multiple spikes and wave complexes originated from the left centrotemporal region followed by marked attenuation of the left hemispheric background [115]. Subclinical rhythmic discharges of spike and wave in the centrotemporal region have been documented by several authors in RE [116, 117]. Saint-Martin et al. in 2001 described a series of patients presenting with typical and also atypical ictal manifestations such as falls, negative myoclonus and observed that positive motor phenomenon correlated to the spike component preceding a negative motor phenomenon, correlated with the slow-wave component of the spike and wave complex [118].

Capovilla et al. recorded 34 seizures in 30 patients with RE and described four electrographic seizure patterns thus emphasizing that ictal pattern for RE is not unique [116]:

- low-voltage activity of fast rhythmic spikes, increasing in amplitude and decreasing in frequency observed in the majority of patients,
- a discharge of spikes intermixed with sharp waves increasing in frequency and amplitude,
- monomorphic theta which progressively formed a discharge increasing in amplitude and decreasing in frequency,
- initial focal depression of the electrical activity, followed by one of the three above described patterns.

Ictal EEG source analysis of 3 patients with RE demonstrated the activation of the opercula-insular area, time-locked to the contralateral focal myoclonic jerks [119].

6. Prognosis

In most cases, children with RE have a good prognosis regarding both seizures and neurodevelopment [120, 121]. The remission of seizures usually occurs before the age of 18 years [11, 98]. The cognitive and behavior problem may happen in an active period of disease which is reversible in most patients [11, 12].

Rolandic seizures occur in a period of significant brain maturation. The dysfunction of neuronal network activities such as focal discharges may be associated with neuropsychological problems, including, linguistic, cognitive, and behavioral impairment [28–30, 122]. The frequent spike discharges in sleep may boost language and attention processing problems [120, 123–125].

Mood and behavioral disorders were present in nearly a third of children (30.9%) with RE [126–128]. Retrospective studies have proposed that early age at onset pretends a more aggressive seizure course [18, 129–131].

Functional MRI study revealed CTS density caused hemodynamic changes even during wakefulness can interfere with the normal brain-language network and the bilateral insular cortex [132].

The neuropsychological tests such as Wechsler Intelligence Scale for Children-III (WISC-3rd), verbal fluency test, Wisconsin card sorting test, attention deficit diagnostic scale, and child behavior checklist scale are usually administered to measure a wide range of skills and cognitive functions of RE patients [35–38, 133].

Many researchers showed a variety of neuropsychological deficits, behavioral and emotional difficulties in a limited cohort of patients with RE range from 19 to 67% [22–40, 134, 135]. The series of reported children with uncomplicated RE were described lower average results on neuropsychological tests involving visuomotor coordination, some executive functions, sustained attention, and language issues like spelling, reading aloud, reading comprehension, memory, and learning of auditory–verbal material, delayed recall, and verbal fluency, compared with controls. However, the Full-Scale Intelligence Quotient (FSIQ) was not significantly low in most of them.

D'Alessandro et al. investigated the neuropsychological data of 44 children with RE who did not have a seizure for more than 6 months without treatment. Attention, language, and visuomotor coordination tasks problems were more severe in children with a bilateral epileptiform discharge. However, in a follow-up assessment for 4 years, a re-examination of 11 children had revealed the normalization of cognitive functions in all [21].

Several studies reported that cognitive abnormalities and behavioral impairments are associated with a high interictal spike frequency [24, 25, 35, 120], the number of interictal abnormalities in wake or sleep [136], activation of interictal spikes during sleep [118, 137], and the presence of non-tangential dipole spikes [73].

Piccinelli et al. [138], investigated the frequency of specific learning disabilities such as reading, writing, and calculation in patients with typical RE and possible related electroclinical findings. They reported children with RE who developed seizures before age 8 years and had epileptiform discharges more than 50% of the sleep EEG recording in several tracings over more than a year were at risk of developing academic difficulties [138].

EEG may predict educational and behavioral impairments in children with RE. The presence of an intermittent slow-wave focus during wakefulness, a high number of spikes in the first hour of sleep (and during whole night sleep), and multiple asynchronous bilateral spike–wave foci in the first hour of sleep are associated with learning problems in children with RE [16, 139].

7. Atypical rolandic epilepsy

RE can present or evolve to an atypical form, characterized by atypical ictal semiology, different EEG findings, and poor neuropsychological outcomes [19, 140, 141].

Massa et al. described 5 interictal EEG patterns that significantly correlated with atypical evolutions of RE: [41] intermittent slow-wave focus; [2] multiple asynchronous spike–wave foci; [3] long spike–wave clusters; [4] generalized 3-c/s "absence-like" spike–wave discharges; [1] conjunction of interictal paroxysms with negative or positive myoclonia, and abundance of interictal abnormalities during wakefulness and sleep [136].

Several studies have shown an association between atypical rolandic epilepsy and known genes (**Table 1**). The identification of de novo or inherited mutations of N-methyl-D-aspartate (NMDA) receptor subunit-encoding genes (GRIN2A and GRIN2B) linked to speech and language, cognitive impairment, and behavioral difficulties have been a significant breakthrough in the understanding of the nature of atypical RE [142–145]. Another relevant gene is elongation factor protein 4 (ELP4), which is associated with language impairment, autism spectrum disorder, mental retardation, and epilepsy with centrotemporal spikes on EEG [146].

Atypical rolandic epilepsy (ARE) is a severe epileptic condition especially with regards to cognitive consequences. The first description of atypical features of RE was published by Aicardi & Chevrie in 1982 showed rolandic epilepsy presenting periods with new types of seizures, mainly atonic and myoclonic, associated with continuous spike-and-waves in slow-sleep EEG (CSWS/ESES), and transitory learning difficulties [147]. Doose and Baier described similar patients with atonic fits leading to daily falls which is the hallmark seizure type for Lennox–Gastaut syndrome and termed the condition "pseudo-Lennox syndrome" to differentiate this two distinct conditions [148]. Patients with ARE have significantly lower full-scale and verbal IQ than the patients with typical RE [149]. Neuropsychological impairment, which may sometimes be present before the onset of the disease, is constantly present during the clinical course, but in contrast to ESES and LKS, the cognitive outcome is always favorable [92, 150]. Clinical semiology consists of typical for RE focal seizures, generalized tonic–clonic seizures, atypical absences, myoclonic seizures, and atonic seizures. The atonic attacks may involve the whole axial musculature or be localized, causing repeated brief (0.5–2.0 s) atonic episodes in the head or a limb (epileptic negative myoclonus) that usually occur for periods lasting one to several weeks, separated by seizure-free intervals of weeks or months [6, 90, 92]. Such atonic attacks are associated with the slow-wave component of spike and wave complexes, and the location of the EEG discharges corresponds to that of the atonic episodes [151, 152]. Interictal awake EEG shows bilateral sharp and sharp-slow wave complexes with higher amplitude in the rolandic area, which increases during sleep with bilateral synchronization [90, 92, 116, 153].

Using carbamazepine may promote the diffusion of spike–wave activity from the rolandic focus to induce atonic seizures, atypical absences in patients with RE [154].

Rolandic status epilepticus refers to status epilepticus that can be convulsive or non-convulsive, and either generalized or focal lasting days or weeks including motor facial seizures, oromotor dyspraxia, anarthria with persistent drooling and swallowing problems [155]. The interictal EEG usually shows focally or bilaterally synchronous sharp waves or sharp and slow wave complexes predominant in the rolandic area with a tendency to become continuous during sleep [146, 155]. The condition can be resolved with a good neurocognitive outcome with appropriate treatment [146]. These seizures can persist for more than 1 month without treatment [156, 157].

8. Treatment

The decision whether to treat children with RE or not requires a particularly careful risk–benefit analysis [2, 158–163]. Many authors suggest that drug treatment is not necessary for typical RE because of its good prognosis, and usually infrequent nocturnal seizures [114, 154]. Moreover, in 40–50% of cases, the seizures are difficult to control with drugs [148]. Besides, the treatment with AED usually does not influence the duration of active epilepsy [163].

However, treatment may be indicated in patients with frequently recurring daytime seizures, generalized tonic–clonic seizures, young age at onset [164], or when the ictal events are disruptive to the patient or family [161, 163]. Furthermore, the presence of cognitive and behavioral disturbances, either transitory or persistent has to be considered [2, 5, 91, 92]. There is no single solution supported by definitive evidence which AED is more effective in the treatment of RE.

Internationally, carbamazepine (CBZ 20-40 mg/kg/d [165]) and valproate (VPA 20-30 mg/kg/d [166]) are the most often prescribed AED for children newly diagnosed RE [167]. However, the possible worsening of EEG in rolandic epilepsy by some drugs and particularly by CBZ, increasing epileptiform abnormalities during sleep, and inducing epileptic negative myoclonus have been reported [154].

Sulthiame, levetiracetam, and gabapentin were studied in a randomized controlled trial [158, 159, 167–169]. Sulthiame administered varied between 3.1 and 5.7 mg/kg/day was effective in controlling seizures in children with RE [159].

A prospective, open-label, pilot trial evaluating the efficacy and tolerability of levetiracetam (LVT 20-30 mg/kg/d) or oxcarbazepine (OXC 20-35 mg/kg/d) as monotherapy in two parallel groups of newly diagnosed RE patients demonstrated effectiveness in controlling seizures a follow-up period up to 2 years [162].

A randomized controlled multicenter trial comparing the effects of either Levetiracetam or Sulthiame on EEG in RE showed a reduction of epileptiform discharges after 12 weeks of treatment [158]. Persistent epileptiform discharges after 12 weeks of treatment are associated with recurrent seizures [158].

When the presence of ESES associated or not with negative myoclonus, clinical status, or acquired aphasia is detected in children with RE, a change of antiepileptic drugs should be considered. Class IV studies suggest that sulthiame, benzodiazepines, ethosuximide, and, in most severe cases, corticosteroids might be useful [91, 92].

Duration of treatment in RE should not exceed 1 year following the last seizure, regardless of EEG changes [2].

Acknowledgements

We are grateful to Dr. Sándor Beniczky for his valuable comments on EEG figures.

Disclosure

None of the authors has any conflict of interest to disclose.

Author details

Ulviyya Guliyeva[1*], Nana Nino Tatishvili[2] and Rauan Kaiyrzhanov[3]

1 MediClub Hospital, Baku, Azerbaijan

2 Neuroscience Department, Central Children Hospital, Tbilisi, Georgia

3 Department of Neurogenetics, Institute of Neurology, UCL, London, England

*Address all correspondence to: doctor.ulya@gmail.com

References

[1] Hauser WA, Annegers JF, Kurland LT. Incidence of epilepsy and unprovoked seizures in Rochester, Minnesota: 1935-1984. Epilepsia. 1993 May-Jun;34(3):453-468. doi: 10.1111/j.1528-1157.1993.tb02586.x. PMID: 8504780.

[2] Federico Vigevano, Nicola Specchio, Natalio Fejerman, Chapter 61 - Idiopathic focal epilepsies, Editor(s): Olivier Dulac, Maryse Lassonde, Harvey B. Sarnat, Handbook of Clinical Neurology, Elsevier, Volume 111, 2013,p. 591-604

[3] Koutroumanidis M, Panayiotopoulos CP. Benign childhood seizure susceptibility syndromes. In: Rugg-Gunn RJ, Smalls JE, editors. From channels to commissioning – a practical guide to epilepsy. London: International League Against Epilepsy (UK Chapter) and Epilepsy Society; 2015. p. 89-113.

[4] Chrysostomos P. Panayiotopoulos, Michelle Bureau Roberto H. Caraballo, Bernardo Dalla Bernardina, Thalia Valeta. Idiopathic childhood focal epilepsies. In: Michelle Bureau, Pierre Genton, Charlotte Dravet, Antonio, Delgado-Escueta, Carlo Alberto Tassinari, Pierre Thomas, Peter Wolf, Epileptic Syndromes in Infancy, Childhood and Adolescence – 5th updated edition, JOHN LIBBEY EUROTEXT,2012. p. 217-224

[5] Panayiotopoulos CP. Benign childhood partial epilepsies: benign childhood seizure susceptibility syndromes. J Neurol Neurosurg Psychiatry. 1993 Jan;56(1):2-5. doi: 10.1136/jnnp.56.1.2. PMID: 8429319; PMCID: PMC1014755.

[6] Guerrini R, Pellacani S. Benign childhood focal epilepsies. Epilepsia. 2012 Sep;53 Suppl 4:9-18. doi: 10.1111/j.1528-1167.2012.03609.x. PMID: 22946717.

[7] Deb.K.PaI et al, Idiopathic focal epilepsies: the “lost tribes”. Epileptic Disorder 2016,18(3):252-288

[8] Shields W, Snead 3rd O. Benign epilepsy with centrotemporal spikes. Epilepsia 2009; 50:10-15. https://doi.org/10.1111/j.1528-1167.2009.02229.x.

[9] Bray PF, Wiser WC. Hereditary characteristics of familial temporal-central focal epilepsy. Pediatrics 1965;36:207-211.

[10] Commission on Classification and Terminology of the International League Against Epilepsy, 1989. Proposal for revised classification of epilepsies and epileptic syndromes Epilepsia 1989;30:389-399

[11] Petra MC.Callenbach et.al, Long term outcome of benign childhood epilepsy with centrotemporal spikes: Dutch study of epilepsy in childhood. Seizure (19) 2010, 501-506

[12] P.Piccinelli et al, Academic performance of children with Rolandic epilepsy. Developmental medicine and Child Neurology, 50; 353-356, 2008

[13] Berg, A. T., Berkovic, S. F., Brodie, M. J., Buchhalter, J., Cross, J. H., van Emde Boas, W., ... Scheffer, I. E. (2010). Revised terminology and concepts for organization of seizures and epilepsies: Report of the ILAE Commission on Classification and Terminology, 2005-2009. Epilepsia, 51(4), 676-685. doi:10.1111/j.1528-1167.2010.02522.x

[14] H. Goldberg-Stern et al, Neuropsychological aspects of benign childhood epilepsy with centrotemporal spikes. Seizure 19 (12-16), 2010

[15] Sabine Völkl-Kernstock et al, Speech and school performance in children with benign partial epilepsy with centro-temporal spikes (BCECTS). Seizure 18 (320-326), 2009

[16] Joost Nicolai et al, EEG Characteristics Related to Educational Impairments in Children with Benign Childhood Epilepsy with Centrotemporal Spikes. Epilepsia, 48(11):2093-2100, 2007

[17] Beaussart M, Faou R. Evolution of epilepsy with rolandic paroxysmal foci: a study of 324 cases. Epilepsia 1978;19:337-342

[18] Loiseau P, Duché B, Cordova S, et al. Prognosis of benign childhood epilepsy with centrotemporal spikes: a follow-up study of 168 patients. Epilepsia 1988;29:229-235.

[19] Piccirilli M, D_Alessandro P, Tiacci C, et al. Language lateralization in children with benign partial epilepsy. Epilepsia 1988;29:19-25.

[20] D_Alessandro P, Piccirilli M, Tiacci C, et al. Neuropsychological features of benign partial epilepsy in children. Ital J Neurol Sci 1990;11:265-269.

[21] D_Alessandro P, Piccirilli M, Sciarma T, et al. Cognition in benign childhood epilepsy: a longitudinal study. Epilepsia 1995;36(Suppl. 3):S124.

[22] Piccirilli M, D_Alessandro P, Sciarma T, et al. Attention problems in epilepsy: possible significance of the epileptic focus. Epilepsia 1994;35:1091-1096.

[23] Morooka K, Arimoto K, Takagi K, et al. Developmental disabilities in benign childhood epilepsy with centrotemporal spikes. Epilepsia 1995;36(Suppl. 3):S127.

[24] Weglage J, Demsky A, Pietsch M, et al. Neuropsychological, intellectual, and behavioral findings in patients with centrotemporal spikes with and without seizures. Dev Med Child Neurol 1997;39:646-651.

[25] Staden U, Isaacs E, Boyd SG, et al. Language dysfunction in children with rolandic epilepsy. Neuropediatrics 1998;29:242-248.

[26] Croona C, Kihlgren M, Lundberg S, et al. Neuropsychological findings in children with benign childhood epilepsy with centrotemporal spikes. Dev Med Child Neurol 1999;41:813-818.

[27] Gunduz E, Demirbilek V, Korkmaz B. Benign rolandic epilepsy: neuropsychological findings. Seizure 1999;8:246-249.

[28] Metz-Lutz MN, Kleitz C, De Saint-Martin A, et al. Cognitive development in benign focal epilepsies of childhood. Dev Neurosci 1999;21:182-190.

[29] Deonna T, Zesiger P, Davidoff V, et al. Benign partial epilepsy of childhood: a longitudinal neuropsychological and EEG study of cognitive function. Dev Med Child Neurol 2000;42:595-603.

[30] Yung AWY, Park YD, Cohen MJ, et al. Cognitive and behavioural problems in children with centrotemporal spikes. Pediatr Neurol 2000;23:391-395.

[31] Chevalier H, Metz-Lutz MN, Segalowitz SJ. Impulsivity and control of inhibition in benign focal childhood epilepsy (BFCE). Brain Cogn 2000;43:86-90.

[32] Schouten A, Oostrom K. Cognition and behaviour of schoolchildren with newly diagnosed idiopathic or cryptogenic epilepsy. Thesis, University Utrecht, 2001.

[33] Nicolai, J., Aldenkamp, A. P., Arends, J., Weber, J. W., & Vles, J. S. H. (2006). *Cognitive and behavioral effects of nocturnal epileptiform discharges in children with benign childhood epilepsy with centrotemporal spikes.* Epilepsy & Behavior, *8(1), 56-70.* doi:10.1016/j.yebeh.2005.08.016

[34] Hommet C, Billard C, Motte J, et al. Cognitive function in adolescents and

young adults in complete remission from benign childhood epilepsy with centro-temporal spikes. Epileptic Disord 2001;3:207-216.

[35] Fonseca LC, Tedrus GM, Tonelotto JM, et al. School performance in children with benign childhood epilepsy with centrotemporal spikes. Arq Neuropsiquiatr 2004;62:459-62. Epub 2004 jul.

[36] Lingren A, Kihlgren M, Melin L, et al. Development of cognitive functions in children with rolandic epilepsy. Epilepsy Behav 2004;5:903-910.

[37] Volkl-Kernstock S, Willinger U, Feucht M. Cognitive disabilities of children with a benign partial epilepsy. Neuropediatrics 2004;35. doi:10.1055/s-2004-819383.

[38] Monjauze C, Tuller L, Hommet C, et al. Language in benign epilepsy with centro-temporal spikes abbreviated form: Rolandic epilepsy and language. Brain Lang 2005;92:300-308.

[39] Papavasiliou A, Mattheou D, Bazigou H, et al. Written language skills in children with benign childhood epilepsy with centrotemporal spikes. Epilepsia Behav 2005;6:50-58.

[40] Northcott E, Connolly AM, Berroya A, et al. The neuropsychological and language profile of children with benign Rolandic epilepsy. Epilepsia 2005;46:924-930.

[41] Ingrid E. Scheffer et al, ILAE classification of the epilepsies: Position paper of the ILAE Commission for Classification and Terminology. Epilepsia, 58(4):512-521, 2017

[42] Bray, P. F., Wiser, W. C., Wood, M. C., & Pusey, S. B. (1964). Evidence for a Genetic Etiology of Temporal-Central Abnormalities in Focal Epilepsy. New England Journal of Medicine, 271(18), 926-933. doi:10.1056/nejm196410292711803

[43] Doose H, Brigger-Heuer B, Neubauer BA: Children with focal sharp waves: clinical and genetic aspects. Epilepsia 1997; 38: 788-796.

[44] Vadlamudi L, Kjeldsen MJ, Corey LA, Solaas MH, Friis ML, Pellock JM, et al. Analyzing the etiology of benign rolandic epilepsy: a multicenter twin collaboration. Epilepsia 2006;47:550-555.

[45] G. Rudolf et al., Exome sequencing in 57 patients with self-limited focal epilepsies of childhood with typical or atypical presentations suggests novel candidate genes, European Journal of Paediatric Neurology, https://doi.org/10.1016/j.ejpn.2020.05.003

[46] Gkampeta A, Fidani L, Clarimon J, Kalinderi K, Katopodi T, Zafeiriou D, et al. Association of brain-derived neurotrophic factor (BDNF) and elongator protein complex 4 (ELP4) polymorphisms with benign epilepsy with centrotemporal spikes in a Greek population. Epilepsy Res 2014;108:1734-1739.

[47] Dibbens LM, de Vries B, Donatello S, Heron SE, Hodgson BL, Chintawar S, et al. Mutations in DEPDC5 cause familial focal epilepsy with variable foci. Nat Genet 2013;45:546-551.

[48] Ishida S, Picard F, Rudolf G, Noe E, Achaz G, Thomas P, et al. Mutations of DEPDC5 cause autosomal dominant focal epilepsies. Nat Genet 2013;45:552-555.

[49] Baulac S. Genetics advances in autosomal dominant focal epilepsies: focus on DEPDC5. Prog Brain Res 2014;213:123-139.

[50] Lal D, Reinthaler EM, Schubert J, Muhle H, Riesch E, Kluger G, et al. DEPDC5 mutations in genetic focal

epilepsies of childhood. Ann Neurol 2014;75:788-792.

[51] van Kranenburg M, Hoogeveen-Westerveld M, Nellist M. Preliminary functional assessment and classification of DEPDC5 variants associated with focal epilepsy. Hum Mutat 2015;36:200-209.

[52] Vears, D. F., Tsai, M.-H., Sadleir, L. G., Grinton, B. E., Lillywhite, L. M., Carney, P. W., ... Scheffer, I. E. (2012). Clinical genetic studies in benign childhood epilepsy with centrotemporal spikes. Epilepsia, 53(2), 319-324. doi:10.1111/j.1528-1167.2011.03368.x

[53] Eeg-Olofsson O, Petersen I, Sellden U. The development of the electroenceph-alogram in normal children from the age of 1 through 15 years. Paroxysmal activity. Neuropadiatrie 1971;2:375-404.

[54] Ballaban-Gil K, Tuchman R. Epilepsy and epileptiform EEG: association with autism and language disorders. Ment Retard Dev Disabil Res Rev 2000;6:300-308.

[55] Heijbel J, Blom S, Rasmuson M. Benign epilepsy of childhood with centrotemporal EEG foci: A genetic study. Epilepsia 1971; 16: 285-293.

[56] Ottman R. Genetics of the partial epilepsies: a review. Epilepsia 1989; 30: 107-111.

[57] L.J. Strug, T. Clarke, T. Chiang, et al., Centrotemporal sharp wave EEG trait in Rolandic epilepsy maps to Elongator Protein Complex 4 (ELP4), Eur. J. Hum. Genet. 17 (2009) 1171e1181, https://doi.org/10.1038/ejhg.2008.267.

[58] Guerrini R, Bonanni P, Nardocci N, Parmeggiani L, Piccirilli M, De Fusco M, et al. Autosomal recessive rolandic epilepsy with paroxysmal exercise-induced dystonia and writer's cramp: delineation of the syndrome and gene mapping to chromosome 16p 12-11.2. Ann Neurol 1999;45:344-352.

[59] Neubauer BA, Fiedler B, Himmelein B, Kampfer F, Lassker U, Schwabe G, et al. Centrotemporal spikes in families with rolandic epilepsy: linkage to chromosome 15q14. Neurology 1998;51:1608-1612.

[60] Bobbili, D. R., Lal, D., May, P., Reinthaler, E. M., Jabbari, K., ... Neubauer, B. A. (2018). Exome-wide analysis of mutational burden in patients with typical and atypical Rolandic epilepsy. European Journal of Human Genetics, 26(2), 258-264. doi:10.1038/s41431-017-0034-x

[61] Xiong, W., & Zhou, D. (2017). Progress in unraveling the genetic etiology of rolandic epilepsy. Seizure, 47, 99-104. doi:10.1016/j.seizure.2017.02.012

[62] Maihara T, Tsuji M, Higuchi Y, Hattori H. Benign familial neonatal convulsions followed by benign epilepsy with centrotemporal spikes in two siblings. Epilepsia 1999;40:110-113.

[63] Coppola G, Castaldo P, Miraglia del Giudice E, Bellini G, Galasso F, Soldovieri MV, et al. A novel KCNQ2 K+ channel mutation in benign neonatal convulsions and centrotemporal spikes. Neurology 2003;61:131-134.

[64] Neubauer BA, Waldegger S, Heinzinger J, Hahn A, Kurlemann G, Fiedler B, et al. KCNQ2 and KCNQ3 mutations contribute to different idiopathic epilepsy syndromes. Neurology 2008;71:177-183.

[65] Roll, P., Rudolf, G., Pereira, S., Royer, B., Scheffer, I. E., Massacrier, A., ... Szepetowski, P. (2006). SRPX2 mutations in disorders of language cortex and cognition. Human Molecular Genetics, 15(7), 1195-1207. doi:10.1093/hmg/ddl035

[66] Lemke JR, Lal D, Reinthaler EM, et al. Mutations in GRIN2A cause idiopathic focal epilepsy with rolandic spikes. Nat Genet 2013;45: 1067-1072.

[67] Lal, D., Reinthaler, E. M., Altmüller, J., Toliat, M. R., Thiele, H., Nürnberg, P., ... Neubauer, B. A. (2013).RBFOX1 and RBFOX3 Mutations in Rolandic Epilepsy. PLoS ONE, 8(9), e73323. doi:10.1371/journal.pone.0073323

[68] Reinthaler, E. M., Dejanovic, B., Lal, D., Semtner, M., Merkler, Y., ... Reinhold, A. (2015). Rare variants in γ-aminobutyric acid type A receptor genes in rolandic epilepsy and related syndromes. Annals of Neurology, 77(6), 972-986. doi:10.1002/ana.24395

[69] Neng, X., Xiao, M., Yuanlu, C., Qinyan, L., Li, S., & Zhanyi, S. (2020). Novel variant in CHRNA4 with benign childhood epilepsy with centrotemporal spikes and contribution to precise medicine. Molecular Genetics & Genomic Medicine. doi:10.1002/mgg3.1264

[70] Scala, M., Bianchi, A., Bisulli, F., Coppola, A., Elia, M., Trivisano, M., ... Gambardella, A. (2020). Advances in genetic testing and optimization of clinical management in children and adults with epilepsy. Expert Review of Neurotherapeutics. Doi:10.1080/14737175.2020.1713101

[71] Holmes GL. Rolandic epilepsy: clinical and electroencephalographic features. Epilepsy Res Suppl. 1992;6:29-43. PMID: 1418488.

[72] Stephani U. Typical semiology of benign childhood epilepsy with centrotemporal spikes (BCECTS). Epileptic Disord. 2000;2 Suppl 1:S3–S4. PMID: 11231216.

[73] Vinayan, K. P., Biji, V., & Thomas, S. V. (2005). Educational problems with underlying neuropsychological impairment are common in children with Benign Epilepsy of Childhood with Centrotemporal Spikes (BECTS). Seizure, 14(3), 207-212. doi:10.1016/j.seizure.2005.01.009

[74] Panayiotopoulos, C. P., Michael, M., Sanders, S., Valeta, T., & Koutroumanidis, M. (2008). Benign childhood focal epilepsies: assessment of established and newly recognized syndromes. Brain, 131(9), 2264-2286. doi:10.1093/brain/awn162

[75] Bouma PA, Bovenkerk AC, Westendorp RG, Brouwer OF. The course of benign partial epilepsy of childhood with centrotemporal spikes: a meta-analysis. Neurology. 1997 Feb;48(2):430-437. doi: 10.1212/wnl.48.2.430. PMID: 9040734.

[76] Ferrari-Marinho, T., Hamad, A. P. A., Casella, E. B., Yacubian, E. M. T., & Caboclo, L. O. (2020). Seizures in self-limited epilepsy with centrotemporal spikes: video-EEG documentation. Child's Nervous System. doi:10.1007/s00381-020-04763-8

[77] Cortesi F, Gianotti F, Ottaviano S. Sleep problems and daytime behavior in childhood idiopathic epilepsy. Epilepsia 1999;40:1557-1565.

[78] Panayiotopoulos, C. P. (2004). Autonomic seizures and autonomic status epilepticus peculiar to childhood: diagnosis and management. Epilepsy & Behavior, 5(3), 286-295. doi:10.1016/j.yebeh.2004.01.013

[79] Yoshinaga, H., Kobayashi, K., Shibata, T., Inoue, T., Oka, M., & Akiyama, T. (2015). Manifestation of both emetic seizures and sylvian seizures in the same patients with benign partial epilepsy. Brain and Development, 37(1), 13-17. doi:10.1016/j.braindev.2014.01.013

[80] Covanis A, Lada C, Skiadas K. Children with Rolandic spikes and ictal vomiting: Rolandic epilepsy or

Panayiotopoulos syndrome? Epileptic Disord. 2003 Sep;5(3):139-143. PMID: 14684348.

[81] Caraballo R, Cersosimo R, Medina C, Fejerman N. Panayiotopoulos-type benign childhood occipital epilepsy: a prospective study. Neurology 2000; 55: 1096-1100.

[82] Ferrie CD, Beaumanoir A, Guerrini R, et al. Early-onset benign occipital seizure susceptibility syndrome. Epilepsia 1997; 38: 285-293.

[83] Guerrini R, Belmonte A, Veggiotti P, Mattia D, Bonanni P. Delayed appearance of interictal EEG abnormalities in early onset childhood epilepsy with occipital paroxysms. Brain 1997; 19: 343-346.

[84] Panayiotopoulos CP. Extraoccipital benign childhood partial seizures with ictal vomiting and excellent prognosis. J Neurol Neurosurg Psychiatry 1999; 66: 82-85.

[85] Panayiotopoulos CP. Benign childhood partial seizures and related epileptic syndromes. London: John Libbey, Company Ltd, 1999.

[86] Chrysostomos P. Panayiotopoulos, The Birth and Evolution of the Concept of Panayiotopoulos Syndrome, Epilepsia 48(6);1041-1043,2007

[87] Colamaria, V., Sgro, V., Caraballo, R., Simeone, M., Zullini, E., Fontana, E., ... Bernardina, B. D. (1991).Status Epilepticus in Benign Rolandic Epilepsy Manifesting as Anterior Operculum Syndrome. Epilepsia, 32(3), 329-334. doi:10.1111/j.1528-1157.1991.tb04659.x

[88] Fejerman N. Atypical rolandic epilepsy. Epilepsia 2009;50 Suppl 7:9-12.

[89] Aicardi J. Atypical semiology of rolandic epilepsy in some related syndromes. Epileptic Disord 2000;2 Suppl 1:S5–S9.

[90] Fejerman N, Caraballo R, Tenembaum SN. (2000) Atypical evolutions of benign localization-related epilepsies in children: are they predictable? Epilepsia 41:380-390.

[91] Fejerman N, Caraballo R, Dalla Bernardina B. (2007a) Benign childhood epilepsy with centrotemporal spikes. In Fejerman N, Caraballo RH (Eds) Benign focal epilepsies in infancy, childhood and adolescence. John Libbey, Montrouge, pp. 77-113.

[92] Fejerman N, Caraballo R, Dalla Bernardina B. (2007b) Atypical evolutions of benign focal epilepsies in childhood. In Fejerman N, Caraballo RH (Eds) Benign focal epilepsies in infancy, childhood and adolescence. John Libbey, Montrouge, pp. 179-220.

[93] Trinka, E., Cock, H., Hesdorffer, D., Rossetti, A. O., Scheffer, I. E., Shinnar, S., ... Lowenstein, D. H. (2015). A definition and classification of status epilepticus - Report of the ILAE Task Force on Classification of Status Epilepticus. Epilepsia, 56(10), 1515-1523. doi:10.1111/epi.13121

[94] Donald Shields W, Snead III C. Benign epilepsy with centrotemporal spikes. Epilepsia 2009;50:10-15

[95] Loiseau P, Duche B, Benign childhood epilepsy with centrotemporal spikes. Cleve Clin J Med 56: 17-22, 1989

[96] Engel J, Fejerman N. Benign childhood epilepsy with centrotemporal spikes. In: J Engel, N Fejerman (Eds.), MedLink Neurology (Section of Epilepsy). MedLink Corporation, San Diego. Available at http://www.medlink.com. 2006

[97] Lombroso CT (1967). Sylvian seizures and midtemporal spike foci in children. Arch Neurol 17: 52-59.

[98] Bouma PAD, Bovenkerk AC, Westendorp RGJ, Brouwer OF. The

course of benign partial epilepsy of childhood with centrotemporal spikes: a meta-analysis. Neurology 1997;48(2):430-437. https://doi.org/10.1212/wnl.48.2.430.

[99] Wong P.K. Stability of source estimates in rolandic spikes. Brain Topogr. 1989; **2**: 31-36

[100] Yoshinaga, H., Amano, R., Oka, E., & Ohtahara, S. (1992). *Dipole tracing in childhood epilepsy with special reference to Rolandic epilepsy.* Brain Topography, *4(3), 193-199.* doi:10.1007/bf01131150

[101] De Marco P, Tassinari CA (1981). Extreme somatosensory evoked potentials (ESEPs): an EEG sign forecasting the possible occurrence of seizures in children. Epilepsia 22: 569-585.

[102] Gelisse, P., Genton, P., Bureau, M., Dravet, C., Guerrini, R., Viallat, D., & Roger, J. (1999). *Are there generalised spike waves and typical absences in benign rolandic epilepsy?* Brain and Development, *21(6), 390-396.* doi:10.1016/s0387-7604(99)00040-6

[103] Ishitobi M, Nakasato N, Yamamoto K, Iinuma K. Opercular to interhemispheric source distribution of benign rolandic spikes of childhood. Neuroimage 2005;25:417-423.

[104] Archer, J.S., Briellman, R.S., Abbott, D.F., Syngeniotis, A., Wellard, R.M., Jackson, G.D., 2003. Benign epilepsy with centro-temporal spikes: spike triggered fMRI shows somato-sensory cortex activity. Epilepsia 44, 200-204.

[105] Kubota M, Oka A, Kin S, Sakakihara Y: Generators of rolandic discharges identified by magnetoencephalography. Electroencephalogr Clin Neurophysiol 1996;(Suppl 47):393-401.

[106] Kubota, M., Takeshita, K., Sakakihara, Y., Yanagisawa, M., 2000. Magnetoencephalographic study of giant somatosensory evoked responses in patients with rolandic epilepsy. J. Child. Neurol. 15, 370-379.

[107] Gregory DL, Wong PKH. Topographic analysis of the centrotemporal discharges in benign rolandic epilepsy of childhood. Epilepsia 1984; 25: 705-711.

[108] Jung, K.-Y., Kim, J.-M., & Kim, D. W. (2003). Patterns of Interictal Spike Propagation across the Central Sulcus in Benign Rolandic Epilepsy. Clinical Electroencephalography, 34(3), 153-157. doi:10.1177/155005940303400309

[109] Cavazutti GB, Cappella L, Nalin A. Longitudinal study of epileptiform EEG patterns in normal children. Epilepsia1980;21:43-55.

[110] Stephani U, Carlsson G. The spectrum from BCECTS to LKS: the rolandic EEG trait—impact on cognition. Epilepsia 2006;47:67-70.

[111] Heijbel J, Blom S, Rasmussen M. Benign epilepsy of childhood with centrotemporal EEG foci: a genetic study. Epilepsia1975;16:285-293.

[112] Mariam Tashkandi, Duaa Baarma, Andrea C. Tricco, Cyrus Boelman, Reem Alkhater, EEG of asymptomatic first-degree relatives of patients with juvenile myoclonic, childhood absence and rolandic epilepsy: a systematic review and meta-analysis, Epileptic Disorders, Vol 21, Issue 1, p 30-41, 2019, https://doi.org/10.1684/epd.2019.1024

[113] Kellaway P. The electroencephalographic features of benign centrotemporal (rolandic) epilepsy of childhood. Epilepsia 2000; 41: 1053-1056.

[114] Dalla Bernardina B, Tassinari CA. EEG of a nocturnal seizure in a patient with "Benign Epilepsy of Childhood

with Rolandic Spikes". Epilepsia 1975;16:497-501.

[115] Gutierrez AR, Brick JF, Bodensteiner J. Dipole reversal: an ictal feature of benign partial epilepsy with centrotemporal spikes.Epilepsia 1990;31:544-548.

[116] Capovilla, G., Beccaria, F., Bianchi, A., Canevini, M. P., Giordano, L., Gobbi, G., ... Pruna, D. (2011). Ictal EEG patterns in epilepsy with centro-temporal spikes. Brain and Development, 33(4), 301-309. doi:10.1016/j.braindev.2010.06.007

[117] Oliveira de Andrade D. Padrao eletrografico ictal subclinico em um caso de epilepsia parcial benigna da infancia com pontascentro-temporais. Arq Neuropsiquiatr 2005;63(2A):360-363.

[118] Saint-Martin AD, Carcangiu R, Arzimanoglou A, Massa R, Thomas P, Motte J, et al. Semiology of typical and atypical Rolandic epilepsy: a video-EEG analysis. Epil Disord 2001;3:173-182.

[119] Alving, J., Fabricius, M., Rosenzweig, I., & Beniczky, S. (2017). Ictal source imaging and electroclinical correlation in self-limited epilepsy with centrotemporal spikes. Seizure, 52, 7-10. doi:10.1016/j.seizure.2017.09.006

[120] Dean P.Sarco et al., Benign Rolandic epileptiform discharges are associated with mood and behavior problems. Epilepsy Behav.2011 Oct.22(2):298-303

[121] Nicolai J. et al., Cognitive and behavioral effects on nocturnal epileptiform discharges in children with benign childhood epilepsy with centrotemporal spikes. Epilepsy Behav.8 2006, 56-70

[122] Garcia-Ramos, C., Dabbs, K., Lin, J. J., Jones, J. E., Stafstrom, C. E., Hsu, D. A., ... Hermann, B. P. (2019). Network analysis of prospective brain development in youth with benign epilepsy with centrotemporal spikes and its relationship to cognition. Epilepsia. doi:10.1111/epi.16290

[123] Baglietto MG, Battaglia FM, Nobili I, et al. Neuropsychological disorders relate to interictal epileptic discharges during sleep in benign epilepsy of childhood with centrotemporal or Rolandic spikes. Dev Med Child Neurol 2001;43:407-412.

[124] Vannest J. Tenney JR.et al. Impact of frequency and lateralization of interictal discharges on neuropsychological and fine motor status in children with benign epilepsy with centrotemporal spikes Epilepsia, 57(8):e161–e167, 2016 doi: 10.1111/epi.13445

[125] Smith AB, Bajomo O, Pal DK. A meta-analysis of literacy and language in children with rolandic epilepsy. Dev Med Child Neurol 2015;57:1019-1026.

[126] Ross, E. E., Stoyell, S. M., Kramer, M. A., Berg, A. T., & Chu, C. J. (2019). The natural history of seizures and neuropsychiatric symptoms in childhood epilepsy with centrotemporal spikes (CECTS). Epilepsy & Behavior, 106437. doi:10.1016/j.yebeh.2019.07.038

[127] Besag FMC. Cognitive and behavioral outcomes of epileptic syndromes: implications for education and clinical practice. Epilepsia 2006;47(s2):119-25. https://doi.org/10.1111/j.1528-1167.2006.00709.x.

[128] Samaitienė R, Norkūnienė J, Jurkevičienė G, Grikinienė J. Behavioral problems in children with benign childhood epilepsy with centrotemporal spikes treated and untreated with antiepileptic drugs. Medicina 2012;48(7):50. https://doi.org/10.3390/medicina48070050.

[129] Hughes JR. Benign epilepsy of childhood with centrotemporal

spikes (CECTS): to treat or not to treat, that is the question. Epilepsy Behav 2010;19(3):197-203. https://doi.org/10.1016/j.yebeh.2010.07.018.

[130] Kramer U, Zelnik N, Lerman-Sagie T, Shahar E. Benign childhood epilepsy with centrotemporal spikes: clinical characteristics and identification of patients at risk for multiple seizures. J Child Neurol 2002;17(1):17-19. https://doi.org/10.1177/ 088307380201700104.

[131] You SJ, Kim DS, Ko TS. Benign childhood epilepsy with centro-temporal spikes (BCECTS): early onset of seizures is associated with poorer response to initial treatment. Epileptic Disord 2006;8(4):285-288. https://doi.org/10.1684/epd. 2006.0049.

[132] Anna Elisabetta Vaudano, Pietro Avanzini, Gaetano Cantalupo, Melissa Filippini, Andrea Ruggieri, Mapping the Effect of Interictal Epileptic Activity Density During Wakefulness on Brain Functioning in Focal Childhood Epilepsies With Centrotemporal Spikes. Front. Neurol. 2019; 10: 131.doi:10.3389/fneur.2019.01316

[133] Kwon, S., Seo, H.-E., & Hwang, S. K. (2012). Cognitive and other neuropsychological profiles in children with newly diagnosed benign rolandic epilepsy. Korean Journal of Pediatrics, 55(10), 383. doi:10.3345/kjp.2012.55.10.383

[134] Wickens S. et al. Cognitive functioning in children with self-limited epilepsy with centrotemporal spikes: A systematic review and meta-analysis, Epilepsia, 58(10):1673-1685, 2017 doi: 10.1111/epi.1385

[135] Carmen Silvia Molleis Galego Miziara et al, Impact of benign childhood epilepsy with centrotemporal spikes (BECTS) on school performance. Seizure 21 (87-91), 2012

[136] Massa R, de Saint-Martin A, Carcangiu R, Rudolf G, Seegmuller C, Kleitz C, et al. EEG criteria predictive of complicated evolution in idiopathic rolandic epilepsy. Neurology 2001;57:1071-1079.

[137] Dalla Bernardina B. Partial epilepsies of childhood, bilateral synchronization continuous spike-wave during slow sleep. In: Manelis J, Bental E, Loeber JN, Dreifuss FE, eds. Advances in Epileptology, New York: Raven Press, 1989; XVII:295-302.

[138] Piccinelli, P., Borgatti, R., Aldini, A., Bindelli, D., Ferri, M., Perna, S., ... Balottin, U. (2008). Academic performance in children with rolandic epilepsy. Developmental Medicine & Child Neurology, 50(5), 353-356. doi:10.1111/j.1469-8749.2008.02040.x

[139] Kim H, Yoo IH et al. Averaged EEG spike dipole analysis may predict atypical outcome in Benign Childhood Epilepsy with Centrotemporal Spikes (BCECTS). 22 January 2018

[140] E.Tovia et al, The prevalence of atypical presentations and comorbidities of benign childhood epilepsy with centrotemporal spikes. Epilepsia 52(8): 1483-1488, 2011

[141] Parisi P, Paolino MC, Raucci U, Ferretti A, Villa MP, Trenite DK. "Atypical forms" of benign epilepsy with centrotemporal spikes (BECTS): How to diagnose and guide these children. A practical/scientific approach. Epilepsy Behav. 2017 Oct;75:165-169. doi: 10.1016/j.yebeh.2017.08.001. Epub 2017 Sep 1. PMID: 28866336.

[142] Kai Gao, Anel Tankovic et al, A de novo loss-of-function GRIN2A mutation associated with childhood focal epilepsy and acquired epileptic aphasia. PLOS ONE | DOI:10.1371 , 2017

[143] Dheeraj R. Bobbili. Exome-wide analysis of mutational burden in

patients with typical and atypical Rolandic epilepsy. European Journal of Human Genetics volume 26, pages 258-264, 2018

[144] Reutlinger, C., Helbig, I., Gawelczyk, B., Subero, J. I. M., Tönnies, H., Muhle, H., ... Caliebe, A. (2010). Deletions in 16p13 including GRIN2A in patients with intellectual disability, various dysmorphic features, and seizure disorders of the rolandic region. Epilepsia, 51(9), 1870-1873. doi:10.1111/j.1528-1167.2010.02555.x

[145] Dimassi S, Labalme A, Lesca G, Rudolf G, Bruneau N, Hirsch E, et al. A subset of genomic alterations detected in rolandic epilepsies contains candidate or known epilepsy genes including GRIN2A and PRRT2. Epilepsia 2014;55:370-378.

[146] Yun Jeong Lee et.al, The clinical spectrum of benign epilepsy with centro-temporal spikes; a challenge in categorization and predictability. Journal of epilepsy research Vol7, N1, 2017

[147] Aicardi J, Chevrie JJ. Atypical benign partial epilepsy of childhood. Dev Med Child Neurol. 1982 Jun;24(3):281-292. doi: 10.1111/j.1469-8749.1982.tb13620.x. PMID: 6807733.

[148] Doose H, Baier WK. Benign partial epilepsy and related conditions: multifactorial pathogenesis with hereditary impairment of brain maturation. Eur J Pediatr. 1989 Dec;149(3):152-158. doi: 10.1007/BF01958268. PMID: 2693093.

[149] Pesántez-Ríos G, Martínez-Bermejo A, Arcas J, Merino-Andreu M, Ugalde-Canitrot A. Las evoluciones atipicas de la epilepsia rolandica son complicaciones predecibles [The atypical developments of rolandic epilepsy are predictable complications]. Rev Neurol. 2015 Aug 1;61(3):106-13. Spanish. PMID: 26178515.

[150] Japaridze, N., Menzel, E., von Ondarza, G., Steinmann, E., & Stephani, U. (2014). Risk factors of cognitive outcome in patients with atypical benign partial epilepsy/pseudo-Lennox syndrome (ABPE/PLS) and continues spike and wave during sleep (CSWS). European Journal of Paediatric Neurology, 18(3), 368-375.

[151] Guerrini, R., Dravet, C., Genton, P., Bureau, M., Roger, J., Rubboli, G. and Tassinari, C.A. Epileptic negative myoclonus. Neurology, 1993, 43: 1078-1083.

[152] Kanazawa, 0. and Kawai, 1. Status epilepticus characterized by repetitive asymmetrical atonia: two cases accompanied by partial seizures. Epilepsia, 1990, 31: 536-543

[153] Tassinari CA, Rubboli G. Cognition and paroxysmal EEG activities: from a single spike to electrical status epilepticus during sleep.Epilepsia 2006;47:40-43.

[154] Caraballo R, Fontana E, Michelizza B, Zullini B, Sgro V, Pajno-Ferrara F, Dalla Bernardina B, Espositio S. (1989) Carbamazepine inducing atypical absences, atonic seizures and continuous spike and waves during slow wave sleep. Boll Lega It Epil 66/67:379-381.

[155] Kramer, U. (2008). Atypical Presentations of Benign Childhood Epilepsy With Centrotemporal Spikes: A Review. Journal of Child Neurology, 23(7), 785-790. doi:10.1177/0883073808316363

[156] Fejerman N, Di Blasi M. Status epilepticus of benign partial epilepsies in children: report of two cases. Epilepsia. 1987;28: 351-355.

[157] Salas-Puig J, Perez-Jimenez A, Thomas P, et al. Opercular epilepsies

with oromotor dysfunction. In: Guerrini R, Aicardi J, Andermann F, Hallet R, eds. Epilepsy and Movement Disorders. London: Cambridge University Press; 2002:251-268

[158] Tacke, M., Borggraefe, I., Gerstl, L., Heinen, F., Vill, K., Bonfert, M., ... Baethmann, M. (2018).Effects of Levetiracetam and Sulthiame on EEG in benign epilepsy with centrotemporal spikes: A randomized controlled trial. Seizure, 56, 115-120. doi:10.1016/j.seizure.2018.01.015

[159] Dietz Rating, Christian Wolf, and Thomas Bast. Sulthiame as monotherapy in children with benign childhood epilepsy with centrotemporal spikes: A 6-month randomized, double-blind, placebo-controlled study. Epilepsia, 41(10):1284-1288, 2000.

[160] Bruria Ben-Zeev, Nathan Watemberg, Pinchas Lerman, Itshak Barash, Nathan Brand, and Tally Lerman-Sagie. Sulthiame in childhood epilepsy. Pediatr. int., 46(5):521-524, 2004.

[161] A Verrotti, G Coppola, R Manco, G Ciambra, P Iannetti, S Grosso, P Balestri, E Franzoni, and F Chiarelli. Levetiracetam monotherapy for children and adolescents with benign rolandic seizures. Seizure, 16(3):271-275, 2007.

[162] Coppola G, Franzoni E, Verrotti A, GaroneC,SarajlijaJ,OpertoFF,PascottoA. Levetiracetam or oxcarbazepine as monotherapy in newly diagnosed benign epilepsy of childhood with centrotemporal spikes (BECTS): an open-label, parallel group trial. Brain Dev. 2007 Jun;29(5):281-284. doi: 10.1016/j.braindev.2006.09.008. Epub 2006 Oct 20. PMID: 17055681.

[163] Hamada Y, Okuno T, Hattori H, Mikawa H. Indication for antiepileptic drug treatment of benign childhood epilepsy with centro-temporal spikes. Brain Dev 1994;16:159—161.

[164] Bourgeois BF. Drug treatment of benign focal epilepsies of childhood. Epilepsia 2000;41:1057-1058

[165] Reed, M. D., & Gilman, J. T. (1991). Carbamazepine Dosing for Pediatric Seizure Disorders: The Highs and Lows. DICP, 25(10), 1109-1112. doi:10.1177/106002809102501017

[166] Guerrini, R. (2006). Valproate as a Mainstay of Therapy for Pediatric Epilepsy. Pediatric Drugs, 8(2), 113-129. doi:10.2165/00148581-200608020-00004

[167] Glauser TA, Ayala R, Elterman RD et al. (2000). Double-blind placebo-controlled trial of adjunctive levetiracetam in pediatric partial seizures. Neurology 66: 1654-1660.

[168] George L. Morris, Gabapentin, Epilepsia, 40 (Suppl 5),1999

[169] Bourgeois B, Brown LW, Pellock JM, et al. Gabapentin monotherapy in children with benign childhood epilepsy with centro-temporal spikes (BECTS): a 36-week, double-blind. placebo-controlled study. Am Proc Epilepsy Soc Meef 1998.

Chapter 4

Review in Autism and Epilepsy

Mashael AlKhateeb and Hesham AlDhalaan

Abstract

Autism is a neurodevelopmental disorder of undefined etiology characterized by social, communication deficits, and restricted interests/repetitive or isolated behaviors. The determination of autism is made in early life as the patients create unusual or decreased social interaction and communication, together with stereotypic movement. In most patients, a delay in verbal and nonverbal communication is watched, whereas a few patients never accomplish valuable language. Patients with autism and epilepsy may develop any type of seizure and maybe all type of seizures. Interestingly, not absolutely understood relationship between each and a lot of research in progress concerning these relations. In patients with autism, some they do not develop seizures; however, abnormal paroxysmal electroencephalographic "EEG" activity can be seen in up to 30%. For that reason, important investigation of patients with autistic spectrum disorders, and any kids with language regression, should always include sleep recording EEG in order to exclude acquired epileptic aphasia (Landau-Kleffner syndrome). The complex relationship between autism and epilepsy provides a bridge to further knowledge of shared neuronal networks for both the autisms and the epilepsies We review the literature to elucidate the relationships between epilepsy and autism.

Keywords: epilepsy, autism, EEG, seizure, syndromes, autistic spectrum disorders

1. Epilepsy and autism

Epilepsy is a neurological disorder not uncommon in children especially with Autism Spectrum Disorder (ASD) [1–4] but little is known about how seizures impact the autism phenotype and the co-occurrence of both conditions leads to opens a lot of windows to speculate that [5]. The etiology of this co-morbidity (autism and epilepsy) is in most cases unclear. In some cases both conditions may be entirely independent and acquired together by chance. In other cases, autistic phenotype and epilepsy are associated with genetic disorder (e.g., fragile-X syndrome, Rett syndrome) or the same acquired early cerebral insult (e.g., congenital rubella).

2. What is the prevalence of autism?

The most recent estimate from the Autism and Developmental Disabilities Monitoring (ADDM) ASD prevalence (1.46%) in 2012, with increase from 0.67% in 2000 to 1.47% in 2010. In a large, nationwide population-based study, the estimated ASD prevalence was 2.47% among US children and adolescents in 2014–2016, with no statistically significant increase over the 3 years [6].

 IntechOpen

3. What is the rate of epilepsy in ASD?

The rate of epilepsy in ASD has long been reported, but prevalence estimates vary from as little as 5% to as much as 46% [1].

4. Is there any connection between autism and epilepsy?

The complex relationship between autism and epilepsy, as reflected in the autism–epilepsy phenotype, provides a bridge to further knowledge of shared neuronal networks for both the autisms and the epilepsies.

The autisms and epilepsies are heterogeneous disorders that have diverse etiologies and pathologies. Some epilepsy syndromes and specific genetic factors involved in those syndromes are associated with a high risk of ASD. For example, patients with tuberous sclerosis, especially TSC2 mutations, Dravet syndrome, caused by mutations in SCN1A, and epilepsy in females mentally challenged or EFMR, found to be auxiliary to PCDH19 mutations that increase the chance to have autistic like features [7].

The increased prevalence of epilepsy and/or epileptiform discharges in individuals with ASD may be an important sign for an underlying neurological abnormality. Until recently, reported rates of interictal epileptiform discharges varied from 6 to 30% of ASD patients. But higher rates of isolated epileptifom EEGs have been reported recently and one study of children referred for video EEG monitoring to evaluate possible seizures found interictal epileptiform abnormalities in 59% [1].

The correlation between ASD and epilepsy suggests an underlying encephalopathy presenting with a combination of neurologic abnormalities.

5. Conceptual framework between autism and epilepsy

Autism includes heterogeneous conditions that affect the developmental trajectory of social cognition and verbal and non-verbal communication. Repetitive behaviors and narrow interests are characteristic of individuals with autism.

The commonly used terms Autism spectrum disorders (ASD) or pervasive developmental disorder (PDD) to incorporate children with autistic disorder, pervasive developmental disorders not otherwise specified (PDD-NOS) and those with Asperger disorder (AS). Children with disintegrative disorder (DD) and Rett disorder (RS) are too included beneath the umbrella term of PDD but have features, particularly when examining the relationship of epilepsy to autism, that recognize them from children with AD, PDD-NOS, and AS. With the exemption of RS, these disorders are all behaviorally characterized and most recent studies utilize the term autism interchangeably with that of ASD to incorporate children with AD, PDD-NOS, AS, and DD, but not RS [8].

There's no single no single etiology for autism or for epilepsy. Both are associated with change in behavior, cognitive, and variable outcomes.

6. Genetics of autism

Autism is not a disease but a syndrome with multiple non-genetic and genetic causes.

According to the Diagnostic and Statistical Manual of Mental Disorders, Fourth Edition, Text Revision (DSMIV-TR)7 and International Classification of Diseases, Tenth Revision (ICD-10).

(The autistic spectrum disorders [ASDs]), characterized by impairments in 3 behavioral domains:

1. Social interaction.

2. Language, communication, and imaginative play and

3. Range of interests and activities [9].

A number of approaches are being used to elucidate the association between specific genes and autism.

7. Cytogenetics and chromosomes 15q and 7q

Cytogenetic assays used for decades to explore chromosomal defects in patients with autism, and a number of cytogenetic abnormalities besides fragile X have been described [9].

Less than 10% of cases of autism are associated with clear chromosomal abnormalities, Cytogenetic abnormalities found at the 15q11-q13 locus are reported most frequently in patients with autism, up to 1–4%.

Analysts have started to look at the glutamatergic framework within the pathogenesis of autism. A few lines of prove recommend the inclusion of glutamate receptors: (1) Indications of hypoglutamatergia mirror the behavioral phenotypes of autism. (2) Serotonin receptor 2A (5-HT2A) agonists cause behavior comparative to autism, maybe through expression of 5HT2A on glutamatergic-inhibiting GABAergic neurons. (3) Association studies have involved the inclusion of GABAA receptors on 15q11-q13 that in turn balance glutamatergic function. (4) Excessive glutamatergic activity is associated with epileptiform activity, which is highly associated with autism.

The inotropic glutamate receptor 6 (GluR6) gene on chromosome 6q21 was associated significantly with autism. Also, the metabotropic glutamate receptor GRM8 in the chromosome 7q31-q33 autism susceptibility locus has exhibited linkage disequilibrium LD with autism. These data highlight the need for additional investigations into the relationship between the glutamate system and autism.

The neuromodulator oxytocin (OT) is also potentially relevant to the impaired sociability of autism [9].

Autism genes have been troublesome to recognize, in spite of the fact that well known the high heritability of autism disorders. Up to 10% of autism cases may be due to uncommon sequence and gene dosage variations, for example, mutations in NRXN1, NLGN3/4X, SHANK3, and copy number variants at 15q11-q13 and 16p11.2 [10].

A number of illnesses of known etiology, including Rett disorder, fragile X disorder, neurofibromatosis, tuberous sclerosis, Potocki-Lupski syndrome and Smith-Lemli-Opitz syndrome, are also related with autism. The remaining 90% of autism spectrum disorders, whereas exceedingly familial, have unknown hereditary etiology [10].

8. Genes implicated in autism and epilepsy

The genetic abnormalities in autism and epilepsy not completely identified.

Cytogenetic studies have identified recurrent, maternally inherited duplications of chromosome 15q11-13 along with other rare chromosomal abnormalities is considered to be an important cause of ASD [8].

Some genes, such as NLGN4, NRXN1, and SHANK3, have been identified by array-based methods. Although they collectively account for an estimated 15% of cases, variants at these and other loci are detected in no more than 1–2% of children with an ASD [8].

In addition to that copy number variants (CNVs; e.g., microdeletions, microduplications, insertions) and single gene disorders have been found to be associated to ASD.

Many disease genes have been described as related to ASD, for example: SCN 1A, SCN2A, KCNMA1, NLGN4X, NRXN1, SYNGAP1, ARX, SHANK3, CNTNAP2, NLGN4X, and play important role in epilepsy [11].

9. Genetic syndromes with ASD and epilepsy

Gene disorders known to be associated with ASD, such as Rett Syndrome (MECP2Fragile X Syndrome (FMR1), 22q13 Deletion Syndrome/Phelan-McDermid Syndrome,), and Tuberous Sclerosis (TSC1, TSC2), and cortical dysplasia focal epilepsy syndrome (CDFE) a recessive nonsense mutation in CNTNAP2 are associated with epilepsy [12].

CNTNAP2 (also known as CASPR2) encodes a neuronal transmembrane protein member of the neurexin superfamily involved in neuron-glia interactions and clustering of K+ channels in myelinated axons. This is supported by the imaging and pathology data in patients with CDFE, in whom nearly half manifest presumed neuronal migration abnormalities on MRI, confirmed by histological analysis of brain tissue resected from patients who underwent surgery for epilepsy.

It is rare disorder resulting in epileptic seizures, language regression, intellectual disability, hyperactivity, and, in nearly two-thirds of the patients, autism [13].

The Continuous Spikes and Waves during Slow-wave Sleep syndrome (CSWSS) and Landau-Kleffner (LKS) syndrome are two epileptic encephalopathies that share common clinical features, including seizures and regression with autistic features. Both LKS and Regressive ASD patients experience an onset of regression. In LKS, the regression is specific to language skills but in Regressive ASD, it is a global. The important difference between both, the age of onset of regression for LKS is between the ages of 3 and 9 years, whereas for Regressive ASD the onset is before 2 years of age.

10. The autism-epilepsy phenotype

The characteristics of the autism-epilepsy phenotype propose that there are fundamental etiologies and pathologies dependable for both the seizures and the socio-cognitive and communicative behaviors that characterize autism. Understanding of neuronal systems and the part of cellular dysfunction, and molecular derangements common to both autism and epilepsy.

10.1 Neural networks in epilepsy and autism

Both epilepsy and autism may be consequences of disorders of large-scale neural networks with alterations in cortical-subcortical systems connectivity.

DOI: http://dx.doi.org/10.5772/intechopen.93424

Alterations in subcortical systems such as basal ganglia-substantia nigra connectivity, may lower the seizure threshold, contribute to cognitive impairments and to the motor stereotypies commonly found in autism.

A disorder in which abnormalities of interneurons are hypothesized and in which both autism and epilepsy commonly coexist is infantile spasm [14].

Malformations of cortical development (MCD), due to focal disruption of normal cortical organization are commonly lead to epilepsy, which also can lead to autism, as is highlighted in tuberous sclerosis in which both autism and epilepsy co-exist [14].

10.2 Biomarker for autism gives hope for future autism treatment

The clinical heterogeneity and molecular complexities of autism spectrum disorders have increasing interest into biomarkers and endophenotypes, measurable quantitative parameters able to facilitate more reliable diagnoses and may help in the treatment of ASD.

'Biomarkers' can be defined as biological variable or cellular alteration associated with the disease and measurable directly using sensitive and reliable quantitative procedures [15].

Elevated blood serotonin (5-HT) levels, and serotonin transporter (SERT) consistently recorded in individuals with ASD [16].

11. Conclusions

The progression of biomarker research in autism mirrors that of other neurologic disorders in that it is still in its infancy and marked largely by discovery rather than validation.

The search for biomarkers for autism will proceed, given the profundity and extend of their potential benefits for individuals with autism and their families. If effective, biomarkers for autism may one day demonstrate important for finding out chance, helping with determination and/or recognizing therapeutic interventions.

Finally, Biomarker research has great heuristic potential in targeting autism diagnosis and treatment.

Author details

Mashael AlKhateeb[1*] and Hesham AlDhalaan[2]

1 Neurology Section, Department of Neurosciences, King Faisal Specialist Hospital and Research Centre, Riyadh, Saudi Arabia

2 Comprehensive Epilepsy Program, Department of Neurosciences, Director Autism Center, King Faisal Specialist Hospital and Research Centre, Riyadh, Saudi Arabia

*Address all correspondence to: kmashael@kfshrc.edu.sa

References

[1] Spence SJ, Schneider MT. The role of epilepsy and epileptiform EEGs in autism spectrum disorders. Pediatric Research. 2009;**65**(**6**):599-606. DOI: 10.1203/PDR.0b013e31819e7168

[2] Baird G, Cass H, Slonims V. Diagnosis of autism. BMJ. 2003;**327**(7413):488-493

[3] Canitano R. Autism with epilepsy: A neurodevelopmental association. OA Autism. 2014;**2**(1):7

[4] Lee BH, Smith T, Paciorkowski AR. Autism spectrum disorder and epilepsy: Disorders with a shared biology. Epilepsy & Behavior. 2015;**47**:191-201

[5] Viscidi EW, Jhonson AL, Spence SJ, Buka SL, Morrow EM, Triche EW. The association between epilepsy and autism symptoms and maladaptive behaviors in children with autism spectrum disorder. Autism. 2013;**18**(8):996-1006

[6] Xu G, Schieve LA, Liu B, Bao W. Prevalence of autism spectrum disorder among US children and adolescents. JAMA. 2014;**319**(5):505

[7] Berg AT, Plioplys S. Epilepsy and autism: Is there a special relationship? Epilepsy & Behavior. 2012;**23**(3): 193-198. DOI: 10.1016/j.yebeh.2012.01

[8] Ghacibeh GA, Fields C. Interictal epileptiform activity and autism. Epilepsy & Behavior. 2015;**47**:158-162. DOI: 10.1016/j.yebeh.2015.02.025

[9] Rebecca Muhle SVT, Rapin I. The genetics of autism. Pediatrics. 2004;**113**(5):e472-e486. DOI: 10.1542/peds.113.5.e472

[10] Wöhr M, Scattoni ML. Neurobiology of autism. Behavioural Brain Research. 2013;**15**:251

[11] Daghsni M, Rima M, Fajloun Z, et al. Autism throughout genetics: Perusal of the implication of ion channels. Brain and Behavior: A Cognitive Neuroscience Perspective. 2018:**8**(8):e00978. DOI: 10.1002/brb3.978

[12] Ornoy A, Weinstein-Fudim L, Ergaz Z. Genetic Syndromes, Maternal Diseases and Antenatal Factors Associated with Autism Spectrum Disorders (ASD). Frontiers in Neuroscience. 2016;**10**:316

[13] OEA P. Absence of CNTNAP2 leads to epilepsy, neuronal migration abnormalities, and core autism-related deficits. Cell. 2011;**147**:1

[14] Tuchman R, Moshé SL, Rapin I. Convulsing toward the pathophysiology of autism. Brain Dev. 2008;**31**(2):95-103

[15] Mayeux R. Biomarkers: Potential uses and limitations. NeuroRx. 2004;**1**(2):182-188

[16] Bdulamir HA, Abdul-Rasheed OF, Abdulghani EA. Serotonin and serotonin transporter levels in autistic children. Saudi Medical Journal. 2018;**39**(5):487-494

Chapter 5

Cerebrovascular Disease; A Leading Cause of Epilepsy

Kaoru Obata, Kazuaki Sato, Hiroya Ohara and Masako Kinoshita

Abstract

Various types of cerebrovascular diseases can result in epilepsy in any age, especially in the elderly. Besides well-known cause of epilepsy as large cerebral infarction involving cerebral cortex and intracerebral hemorrhage, there are growing evidences of roles of subcortical infarction, chronic subdural hematoma, and superficial siderosis of the central nervous system in the pathogenesis of epilepsy. We review here the epidemiology and possible predictors of epilepsy in each type of cerebrovascular lesions and summarize the characteristics of semiology and electroencephalography findings in order to take early treatment strategy. Additionally, relevance of acute-symptomatic seizures and status epilepticus to epilepsy is discussed.

Keywords: epilepsy, cerebrovascular diseases, cerebral infarction, intracranial hemorrhage, stroke, provoked seizures, acute symptomatic seizures, early seizures, late seizures

1. Introduction

Various kinds of brain insults are associated with an increased risk for development of seizures and epilepsy. In adults, a probable etiology of approximately 50% of new-onset seizures can be determined. Cerebrovascular diseases are the most common risk factors of epilepsy (21%), followed by tumors (11%) and traumatic brain injury (7%) [1]. In children and adolescents of 0–19 years of age, the leading epilepsy etiologies are static encephalopathies (38.2%), stroke (12.1%), traumatic brain injury (11.4%), and infection (8.6%) [2].

The traditional definition of stroke is based on clinical characteristics of the sudden onset of loss of focal neurological dysfunction due to infarction or hemorrhage in the relevant part of the brain, retina, or spinal cord, lasting longer than 24 hours [3]. Stroke is classified into cerebral infarction, intracerebral hemorrhage, and subarachnoid hemorrhage (SAH).

Post-stroke seizures have been classified as either early seizures or late seizures, depending on the interval from stroke onset to seizure onset. In the field of stroke, the latent period of two weeks has been most commonly used to distinguish between early seizures and late seizures [4]. Approximately 5–10% of patients with stroke present early seizures within the first two weeks and about half of them occur during the first day after the stroke [5, 6]. In the field of epilepsy, the International League Against Epilepsy (ILAE) proposes a recommendation to define acute symptomatic seizures as seizures occurring within one week subsequent to acute damage to the brain, caused by such as stroke, traumatic brain injury, anoxic encephalopathy, and intracranial surgery [7]. Seizures occurring at least two weeks after stroke are called late or remote symptomatic seizures [4, 8]. Epilepsy is a brain disorder with an enduring preposition to generate epileptic seizures, usually applicable to patients having two or more unprovoked seizures occurring at least 24 hours apart. In addition, ILAE updated the practical definition of epilepsy in 2014 to apply also to a condition of one unprovoked (or reflex) seizure and a probability of further seizures similar to the general recurrence risk (at least 60%) after two unprovoked seizures, occurring over the next 10 years [9]. Therefore, occurrence of an unprovoked late seizure is necessary and sufficient for the diagnosis of post-stroke epilepsy (PSE) because of a high risk of recurrence; such patients are recommended to be treated with antiepileptic medication under the diagnosis of epilepsy [9].

Depending on the type of underlying cerebrovascular disease, 3–30% of patients who experience stroke may develop PSE [10]. The risk to develop epilepsy after stroke is the highest during the first two years, but still elevated even 10 years after stroke [11].

Status epilepticus is a medical emergency that has high mortality rate (approximately 20%) [12]. Classically status epilepticus was defined as a condition characterized by an epileptic seizure sufficiently prolonged or repeated at sufficiently brief intervals so as to produce an unvarying and enduring epileptic condition. In 2015, ILAE proposed the new definition of status epilepticus as follows. Status epilepticus is a condition resulting either from the failure of the mechanisms responsible for seizure termination or from the initiation of mechanisms, which lead to abnormally, prolonged seizures (after time point t1). It is a condition, which can have long-term consequences (after time point t2), including neuronal death, neuronal injury, and alteration of neuronal networks, depending on the type and duration of seizures. Because of incomplete evidence, each time point should be considered as the best estimates currently available. In the case of convulsive status epilepticus, t1 at 5 minute and t2 at 30 minutes are suggested based on animal experiments and clinical research [13]. Patients with status epilepticus rarely recover spontaneously; therefore they should be treated with antiepileptic drugs as soon as possible.

Status epilepticus occurs in 1.5–2.8% of stroke patients [14, 15]. In the older adults (≧65 years of age), 52.3% of status epilepticus are caused by stroke [16]. In the older adults (≧60 years of age), semiology of status epilepticus is less frequently generalized tonic–clonic seizures compared to younger adults (33% vs. 63%, $p = 0.001$); on the other side, non-convulsive status epilepticus with coma are exclusively seen in older patients (10.3% vs. 0%, $p = 0.02$) [17]. In this chapter, we reviewed the epidemiology and possible predictors of epilepsy in each type of cerebrovascular diseases. The characteristics of semiology and electroencephalography (EEG) findings which enable us to take early treatment strategy are summarized. Relevance of acute-symptomatic seizures and status epilepticus to epilepsy is also discussed.

2. What kinds of vascular lesions can cause epilepsy?

2.1 General risk factors of poststroke seizures and epilepsy

Cerebrovascular disease is the most common etiology of acute symptomatic seizures and secondary epilepsy in adults, accounting for approximately 11% of epilepsy diagnosis [18].

All types of cerebrovascular diseases can cause early or late seizures. Among them, the common causes of epilepsy are cerebral infarction, intracerebral hemorrhage, and SAH (**Table 1**). As a genetic risk factor of PSE, the relationship between PSE and the ALDH2 (aldehyde dehydrogenase 2) rs671 polymorphism is known [48].

The risk factors for early seizures after stroke include intracerebral hemorrhage, cerebral infarction with hemorrhagic transformation, stroke severity, and alcoholism [49].

The risk factors for PSE include cortical involvement (visual neglect, dysphagia, field defect, and so on), stroke severity indies at presentation, including low Glasgow Coma Scale, incontinence, or poor Barthel Index, hemorrhagic lesions, young age (< 65 years), and stroke subtype, particularly total anterior circulation infarcts [11]. Abraira et al. pointed that NIHSS score more than 4 at the stroke presentation and post-stroke status epilepticus duration more than 16 hours might predict of PSE in patients with early-onset post-stroke status epilepticus [50].

2.2 Cerebral infarction

Cerebral infarction can occur at any age, with the greatest risk being during the first week after birth. In adults, about 70–85% of cerebrovascular diseases are ischemic. Etiological subtypes of cerebral infarction are classified according to the TOAST classification (**Table 2**) [51], the ASCOD phenotyping system [52], and the Causative Classification System [53]. Most cases of PSE are due to arterial ischemic stroke [54], accounting for up to 9% of incident cases of epilepsy [55].

In ASCOD, every patient should be graded using 5 categories: A (atherosclerosis); S (small-vessel disease); C (cardiac pathology); O (other cause), and D (dissection) [52]. With the Causative Classification System classification of ischemic stroke etiology, ischemic stroke is classified as the following; large artery atherosclerosis, cardio-aortic embolism, small artery occlusion, other causes, and undetermined causes [53].

	Early seizure	Late seizure	Epilepsy
Cerebral infarction	4.8% [6]	3.8% [6]	2.0–4.0% [5, 19–21]
Intracerebral hemorrhage	31% [22]	4.0–11.8% [23, 24]	8.1–13.5% [4, 25]
Subarachnoid hemorrhage	Up to 20% [26]	2.0–5.5% [27]	3.1–25% [28–30],
Acute subdural hematoma[a]	24–36% [31–33]	42–44% [31–33]	58.3% [34]
Chronic subdural hematoma	3.6–42% [33]	1.6–30.7% [33, 35, 36]	4.3–6.9% [37, 38]
Acute epidural hematoma[a]	41% [39]	0% [39]	71.4% [34]
Cerebral venous thrombosis	34.0–46.7% [40–42]	11% [43]	5.2% [42]
Arteriovenous malformation	26.2%[b] [44]	26–35% [44]	67–72% [44]
Arteriovenous fistula	NA	NA	2.7%[c] [45]
Cavernous angioma	NA	NA	32.1%[d] [46]
Moyamoya disease	NA	NA	7.7% [47]

NA: not available.
[a]Post-traumatic seizure/epilepsy.
[b]Seizures with hemorrhage at presentation.
[c]Ratio of convulsion.
[d]Ratio of seizures.

Table 1.
Prevalence of early seizure, late seizure, and epilepsy in each cerebrovascular disease.

Large-artery atherosclerosis (embolus/thrombosis)*
Cardioembolism
Small-vessel occlusion (lacune)*
Stroke of other determined etiology
Stroke of undetermined etiology
a. Two or more causes identified
b. Negative evaluation
c. Incomplete evaluation

**Possible or probable depending on results of ancillary studies.*

Table 2.
The TOAST classification of subtypes of acute ischemic stroke [51].

Early seizure occurrence is associated with hemorrhagic transformation and stroke severity. Late seizure is associated with cortical involvement and stroke severity [56]. The SeLECT score is proposed to predict the risk of late seizures after ischemic stroke, using only five well-defined parameters (Severity of stroke, Large-artery atherosclerotic etiology, Early seizures, Cortical involvement, and Territory of middle cerebral artery involvement) [57]. The overall risk of late seizures was 4% at 1 year and 8% at 5 years after stroke. Based on the estimation, patients with the SeLECT value of 7 points or more have more than 60% risk of seizures within 5 years after stroke, which is higher than the practical definition of epilepsy by ILAE (at least 60% over the next 10 years) [9], even though the patients have no unprovoked seizures. The risk factors for epilepsy after ischemic stroke include early seizures, stroke severity, stroke subtype, stroke location (anterior circulation infarct and cortical involvement), stroke recurrence, artery dissection and established coronary disease [56, 58]. Patients receiving thrombolytic or intra-arterial reperfusion therapies for acute ischemic stroke are at higher risk of epilepsy [59]. Post-stroke seizures can be sometimes associated with small vessel disease. The risk of developing seizures is more strongly related to the localization of lacunar infarctions in the hemispheric white matter (leukoaraiosis) than in the basal ganglia or in the brain stem [60]. Branch atheromatous disease could also have an association with late seizures [61].

2.3 Intracerebral hemorrhage

Early seizures were seen in 31% of patients with spontaneous intracerebral hemorrhage who were evaluated with continuous electroencephalographic monitoring and over half had purely electrographic seizures only [22]. The incidence of PSE after intracerebral hemorrhage is between 8.1 and 13.5% [4, 25]. Seizures secondary to intracerebral hemorrhage are relatively common like this and likely underdiagnosed event that may have little impact on in-hospital mortality and morbidity [62]. Nonconvulsive electrographic seizures may be associated with hematoma expansion [22].

The risk factors for seizures following intracerebral hemorrhage are associated with hemorrhage volume, hemorrhage location within the cerebrum, cortical involvement and the severity of neurological deficits [10]. Surgery for an intracerebral hemorrhage is an additional risk for the development of late seizures [63].

For patients with spontaneous intracerebral hemorrhage, clinical early seizures should be treated with antiepileptic drugs [64]. When the patients have a change in mental status, the evaluation with EEG is recommended. If the patients have electrographic seizures on EEG, they should be treated with antiepileptic drugs [64].

Current clinical guidelines do not recommend the routine use of prophylactic antiepileptic drugs for spontaneous intracerebral hemorrhage [64] because there is no evidence to improve neurological function [65].

Periodic discharges on EEG could be associated with cortical intracerebral hemorrhage and poor outcome [22].

2.4 Subarachnoid hemorrhage

Early seizures may be seen in up to 20% of patients after aneurysmal SAH, and more commonly in association with intracerebral hemorrhage, hypertension, and middle cerebral and anterior communicating artery aneurysms [26]. Early seizures after SAH occur most commonly in the first 24 hours [26]. The actuarial risk of epilepsy after SAH was 18% by the first year, 23% by the second year, and 25% by the fifth year in the survivors of SAH [28]. Aneurysm location most associated with the development of SAH-related epilepsy is middle cerebral artery at the M1 branch and artery bifurcation [66]. The risk factors for epilepsy after aneurysmal SAH include the rupture of aneurysms in the anterior circulation, a young age, intracerebral hemorrhage, a poor neurological outcome, and hemosiderosis [29, 66]. Severe Hunt and Hess score as well as intraventricular hemorrhage elevate the risk of having a seizure after SAH [67]. The degree of neurological impairment and presence of an early seizure soon after the time of SAH have been identified as a risk factor for post-SAH epilepsy [68].

Nonconvulsive seizures following SAH cause transient brain hypoxia, increased intracranial pressure, and increased blood pressure [69]. Although evidence is not sufficient yet, guidelines recommend to consider the prophylactic use of antiepileptic medication except phenytoin (PHT) in the immediate post-hemorrhagic period and to consider the routine use of antiepileptic medication for patients with known risk factors for late seizures such as prior seizure, intracerebral hematoma, intractable hypertension, infarction, or aneurysm at the middle cerebral artery, though long-term use is not recommended [26]. Importantly, PHT should be avoided for the prophylaxis of early seizure following aneurysmal SAH because of known association with vasospasm, worsening of cognitive outcomes, and infarctions [70]. Recently, levetiracetam (LEV) is increasingly used for the prophylaxis of early seizures [26, 70].

2.5 Cerebral venous thrombosis

In patients with cerebral venous thrombosis (CVT), early seizures were seen in 6.9–76% [71], status epilepticus in 6% [40], late seizures in 11% [43], and post-CVT epilepsy in 4–16% [71]. Risk factors for early seizures following cerebral sinus thrombosis include brain parenchymal lesions, focal neurological deficits, supratentorial parenchymal lesions, intracerebral hemorrhage, focal edema/ischemic infarction, superior sagittal sinus thrombosis, cortical venous thrombosis, and pregnancy/puerperium [72–77]. Known risk factors for late seizures after CVT are early seizures, baseline intracerebral hemorrhage, decompressive hemicraniectomy, sigmoid sinus thrombosis, loss of consciousness at presentation, and genetic thrombophilia [43, 75, 78].

In the absence of previous early seizure following cerebral venous thrombosis, there is no evidence to prescribe prophylactic antiepileptic drugs during acute phase [40]. European and American guidelines recommend antiepileptic drug treatment on CVT for patients with early seizures and supratentorial lesions in order to prevent further seizures [79, 80].

Due to the high recurrence risk of late seizures, epilepsy diagnosis and commencement of antiepileptic drugs following a first late seizure after CVT is reasonable [43].

3. How vascular lesions acquire epileptogenicity?

3.1 Epileptogenicity

Epileptogenicity is the development and extension of tissue capable of generating spontaneous seizures, resulting in the development of an epileptic disorder or progression after the disorder is established [81]. In general, there are three phases to acquire epileptogenicity. First, brain-damaging insult (stroke, traumatic brain injury and central nervous system infections etc.) occurs (acute phase). Second, brain acquires epileptogenicity during a certain period of time (latent period), and third, as a result spontaneous recurrent seizures occur (chronic phase). In order to elucidate the mechanism of acquiring epileptogenicity, it is very important to study what occurs in the brain during latent period.

Risk factors, especially relevant to clinical practice, for acquiring epileptogenicity and subsequent development of PSE are summarized in **Table 3**.

PSE: post-stroke epilepsy, PET: positron emission tomography.

Animal experiment of stroke model is very helpful to elucidate epileptogenicity. Several studies directly evaluate neuronal and glial activities after stroke by using electrophysiological and histological measures. Early seizures evoked by traumatic brain injury and stroke can be suppressed by short-term prophylactic administration of antiepileptic drugs but it doesn't alter the incidence of PSE [83]. Therefore, targeting only neurons may be insufficient to prevent epileptogenicity; the glial involvement in the process of epileptogenesis after experimental stroke should be reviewed. Changes in neuro-glial syncytium during the course of acquiring epileptogenesis are shown in **Figure 1**.

Astrocytes form extensive gap junctions composed of connexin (Cx) 43 with other astrocytes and play a central role of neuron–glia syncytium [84]. Astrocyte regulates neural activities by removing excessive extracellular potassium at synapses and transports them into regions of low potassium concentration via gap junction [85]. Cx 43 also forms hemichannels in the astrocyte. Hemichannels allow the exchange of ions and molecules between the cytoplasm and the

Symptom severity	Clinical stroke severity is a major factor in the development of PSE
Lesion size	Post-stroke seizures were more likely to develop in patients with larger lesions involving multiple lobes of the brain than in those with single lobar involvement Total anterior circulation infarct is a particularly strong risk factor for PSE compared with other ischemic stroke subtypes
Lesion location	Extent of cortical involvement is a significant risk factor for PSE Involvement of the parieto-temporal cortex, supramarginal gyrus, and superior temporal gyrus associates with post-stroke epileptogenesis
Stroke subtype	PSE occurred more frequently with hemorrhagic stroke than with ischemic stroke, with about 10–20% of patients developing PSE after hemorrhagic stroke compared with 2–14% after ischemic stroke
Cortical blood flow	A PET study revealed reduced cortical blood flow and oxygen consumption are related to late-onset epilepsy in patients with leukoaraiosis
Vascular risk factors	Vascular risk factors including history of myocardial infarction, peripheral vascular disease, hypertension, total serum cholesterol, and left ventricular hypertrophy, are associated with PSE
Other factors	Genetic factors, peri-injury exposome, etc.

Table 3.
Risk factors for acquiring epileptogenicity after stroke [7, 10, 25, 31, 32, 82].

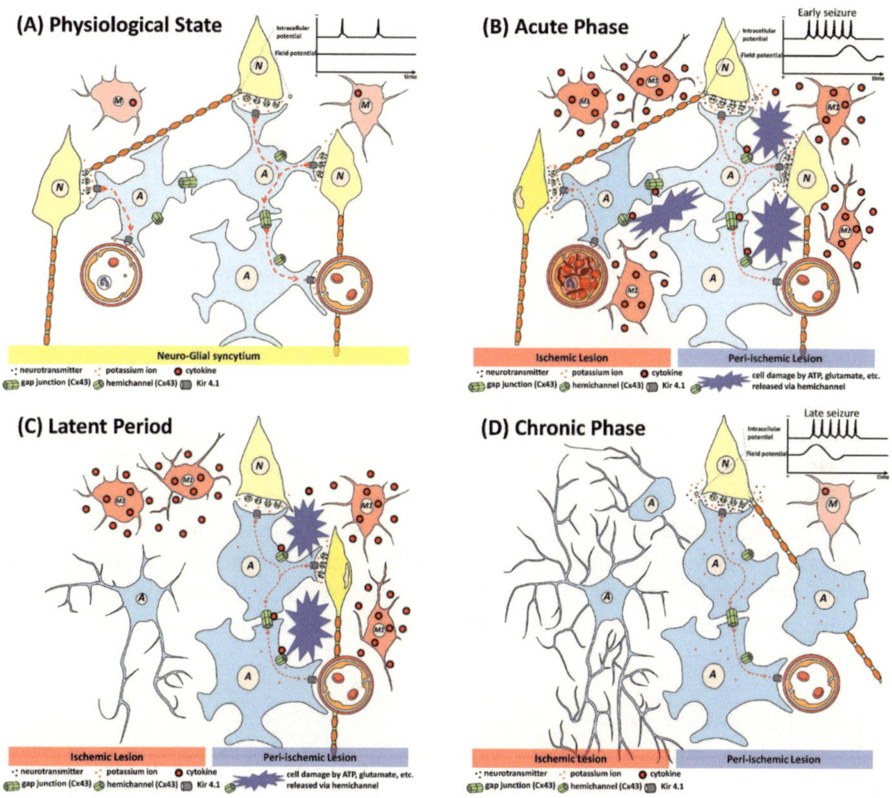

Figure 1.
Neuro-glial syncytium in the course of acquiring epileptogenesis. (A) Physiological state. A neuron generates physiological action potentials in neuro-glial syncytium. As a result of neural firing, extracellular potassium concentration is elevated. Kir 4.1 channels in the astrocyte mediate spatial potassium burring and regulates neural activities by transporting them into regions of low potassium concentration such as blood vessels. (B) Acute phase. In the acute phase of ischemic stroke, ischemic changes of neuron and glia gradually appear in the ischemic lesion. Neurons and astrocyte/microglia cells in the peri-ischemic lesion are activated. Activated microglia called M1 secretes cytokines (e.g. TNF-α, IL-1β), which in turn inhibit gap junctional communication and increase hemichannel activity in astrocytes. The release of molecules, such as ATP and glutamate, damages adjacent neurons and glia cells. Inhibition of gap junction leads to dysfunction of spatial potassium buffering, which further provokes neural firing. Electrophysiologically, neuronal activities lead to increase of spatial potassium, and DC shifts appear as a result of exceeding the capacity of buffering. (C) Latent period. Necrotic region in the ischemic lesion is cleaned by microglia and gliosis occurs in per-ischemic lesion. Inflammation, mainly caused by M1 phenotype, continues in this period and further damages neurons and astrocytes. (D) Chronic phase. In the chronic phase of ischemic stroke, inflammation subsides, and epileptogenicity is acquired. Ischemic lesion is replaced by fibrillary astrocyte and peri-ischemic lesion is occupied by gliosis. Dysfunction of neuro-glial syncytium reaches the pathological state which generates spontaneous epileptic activities. Electrophysiologically, DC shifts precede neural firing. N: neuron, A: astrocyte, M: microglia, TNF-α: tumor necrosis factor-alpha, IL-1β: interleukin 1 beta, ATP: adenosine triphosphate, DC: direct current, Cx43: connexin 43.

extracellular medium, which physiologically regulate neuronal activity as well as synaptic strength and plasticity [86] and also pathologically be activated by inflammation [87].

3.2 Acute phase

Epileptiform activities after middle cerebral artery (MCA) occlusion were first recorded using surface conventional EEG in the rat experiment by Hartings et al. [88]. 55–90% of animals had epileptiform activities 33–50 minutes after stroke which exacerbated brain injury [89–91]. High frequency oscillations (HFOs) are involved with epileptogenic region in intractable epileptic patients (e.g. focal cortical dysplasia) and rat pilocarpine model of temporal lobe epilepsy [92]. In rat stroke model, HFOs were also observed 5–15 seconds before run of theta activities consisted of sharp positive spikes followed by longer negative waves and terminated at the onset of the discharge after ischemia [93]. Direct current (DC) shifts are associated with a steady increase of the extracellular potassium concentration, which matches to the intracellular voltage variations of glial cells [94]. In rat MCA occlusion model, a highly significant linear correlation is reported between the number of depolarization and the infarct size at peri-infarct region, and DC shifts are also recorded [95], which may indicate exceeding of potassium concentration to the buffering capacity of astrocyte.

Histological changes immediately after stroke are reported by Ramírez-Sánchez et al. [96]. When rats were subjected to 90 minutes MCA occlusion followed by 23 hours of reperfusion, neuronal cells in the peri-infart cortex, cornu ammonis (CA) 1, and dentate gyrus (DG) areas were decreased, and widespread reactive astrogliosis in both of the cortex and the hippocampus (CA1, CA3, and DG areas) was observed 24 hours after ischemia.

Therefore, in acute phase of epileptogenesis, stroke immediately damages neurons and glia cells, and provokes neuronal epileptic activity. Furthermore, as a result of destruction of cells and excessive neural firing, the extracellular potassium concentration increases beyond glial potassium buffering capacity, which may lead to a vicious circle of further neural firing.

3.3 Latent period and chronic phase

Chronic phase of the aged rat post-stroke brain is reported by Titova et al. [97]. They evaluated ischemic lesions at 28 days induced by 5o minutes right MCA occlusion in aged rat (18 month-old). In ischemic lesion, extensive glial scar and apoptotic neurons were found and phagocytic macrophages/microglia cells were seen in the peri-lesional rim. The brain irradiation possibly affects normal post-stroke microglia signaling and prevents following activation of inflammatory cascade mechanisms [98]. When proton irradiation was performed at the heads of aged rat ten days prior to right MCA occlusion, chronic phagocytosis and T-lymphocyte infiltration in the brain were reduced, and formation of glio-vascular complexes, neuronal viability, neovascularization were improved in the peri-lesional zone, and neurological severity scoring were improved [97]. These data clearly demonstrated that, in addition to direct damage to brain by stroke itself, subsequent inflammation also damages neuron, astrocyte, vessel and neural function.

In the central nervous system, microglia is a major player in the brain inflammation. Stroke activates microglia which is called M1 phenotype, which secretes inflammatory cytokine like interleukin (IL) and tumor necrosis factor (TNF)-α [99]. Astrocyte also secretes inflammatory cytokines (e.g. TNF-α, IL-1β) via Cx43-hemichannel in the MCA occlusion model [100], whereas Gap19, a selective Cx43-hemichannel inhibitor, exhibits neuroprotective effects on cerebral ischemia/reperfusion via suppression of the expression of Cx43 and toll-like receptor 4 pathway-relevant proteins, and prevention of the overexpression of TNF-α and IL-1β in astrocyte. An obvious improvement in neurological scores and infarct volume reduction were observed in Gap19-treated mice after brain ischemia induced by MCA occlusion [100].

Inflammatory cytokines, specifically IL-1β and TNF-α, are involved in inhibition of gap junctional communication and increase of hemichannel activity in astrocytes [87]. Inhibition of gap junction communication impedes potassium buffering which promotes neural firing. Increased hemichannel activity allows the release of molecules such as adenosine triphosphate, glutamate, nicotinamide adenine dinucleotide, glutathione, and prostaglangin E2 [101–105]. These molecules are toxic to adjacent cells and finally lead to neuronal and glial death [106, 107]. These insults to the central nervous system tissue trigger a range of molecular, morphological, and functional changes of astrocytes called reactive gliosis [108], which is one of the most important pathogenic steps of spontaneous seizure [92].

As for electrophysiological study of PSE model, few data are available because only 10–20% of post-stroke rats develop spontaneous seizure [109]. Brain damage induced by brain injury, axotomy, or toxic substance in addition to stroke also activates microglia [99], therefore, electrophysiological pathology induced by inflammation of other causes is probably plausible as that is induced by stroke. The mechanism of epileptogenesis after status epilepticus model is well studied. Pilocarpine, a muscarinic acetylcholine agonist, induces status epilepticus, and after a certain latent period surviving rats acquire epileptogenesis [110]. This rat model also shows HFOs and DC shifts during seizure at acute phase [92]. Gliosis occurs in 8–12 weeks after pilocarpine injection [111], and spatial potassium buffering function at hippocampus is impaired [112]. EEG recording during epileptic seizures at chronic phase of this model rat showed DC shifts preceding HFOs and conventional ictal EEG patterns, which may be the result of dysfunction of astrocyte extracellular potassium buffering [92]. Minocycline is a second-generation tetracycline and has potent anti-inflammatory effects independent of its antimicrobial action. Minocycline attenuates spontaneous recurrent seizures following pilocarpine-induced status epilepticus, and inhibits the status epilepticus-induced microglial activation and overproduction of IL-1β and TNF-α in the hippocampal CA1 and the adjacent cortex, without affecting astrocyte activation. In addition, minocycline prevents the status epilepticus-induced neuronal loss [113].

4. Neurological examination, electroencephalography, and imaging findings

4.1 Neurological examination

Post-stroke epilepsy is common among the elderly. Nonconvulsive seizures are common in elderly patient with epilepsy, and clinical presentation of elderly patients with epilepsy differs considerably from younger patients; less common and nonspecific auras (e.g. dizziness); less frequent automatisms; prolonged post-ictal confusion; common complaints with altered mental status, confusion, and memory disturbance [114].

These characteristics hinder and delay the diagnosis of epilepsy in the elderly. Co-morbid diseases such as hypertension, dementia, transient ischemic attack (TIA), and cardiac diseases can mislead to attribute these symptoms as one of the manifestations of pre-existing conditions in an elderly patient with new-onset epilepsy [114]. It is necessary and important, for example, to evaluate stroke or TIA immediately for patient with new-onset motor aphasia with brain imaging examinations; however, the symptom can be of aphasic seizures per se or in association with various neurological emergencies, especially if the duration of aphasia is brief, severity of aphasia is fluctuating, or other concomitant neurological findings exist. Clinical presentation of elderly patients with new-onset epilepsy is commonly nonspecific, and thus, EEG should be utilized for the diagnosis of epilepsy in the elderly.

Status epilepticus occurs in 9–19% of patients with post-stroke seizures, while status epilepticus following stroke accounted for 14–27% of all status epilepticus in adults [115]. Tomari et al. reported that 24% of post-stroke seizures with status epilepticus are nonconvulsive status epilepticus [115]. The initiation of treatments for nonconvulsive status epilepticus is commonly delayed compared with convulsive status epilepticus because the diagnosis is often difficult without EEG. The evaluation with EEG is mandatory for patients with nonspecific symptoms such as depressed level of consciousness. Subtle neurological manifestations (e.g. myoclonus, rigidity/spasticity, saccadic eye movement, eye/head turning, abnormal reflexes), their fluctuation, and repetitions of their combination (e.g. myoclonus - > rigidity/spasticity - > paresis - > hyperreflexia, tachypnea - > eyelid twitch - > eye open - > pupil dilation - > eye/head turning) are worthwhile to further evaluation for status epilepticus.

4.2 Electroencephalography

Epileptiform discharges (spikes and sharp waves) in conventional EEG are highly specific to seizure recurrence but not sensitive enough in adult patients (sensitivity 17.3%, specificity 94.7%) [116]. Therefore, lack of epileptiform discharges does not simply exclude the possibility of epileptic seizures. Other nonspecific findings represent both neuronal damage and epileptic activities; amplitude decrease of background activities (e.g. posterior dominant rhythm, fast waves, sleep spindles) and presence of focal slow activities should be serially evaluated.

Recently, long-term, continuous EEG monitoring with video record is increasingly utilized in intensive care unit for early diagnosis of nonconvulsive status epilepticus. Besides conventional EEG seizure patterns (i.e. rhythmic activities with evolution in frequency and amplitude), lateralized periodic discharges, evolving/fluctuating activities, and abnormal rhythmic fast activities superimposed to rhythmic/periodic activities should be evaluated [117–119]. The Salzburg EEG criteria for diagnosis of nonconvulsive status epilepticus include improvement of EEG after intravenous antiepileptic drugs [120].

4.3 Brain imaging

Brain computer tomography is a well-established measure to evaluate intracranial hemorrhage, edema, and mass lesions, and has been utilized for deciding the indication of thrombolytic therapy in acute ischemic stroke.

Initial use of brain magnetic resonance imaging is useful not only to detect cerebrovascular disorders and other neurological conditions but also to evaluate seizure foci and spread of seizures via neural network. Hyperintensity of diffusion-weighted imaging especially in the cortex and hyperperfusion of arterial spin labeling can help early diagnosis of nonconvulsive status epilepticus [118, 119, 121, 122].

5. Treatment strategy: adults in general, and in elderly

5.1 Prevention of post-stroke seizures and epilepsy

The prevalence of post-stroke early seizure is high; 4.8% for ischemic stroke and 7.9% for hemorrhagic stroke [5]. Current clinical guidelines recommend against the routine use of prophylactic antiepileptic drugs for spontaneous intracerebral hemorrhage [64], because primary prevention of seizures with antiepileptic drugs does not improve neurological function during follow up (up to 90 days) [65]. For SAH, guidelines state that a short course (3 to 7 days) of prophylaxis with antiepileptic drugs may be started in the immediate post-bleeding period, although this prophylaxis has a low level of evidence [70]. PHT, which can cause worse cognitive outcomes, vasospasm, and infarctions, should be avoided to use for prophylaxis after SAH, and LEV is increasingly being used [70].

The prevalence of post-stroke late seizure is 3.8% for ischemic stroke and 2.6% for hemorrhagic stroke [5]. As the risk of recurrence after a first unprovoked late seizure can be as high as 71.5% over the next 10 years, the occurrence of a single late post-stroke seizure is consistent with a diagnosis of epilepsy. The risk factors for seizures after ischemic stroke were cortical involvement of infarction and stroke disability. For hemorrhagic stroke, the risk factor of seizures was cortical location. The risk factors in general for post-stroke early seizures during the first 48 hours include advanced age, confusional syndrome, hemorrhagic stroke, large lesions, involvement of parietal and temporal lobes, and occurrence of neurologic and medical complications [6].

None of the currently available antiepileptic medication has been shown to prevent PSE [123–125]. Immediate initiation of continuous antiepileptic medication treatment of the first early seizure after cerebral infarctions decreased the risk of recurrent seizure during the first 2 years but has no influence on the development of recurrent seizures after discontinuing antiepileptic medication in 2 years [124].

As mentioned in Chapter 4, anti-inflammatory therapy is the most expected strategy in order to prevent epileptogenesis. Statins, 3-hydroxy-3-methylglutaryl coenzyme A (HMG-CoA) reductase inhibitors, which are approved for cholesterol reduction, may also be beneficial in the treatment of inflammatory diseases. In animal experiment, atorvastatin reverses paralysis in central nervous system autoimmune disease via suppressing secretion of type 1 helper T cell (Th1) cytokines (IL-2, IL-12, interferon-Γ, and TNF-α) and promoting secretion of Th2 cytokines (IL-4, IL-5 and IL-10) and transform of growth factor-β, in Th1-mediated central nervous system demyelinating disease model of multiple sclerosis [126]. In patients with epilepsy, statin use, especially in the acute phase of ischemic stroke, may reduce the risk of post-stroke early-onset seizures [127]. Adequate statin treatment after ischemic stroke may lower the risk of PSE [128].

In the future, periodic measurement of inflammatory biomarker in the stroke patients having the risk factors as mentioned above and evaluation of the effect of anti-inflammatory agents such as statin to epileptogenicity are warranted.

5.2 Treatment of post-stroke seizures and epilepsy

The decision to initiate antiepileptic medication treatment after a first unprovoked seizure should be individualized and based on age, preference of a patient, and clinical, legal, and socio-cultural factors [129]. Upon commencement of treatment with antiepileptic medication, monotherapy is recommended, among various kinds of antiepileptic medication available. For patients with PSE especially with cerebral infarction, possible adverse event of lipid abnormalities should be avoided to prevent recurrent stroke. High tolerability, which is associated with minimum side effects such as sleepiness or dizziness, is important in elderly patients in terms of safety against falling as well as adherence improvement. In addition, drug interaction is a matter of concern in patients undergoing polypharmacy.

Patients who are treated with enzyme-inducing antiepileptic drugs such as carbamazepine (CBZ), PHT, and phenobarbital (PB) show higher levels of total cholesterol, triglycerides and LDL-cholesterol, although the effects of valproate (VPA) on lipid profiles remain unclear [130]. On the other hand, patients who are treated with enzyme-inhibiting antiepileptic drugs and non-enzyme-inducing antiepileptic drugs are not significantly affected their lipid profile, whereas several reports showed LEV could be associated with higher LDL-cholesterol levels [130]. Due to the side effects of antiepileptic drugs, treatment with non-enzyme-inducing antiepileptic drugs such as lamotrigine (LTG) and LEV is a reasonable treatment strategy in terms of lipid control [130]. In post-stroke seizures and epilepsy, LEV and LTG show higher tolerability than controlled-release CBZ [131].

Weight gain and obesity are associated with hypertension and atherosclerosis. It is well known that VPA, CBZ, PHT, gabapentin, vigabatrin, and pregabalin are associated with weight gain [132–134] while LTG and LEV are not [135, 136], and felbamate, topiramate (TPM), and zonisamide cause weight loss [137, 138].

Carotid-artery intima media thickness (CA-IMT) is an early marker of cerebral atherosclerosis [139]. The old-generation antiepileptic drugs such as CBZ, PHT and VPA are associated with significant increase of CA-IMT in adult patients with epilepsy [139, 140]. On the other hand, the new-generation antiepileptic drugs such as LTG and oxcarbazepine (OXC) have no effects on CA-IMT in adults and children [140, 141].

Hyperhomocysteinemia is an independent risk factor for stroke [142]. OXC, TPM, CBZ, and PB are associated with higher plasma total homocysteine level; adult epilepsy patients treated with LTG and LEV as monotherapy had normal total homocysteine level [143].

Currently, patients with PSE are rarely underwent pre-surgical evaluation even though their seizures are intractable. Good seizure outcome is reported in young generation under 50 years old whose epilepsy onset is at age 20 years or younger, who underwent tailored hemispherectomy based on the findings of stereoelectroencephalography recordings [144]. Approximately 3% of patients with cerebral dural arteriovenous fistula experience seizures [45]. Although status epilepticus is not common among patients with cerebral dural arteriovenous fistula, there is a case report that endovascular intervention improved the seizure control of patients with cerebral dural arteriovenous fistula who present with status epilepticus [145].

Conflict of interest

The authors declare no conflict of interest.

DOI: http://dx.doi.org/10.5772/intechopen.95119

Author details

Kaoru Obata[1], Kazuaki Sato[2], Hiroya Ohara[3] and Masako Kinoshita[4*]

1 Kurashiki Central Hospital, Okayama, Japan

2 Department of Neurology, Ijinkai Takada General Hospital, Kyoto, Japan

3 Department of Neurology, Minaminara General Medical Center, Nara, Japan

4 Department of Neurology, National Hospital Organization Utano National Hospital, Kyoto, Japan

*Address all correspondence to: machak@kuhp.kyoto-u.ac.jp

References

[1] Herman ST. Epilepsy after brain insult: targeting epileptogenesis. Neurology. 2002 Nov 12;**59**(9 Suppl 5):S21-S26. DOI: 10.1212/wnl.59.9_suppl_5.s21

[2] Thurman DJ, Faught E, Helmers S, Kim H, Kalilani L. New-onset lesional and nonlesional epilepsy in the US population: Patient characteristics and patterns of antiepileptic drug use. Epilepsy Research. 2019 Nov;**157**:106210. DOI: 10.1016/j.eplepsyres.2019.106210

[3] Hankey GJ. Stroke. Lancet. 2017 Feb 11;**389**(10069):641-654. DOI: 10.1016/S0140-6736(16)30962-X

[4] Camilo O, Goldstein LB. Seizures and epilepsy after ischemic stroke. Stroke. 2004 Jul;**35**(7):1769-1775. DOI: 10.1161/01.STR.0000130989.17100.96

[5] Bladin CF, Alexandrov AV, Bellavance A, Bornstein N, Chambers B, Cote R, et al. Seizures after stroke: a prospective multicenter study. Archives of Neurology. 2000 Nov;**57**(11):1617-1622. DOI: 10.1001/archneur.57.11.1617

[6] Arboix A, Comes E, Massons J, García L, Oliveres M. Relevance of early seizures for in-hospital mortality in acute cerebrovascular disease. Neurology. 1996 Dec;**47**(6):1429-1435. DOI: 10.1212/wnl.47.6.1429

[7] Beghi E, Carpio A, Forsgren L, Hesdorffer DC, Malmgren K, Sander JW, et al. Recommendation for a definition of acute symptomatic seizure. Epilepsia. 2010 Apr;**51**(4):671-675. DOI: 10.1111/j.1528-1167.2009.02285.x

[8] Annegers JF, Rocca WA, Hauser WA. Causes of epilepsy: contributions of the Rochester epidemiology project. Mayo Clinic Proceedings. 1996 Jun;**71**(6): 570-575. DOI: 10.4065/71.6.570

[9] Fisher RS, Acevedo C, Arzimanoglou A, Bogacz A, Cross JH, Elger CE, et al. ILAE official report: a practical clinical definition of epilepsy. Epilepsia. 2014 Apr;**55**(4):475-482. DOI: 10.1111/epi.12550

[10] Zhao Y, Li X, Zhang K, Tong T, Cui R. The progress of epilepsy after stroke. Current Neuropharmacology. 2018;**16**(1):71-78. DOI: 10.2174/1570159X15666170613083253

[11] Graham NS, Crichton S, Koutroumanidis M, Wolfe CD, Rudd AG. Incidence and associations of poststroke epilepsy: the prospective South London Stroke Register. Stroke. 2013 Mar;**44**(3):605-611. DOI: 10.1161/STROKEAHA.111.000220

[12] Betjemann JP, Lowenstein DH. Status epilepticus in adults. Lancet Neurology. 2015 Jun;**14**(6):615-624. DOI: 10.1016/S1474-4422(15)00042-3

[13] Trinka E, Cock H, Hesdorffer D, Rossetti AO, Scheffer IE, Shinnar S, et al. A definition and classification of status epilepticus--Report of the ILAE Task Force on Classification of Status Epilepticus. Epilepsia. 2015 Oct;**56**(10):1515-1523. DOI: 10.1111/epi.13121

[14] Velioğlu SK, Ozmenoğlu M, Boz C, Alioğlu Z. Status epilepticus after stroke. Stroke. 2001 May;**32**(5):1169-1172. DOI: 10.1161/01.str.32.5.1169

[15] Afsar N, Kaya D, Aktan S, Sykut-Bingol C. Stroke and status epilepticus: stroke type, type of status epilepticus, and prognosis. Seizure. 2003 Jan;**12**(1):23-27. DOI: 10.1016/s1059131102001437

[16] Legriel S, Brophy GM. Managing status epilepticus in the older adult. Journal of Clinical Medicine. 2016 May 11;**5**(5):53. DOI: 10.3390/jcm5050053

[17] Malter MP, Nass RD, Kaluschke T, Fink GR, Burghaus L, Dohmen C. New onset status epilepticus in older patients: Clinical characteristics and outcome. Seizure. 2017 Oct;**51**:114-120. DOI: 10.1016/j.seizure.2017.08.006

[18] Hauser WA, Annegers JF, Kurland LT. Incidence of epilepsy and unprovoked seizures in Rochester Minnesota: 1935-1984. Epilepsia. May-Jun 1993:34;453-468. doi: 10.1111/j.1528-1157.1993.tb02586.x.

[19] Lamy C, Domigo V, Semah F, Arquizan C, Trystram D, Coste J, et al. Early and late seizures after cryptogenic stroke in young adults. Neurology. 2003 Feb 11;**60**(3):400-404. DOI: 10.1212/wnl.60.3.400

[20] Burn J, Dennis M, Bamford J, Sandercock P, Wade D, Warlow C. Epileptic seizures after a first stroke: the Oxfordshire Community Stroke Project. BMJ. 1997 Dec 13;**315**(7122):1582-1587. DOI: 10.1136/bmj.315.7122.1582

[21] So EL, Annegers JF, Hauser WA, O'Brien PC, Whisnant JP. Population-based study of seizure disorders after cerebral infarction. Neurology. 1996 Feb;**46**(2):350-355. DOI: 10.1212/wnl.46.2.350

[22] Claassen J, Jetté N, Chum F, Green R, Schmidt M, Choi H, et al. Electrographic seizures and periodic discharges after intracerebral hemorrhage. Neurology. 2007 Sep 25;**69**(13):1356-1365. DOI: 10.1212/01.wnl.0000281664.02615.6c

[23] Haapaniemi E, Strbian D, Rossi C, Putaala J, Sipi T, Mustanoja S, et al. The CAVE score for predicting late seizures after intracerebral hemorrhage. Stroke. 2014 Jul;**45**(7):1971-1976. DOI: 10.1161/STROKEAHA.114.004686

[24] Rossi C, De Herdt V, Dequatre-Ponchelle N, Hénon H, Leys D, Cordonnier C. Incidence and predictors of late seizures in intracerebral hemorrhages. Stroke. 2013 Jun;**44**(6):1723-1725. DOI: 10.1161/STROKEAHA.111.000232

[25] Lahti AM, Saloheimo P, Huhtakangas J, Salminen H, Juvela S, Bode MK, et al. Poststroke epilepsy in long-term survivors of primary intracerebral hemorrhage. Neurology. 2017 Jun 6;**88**(23):2169-2175. DOI: 10.1212/WNL.0000000000004009

[26] Connolly ES Jr, Rabinstein AA, Carhuapoma JR, Derdeyn CP, Dion J, Higashida RT, et al. Guidelines for the management of aneurysmal subarachnoid hemorrhage: A guideline for healthcare professionals from the American Heart Association/American Stroke Association. 2012 Jun;**43**(6):1711-1737. DOI: 10.1161/STR.0b013e3182587839

[27] Murphy-Human T, Welch E, Zipfel G, Diringer MN, Dhar R. Comparison of short-duration levetiracetam with extended-course phenytoin for seizure prophylaxis after subarachnoid hemorrhage. World Neurosurgery. 2011 Feb;**75**(2):269-274. DOI: 10.1016/j.wneu.2010.09.002

[28] Boling W, Kore L. Subarachnoid hemorrhage-related epilepsy. Acta Neurochirurgica. Supplement. 2020;**127**:21-25. DOI: 10.1007/978-3-030-04615-6_4

[29] Hirano T, Enatsu R, Iihoshi S, Mikami T, Honma T, Ohnishi H, et al. Effects of hemosiderosis on epilepsy following subarachnoid hemorrhage. Neurologia Medico-Chirurgica (Tokyo). 2019 Jan 15;**59**(1):27-32. DOI: 10.2176/nmc.oa.2018-0125

[30] Choi KS, Chun HJ, Yi HJ, Ko Y, Kim YS, Kim JM. Seizures and epilepsy following aneurysmal subarachnoid hemorrhage: Incidence and risk factors. Journal of Korean Neurosurgical Association. 2009 Aug;**46**(2):93-98. DOI: 10.3340/jkns.2009.46.2.93

[31] Jennett B. Epilepsy and acute traumatic intracranial haematoma. Journal of Neurology, Neurosurgery, and Psychiatry. 1975 Apr;**38**(4):378-381. DOI: 10.1136/jnnp.38.4.378

[32] Temkin NR. Risk factors for posttraumatic seizures in adults. Epilepsia. 2003;**44**(s10):18-20. DOI: 10.1046/j.1528-1157.44.s10.6.x

[33] Won SY, Konczalla J, Dubinski D, Cattani A, Cuca C, Seifert V, et al. A systematic review of epileptic seizures in adults with subdural haematomas. Seizure. 2017 Feb;**45**:28-35. DOI: 10.1016/j.seizure.2016.11.017

[34] Kim JA, Boyle EJ, Wu AC, Cole AJ, Staley KJ, Zafar S, et al. Epileptiform activity in traumatic brain injury predicts post-traumatic epilepsy. Annals of Neurology. 2018 Apr;**83**(4):858-862. DOI: 10.1002/ana.25211

[35] Neshige S, Sekihara Y, Ishii N, Sato M, Ota S, Kuriyama M. Clinical and radiological studies of seizure in chronic subdural hematoma--case control study. Rinshō Shinkeigaku. 2014;**54**(11):869-875. DOI: 10.5692/clinicalneurol.54.869. (Japanese)

[36] Yoon SY, Choi YJ, Park SH, Hwang JH, Hwang SK. Traumatic brain injury in children under age 24 months: Analysis of demographic data, risk factors, and outcomes of post-traumatic seizure. Journal of Korean Neurosurgical Association. 2017 Sep;**60**(5):584-590. DOI: 10.3340/jkns.2016.0707.008

[37] Rubin G, Rappaport ZH. Epilepsy in chronic subdural haematoma. Acta Neurochirurgica. 1993;**123**(1-2):39-42. DOI: 10.1007/BF01476283

[38] Kotwica Z, Brzeiński J. Epilepsy in chronic subdural haematoma. Acta Neurochirurgica. 1991;**113**(3-4):118-120. DOI: 10.1007/BF01403195

[39] Beslow LA, Licht DJ, Smith SE, Storm PB, Heuer GG, Zimmerman RA, et al. Predictors of outcome in childhood intracerebral hemorrhage: a prospective consecutive cohort study. Stroke. 2010 Feb;**41**(2):313-318. DOI: 10.1161/STROKEAHA.109.568071

[40] Lindgren E, Silvis SM, Hiltunen S, Heldner MR, Serrano F, de Scisco M, et al. Acute symptomatic seizures in cerebral venous thrombosis. Neurology. 2020 Sep 22;**95**(12):e1706-e1715. DOI: 10.1212/WNL.0000000000010577

[41] Kalita J, Chandra S, Misra UK. Significance of seizure in cerebral venous sinus thrombosis. Seizure. 2012 Oct;**21**(8):639-642. DOI: 10.1016/j.seizure.2012.07.005

[42] Preter M, Tzourio C, Ameri A, Bousser MG. Long-term prognosis in cerebral venous thrombosis. Follow-up of 77 patients. Stroke. 1996 Feb;**27**(2):243-246. DOI: 10.1161/01.str.27.2.243

[43] Sánchez van Kammen M, Lindgren E, Silvis SM, Hiltunen S, Heldner MR, Serrano F, et al. Late seizures in cerebral venous thrombosis. Neurology. 2020 Sep 22;**95**(12):e1716-e1723. DOI: 10.1212/WNL.0000000000010576

[44] Josephson CB, Bhattacharya JJ, Counsell CE, Papanastassiou V, Ritchie V, Roberts R, et al. Seizure risk with AVM treatment or conservative management: prospective, population-based study. Neurology. 2012 Aug 7;**79**(6):500-507. DOI: 10.1212/WNL.0b013e3182635696

[45] Hiramatsu M, Sugiu K, Hishikawa T, Haruma J, Tokunaga K, Date I, et al. Epidemiology of dural arteriovenous fistula in Japan: Analysis of Japanese Registry of Neuroendovascular Therapy (JR-NET2). Neurologia

Medico-Chirurgica (Tokyo). 2014;**54**(1):63-71. DOI: 10.2176/nmc.st.2013-0172

[46] Kang K, Ju Y, Wang D, Li H, Sun L, Ma K, et al. Cerebral venous malformations in a Chinese population: Clinical manifestations, radiological characteristics, and long-term prognosis. World Neurosurgery. 2018 Dec;**120**:e472-e479. DOI: 10.1016/j.wneu.2018.08.106

[47] Tamogami R, Oi S, Nonaka Y, Miwa T, Abe T. Clinical prognosis and therapeutic aspects in management of pediatric moyamoya disease. Nihon Rinsho. 2010 Jan;68(1):45-52. (Japanese)

[48] Yang H, Song Z, Yang GP, Zhang BK, Chen M, Wu T, et al. The ALDH2 rs671 polymorphism affects post-stroke epilepsy susceptibility and plasma 4-HNE levels. PLoS One. 2014 Oct 14;**9**(10):e109634. DOI: 10.1371/journal.pone.0109634

[49] Zhang C, Wang X, Wang Y, Zhang JG, Hu W, Ge M, et al. Risk factors for post-stroke seizures: a systematic review and meta-analysis. Epilepsy Research. 2014 Dec;**108**(10):1806-1816. DOI: 10.1016/j.eplepsyres.2014.09.030

[50] Abraira L, Toledo M, Guzmán L, Sueiras M, Quintana M, Fonseca E, et al. Long-term epilepsy after early post-stroke status epilepticus. Seizure. 2019 Jul;**69**:193-197. DOI: 10.1016/j.seizure.2019.04.022

[51] Adams HP Jr, Bendixen BH, Kappelle LJ, Biller J, Love BB, Gordon DL, et al. Classification of subtype of acute ischemic stroke. Definitions for use in a multicenter clinical trial. TOAST. Trial of Org 10172 in Acute Stroke Treatment. Stroke. 1993 Jan;**24**(1):35-41. DOI: 10.1161/01.str.24.1.35

[52] Amarenco P, Bogousslavsky J, Caplan LR, Donnan GA, Wolf ME, Hennerici MG. The ASCOD phenotyping of ischemic stroke (Updated ASCO Phenotyping). Cerebrovascular Diseases. 2013;**36**(1):1-5. DOI: 10.1159/000352050

[53] Ay H, Benner T, Arsava EM, Furie KL, Singhal AB, Jensen MB, et al. Computerized algorithm for etiologic classification of ischemic stroke: The causative classification of stroke system. Stroke. 2007 Nov;**38**(11):2979-2984. DOI: 10.1161/STROKEAHA.107.490896

[54] Feigin VL, Lawes CMM, Bennett DA, Barker-Collo SL, Parag V. Worldwide stroke incidence and early case fatality reported in 56 population-based studies: a systematic review. Lancet Neurology. 2009 Apr;**8**(4):355-369. DOI: 10.1016/S1474-4422(09)70025-0

[55] Adelow C, Andersson T, Ahlbom A, Tomson T. Prior hospitalization for stroke, diabetes, myocardial infarction, and subsequent risk of unprovoked seizures. Epilepsia. 2011 Feb;**52**(2):301-307. DOI: 10.1111/j.1528-1167.2010.02757.x

[56] Wang JZ, Vyas MV, Saposnik G, Burneo JG. Incidence and management of seizures after ischemic stroke: systematic review and meta-analysis. Neurology. 2017 Sep 19;**89**(12):1220-1228. DOI: 10.1212/WNL.0000000000004407

[57] Galovic M, Döhler N, Erdélyi-Canavese B, Felbecker A, Siebel P, Conrad J, et al. Prediction of late seizures after ischaemic stroke with a novel prognostic model (the SeLECT score): a multivariable prediction model development and validation study. Lancet Neurology. 2018 Feb;**17**(2):143-152. DOI: 10.1016/S1474-4422(17)30404-0

[58] Redfors P, Holmegaard L, Pedersen A, Jern C, Malmgren K. Long-term follow-up of post-stroke epilepsy after ischemic stroke: Room for improved epilepsy treatment. Seizure. 2020 Jan 21;**76**:50-55. DOI: 10.1016/j.seizure.2020.01.009

[59] Naylor J, Thevathasan A, Churilov L, Guo R, Xiong Y, Koome M, et al. Association between different acute stroke therapies and development of post stroke seizures. BMC Neurology. 2018 May 3;**18**(1):61. DOI: 10.1186/s12883-018-1064-x

[60] Schreiner A, Pohlmann-Eden B, Schwartz A, Hennerici M. Epileptic seizures in subcortical vascular encephalopathy. Journal of the Neurological Sciences. 1995 Jun;**130**(2):171-177. DOI: 10.1016/0022-510x(95)00020-3

[61] Obata K, Kinoshita M, Sato K, Chin M, Yamagata S, Ikeda A, et al. Branch atheromatous disease has a stronger association with late-onset epileptic seizures than lacunar infarction in Japanese patients. The Journal of International Medical Research. 2020 Jan;**48**(1):300060519831572. DOI: 10.1177/0300060519831572

[62] Mehta A, Zusman BE, Choxi R, Shutter LA, Yassin A, Antony A, et al. Seizures After Intracerebral Hemorrhage: Incidence, Risk Factors, and Impact on Mortality and Morbidity. World Neurosurgery. 2018 Apr;**112**:e385-e392. DOI: 10.1016/j.wneu.2018.01.052

[63] Pohlmann-Eden B, Bruckmeir J. Predictors and dynamics of posttraumatic epilepsy. Acta Neurologica Scandinavica. 1997 May;**95**(5):257-262. DOI: 10.1111/j.1600-0404.1997.tb00206.x

[64] Hemphill JC 3rd, Greenberg SM, Anderson CS, Becker K, Bendok BR, Cushman M, et al. Guidelines for the management of spontaneous intracerebral hemorrhage: A guideline for healthcare professionals from the American Heart Association/American Stroke Association. Stroke. 2015 Jul;46(7):2032-2060. doi: 10.1161/STR.0000000000000069.

[65] Angriman F, Tirupakuzhi Vijayaraghavan BK, Dragoi L, Lopez Soto C, Chapman M, Scales DC. Antiepileptic drugs to prevent seizures after spontaneous intracerebral hemorrhage. Stroke. 2019 May;**50**(5):1095-1099. DOI: 10.1161/STROKEAHA.118.024380

[66] Huttunen J, Kurki MI, von Und Zu Fraunberg M, Koivisto T, Ronkainen A, Rinne J, et al. Epilepsy after aneurysmal subarachnoid hemorrhage: A population-based, long-term follow-up study. Neurology. 2015 Jun 2;**84**(22):2229-2237. DOI: 10.1212/WNL.0000000000001643

[67] Panczykowski D, Pease M, Zhao Y, Weiner G, Ares W, Crago E, et al. Prophylactic antiepileptics and seizure incidence following subarachnoid hemorrhage: A propensity score-matched analysis. Stroke. 2016 Jul;**47**(7):1754-1760. DOI: 10.1161/STROKEAHA.116.013766

[68] Olafsson E, Gudmundsson G, Hauser WA. Risk of epilepsy in long-term survivors of surgery for aneurysmal subarachnoid hemorrhage: a population-based study in Iceland. Epilepsia. 2000 Sep;**41**(9):1201-1205. DOI: 10.1111/j.1528-1157.2000.tb00326.x

[69] Claassen J, Perotte A, Albers D, Kleinberg S, Schmidt JM, Tu B, et al. Nonconvulsive seizures after subarachnoid hemorrhage: Multimodal detection and outcomes. Annals of Neurology. 2013 Jul;**74**(1):53-64. DOI: 10.1002/ana.23859

[70] Rouanet C, Silva GS. Aneurysmal subarachnoid hemorrhage:

current concepts and updates. Arquivos de Neuro-Psiquiatria. 2019 Nov;**77**(11):806-814. DOI: 10.1590/0004-282X20190112

[71] Mehvari Habibabadi J, Saadatnia M, Tabrizi N. Seizure in cerebral venous and sinus thrombosis. Epilepsia Open. 2018 Jun 8;**3**(3):316-322. DOI: 10.1002/epi4.12229

[72] Masuhr F, Busch M, Amberger N, Ortwein H, Weih M, Neumann K, et al. Risk and predictors of early epileptic seizures in acute cerebral venous and sinus thrombosis. European Journal of Neurology. 2006 Aug;**13**(8):852-856. DOI: 10.1111/j.1468-1331.2006.01371.x

[73] Ferro JM, Canhao P, Bousser MG, Stam J, Barinagarrementeria F, Investigators I. Early seizures in cerebral vein and dural sinus thrombosis: risk factors and role of antiepileptics. Stroke. 2008;**39**(4):1152-1158. DOI: 10.1161/STROKEAHA.107.487363

[74] Ferro JM, Correia M, Rosas MJ, Pinto AN, Neves G. Cerebral Venous Thrombosis Portuguese Collaborative Study Group [Venoport]. Seizures in cerebral vein and dural sinus thrombosis. Cerebrovascular Diseases. 2003;**15**(1-2):78-83. DOI: 10.1159/000067133

[75] Davoudi V, Keyhanian K, Saadatnia M. Risk factors for remote seizure development in patients with cerebral vein and dural sinus thrombosis. Seizure. 2014 Feb;**23**(2):135-139. DOI: 10.1016/j.seizure.2013.10.011

[76] Mahale R, Mehta A, John AA, Buddaraju K, Shankar AK, Javali M, et al. Acute seizures in cerebral venous sinus thrombosis: What predicts it? Epilepsy Res. Jul. 2016;**123**:1-5. DOI: 10.1016/j.eplepsyres.2016.01.011

[77] Li H, Cui L, Chen Z, Chen Y. Risk factors for early-onset seizures in patients with cerebral venous sinus thrombosis: A meta-analysis of observational studies. Seizure. 2019 Nov;**72**:33-39. DOI: 10.1016/j.seizure.2019.09.006

[78] Ferro JM, Canhao P, Stam J, Bousser MG, Barinagarrementeria F, Investigators I. Prognosis of cerebral vein and dural sinus thrombosis: results of the International Study on Cerebral Vein and Dural Sinus Thrombosis (ISCVT). Stroke. 2004 Mar;**35**(3):664-670. DOI: 10.1161/01.STR.0000117571.76197.26

[79] Ferro JM, Bousser MG, Canhão P, Coutinho JM, Crassard I, Dentali F, et al. European Stroke Organisation guideline for the diagnosis and treatment of cerebral venous thrombosis - endorsed by the European Academy of Neurology. European Journal of Neurology. 2017 Oct;**24**(10):1203-1213. DOI: 10.1111/ene.13381

[80] Saposnik G, Barinagarrementeria F, Brown RD Jr, Bushnell CD, Cucchiara B, Cushman M, et al. Diagnosis and management of cerebral venous thrombosis: a statement for healthcare professionals from the American Heart Association/American Stroke Association. Stroke. 2011 Apr;**42**(4):1158-1192. DOI: 10.1161/STR.0b013e31820a8364

[81] Pitkänen A, Nehlig A, Brooks-Kayal AR, Dudek FE, Friedman D, Galanopoulou AS, et al. Issues related to development of antiepileptogenic therapies. Epilepsia. 2013 Aug;54 Suppl 4(0 4):35-43. doi: 10.1111/epi.12297.

[82] Pitkänen A, Roivainen R, Lukasiuk K. Development of epilepsy after ischaemic stroke. Lancet Neurology. 2016 Feb;**15**(2):185-197. DOI: 10.1016/S1474-4422(15)00248-3

[83] Temkin NR. Antiepileptogenesis and seizure prevention trials with antiepileptic drugs: meta-analysis

of controlled trials. Epilepsia. 2001 Apr;**42**(4):515-524. DOI: 10.1046/j.1528-1157.2001.28900.x

[84] Altevogt BM, Paul DL. Four classes of intercellular channels between glial cells in the CNS. The Journal of Neuroscience. 2004 May 5;**24**(18):4313-4323. DOI: 10.1523/JNEUROSCI.3303-03.2004

[85] Walz W. Role of astrocytes in the clearance of excess extracellular potassium. Neurochemistry International. 2000 Apr;**36**(4-5):291-300. DOI: 10.1016/s0197-0186(99)00137-0

[86] Haydon PG, Carmignoto G. Astrocyte control of synaptic transmission and neurovascular coupling. Physiological Reviews. 2006 Jul;**86**(3):1009-1031. DOI: 10.1152/physrev.00049.2005

[87] Même W, Calvo C, Froger N, Ezan P, Amigou E, Koulakoff A, et al. Proinflammatory cytokines released from microglia inhibit gap junctions in astrocytes: potentiation by beta-amyloid. The FASEB Journal. 2006 Mar;**20**(3):494-496. DOI: 10.1096/fj.05-4297fje

[88] Hartings JA, Williams AJ, Tortella FC. Occurrence of nonconvulsive seizures, periodic epileptiform discharges, and intermittent rhythmic delta activity in rat focal ischemia. Experimental Neurology. 2003 Feb;**179**(2):139-149. DOI: 10.1016/s0014-4886(02)00013-4

[89] Williams AJ, Bautista CC, Chen RW, Dave JR, Lu XC, Tortella FC, et al. Evaluation of gabapentin and ethosuximide for treatment of acute nonconvulsive seizures following ischemic brain injury in rats. The Journal of Pharmacology and Experimental Therapeutics. 2006 Sep;**318**(3):947-955. DOI: 10.1124/jpet.106.105999

[90] Williams AJ, Tortella FC, Gryder D, Hartings JA. Topiramate reduces non-convulsive seizures after focal brain ischemia in the rat. Neuroscience Letters. 2008 Jan 3;**430**(1):7-12. DOI: 10.1016/j.neulet.2007.09.052

[91] Williams AJ, Tortella FC, Lu XM, Moreton JE, Hartings JA. Antiepileptic drug treatment of nonconvulsive seizures induced by experimental focal brain ischemia. The Journal of Pharmacology and Experimental Therapeutics. 2004 Oct;**311**(1):220-227. DOI: 10.1124/jpet.104.069146

[92] Ikeda A, Takeyama H, Bernard C, Nakatani M, Shimotake A, Daifu M, et al. Active direct current (DC) shifts and "Red slow": two new concepts for seizure mechanisms and identification of the epileptogenic zone. Neuroscience Research. 2020 Jul;**156**:95-101. DOI: 10.1016/j.neures.2020.01.014

[93] Srejic LR, Valiante TA, Aarts MM, Hutchison WD. High-frequency cortical activity associated with postischemic epileptiform discharges in an in vivo rat focal stroke model. Journal of Neurosurgery. 2013 May;**118**(5):1098-1106. DOI: 10.3171/2013.1.JNS121059

[94] Amzica F, Steriade M. Neuronal and glial membrane potentials during sleep and paroxysmal oscillations in the neocortex. The Journal of Neuroscience. 2000 Sep 1;**20**(17):6648-6665. DOI: 10.1523/JNEUROSCI.20-17-06648.2000

[95] Mies G, Iijima T, Hossmann KA. Correlation between peri-infarct DC shifts and ischaemic neuronal damage in rat. Neuroreport. 1993 Jun;**4**(6):709-711. DOI: 10.1097/00001756-199306000-00027

[96] Ramírez-Sánchez J, Pires ENS, Meneghetti A, Hansel G, Nuñez-Figueredo Y, Pardo-Andreu GL, et al. JM-20 treatment after MCAO reduced astrocyte reactivity and neuronal death on peri-infarct regions of the

rat brain. Molecular Neurobiology. 2019 Jan;**56**(1):502-512. DOI: 10.1007/s12035-018-1087-8

[97] Titova EM, Ghosh N, Valadez ZG, Zhang JH, Bellinger DL, Obenaus A. The late phase of post-stroke neurorepair in aged rats is reflected by MRI-based measures. Neuroscience. 2014 Dec 26;**283**:231-244. DOI: 10.1016/j.neuroscience.2014.09.028

[98] Titova E, Ostrowski RP, Adami A, Badaut J, Lalas S, Ghosh N, et al. Brain irradiation improves focal cerebral ischemia recovery in aged rats. Journal of the Neurological Sciences. 2011 Jul 15;**306**(1-2):143-153. DOI: 10.1016/j.jns.2011.02.034

[99] Block ML, Hong JS. Microglia and inflammation-mediated neurodegeneration: Multiple triggers with a common mechanism. Progress in Neurobiology. 2005 Jun;**76**(2):77-98. DOI: 10.1016/j.pneurobio.2005.06.004

[100] Chen Y, Wang L, Zhang L, Chen B, Yang L, Li X, et al. Inhibition of connexin 43 hemichannels alleviates cerebral ischemia/reperfusion injury via the TLR4 signaling pathway. Frontiers in Cellular Neuroscience. 2018 Oct 17;**12**:372. DOI: 10.3389/fncel.2018.00372

[101] Bruzzone S, Guida L, Zocchi E, Franco L, De Flora A. Connexin 43 hemi channels mediate Ca2+–regulated transmembrane NAD+ fluxes in intact cells. The FASEB Journal. 2001 Jan;**15**(1):10-12. DOI: 10.1096/fj.00-0566fje

[102] Stout CE, Costantin JL, Naus CC, Charles AC. Intercellular calcium signaling in astrocytes via ATP release through connexin hemichannels. The Journal of Biological Chemistry. 2002 Mar 22;**277**(12):10482-10488. DOI: 10.1074/jbc.M109902200

[103] Ye ZC, Wyeth MS, Baltan-Tekkok S, Ransom BR. Functional hemichannels in astrocytes: a novel mechanism of glutamate release. The Journal of Neuroscience. 2003 May 1;**23**(9):3588-3596. DOI: 10.1523/JNEUROSCI.23-09-03588.2003

[104] Cherian PP, Siller-Jackson AJ, Gu S, Wang X, Bonewald LF, Sprague E, et al. Mechanical strain opens connexin 43 hemichannels in osteocytes: a novel mechanism for the release of prostaglandin. Molecular Biology of the Cell. 2005 Jul;**16**(7):3100-3106. DOI: 10.1091/mbc.e04-10-0912

[105] Rana S, Dringen R. Gap junction hemichannel-mediated release of glutathione from cultured rat astrocytes. Neuroscience Letters. 2007 Mar 19;**415**(1):45-48. DOI: 10.1016/j.neulet.2006.12.043

[106] Orellana JA, Froger N, Ezan P, Jiang JX, Bennett MV, Naus CC, et al. ATP and glutamate released via astroglial connexin 43 hemichannels mediate neuronal death through activation of pannexin 1 hemichannels. Journal of Neurochemistry. 2011 Sep;**118**(5):826-840. DOI: 10.1111/j.1471-4159.2011.07210.x

[107] Chen CJ, Liao SL, Kuo JS. Gliotoxic action of glutamate on cultured astrocytes. Journal of Neurochemistry. 2000 Oct;**75**(4):1557-1565. DOI: 10.1046/j.1471-4159.2000.0751557.x

[108] Pekny M, Pekna M. Reactive gliosis in the pathogenesis of CNS diseases. Biochimica et Biophysica Acta. 2016 Mar;**1862**(3):483-491. DOI: 10.1016/j.bbadis.2015.11.014

[109] Löscher W, Brandt C. Prevention or modification of epileptogenesis after brain insults: experimental approaches and translational research. Pharmacological Reviews. 2010 Dec;**62**(4):668-700. DOI: 10.1124/pr.110.003046

[110] Turski WA, Cavalheiro EA, Schwarz M, Czuczwar SJ, Kleinrok Z,

Turski L. Limbic seizures produced by pilocarpine in rats: behavioural, electroencephalographic and neuropathological study. Behavioural Brain Research. 1983 Sep;**9**(3):315-335. DOI: 10.1016/0166-4328(83)90136-5

[111] Nagao Y, Harada Y, Mukai T, Shimizu S, Okuda A, Fujimoto M, et al. Expressional analysis of the astrocytic Kir4.1 channel in a pilocarpine-induced temporal lobe epilepsy model. Frontiers in Cellular Neuroscience. 2013 Jul 5;7:104. doi: 10.3389/fncel.2013.00104.

[112] Heinemann U, Gabriel S, Jauch R, Schulze K, Kivi A, Eilers A, et al. Alterations of glial cell function in temporal lobe epilepsy. Epilepsia. 2000;**41**(Suppl 6):S185-S189. DOI: 10.1111/j.1528-1157.2000.tb01579.x

[113] Wang N, Mi X, Gao B, Gu J, Wang W, Zhang Y, et al. Minocycline inhibits brain inflammation and attenuates spontaneous recurrent seizures following pilocarpine-induced status epilepticus. Neuroscience. 2015 Feb 26;**287**:144-156. DOI: 10.1016/j.neuroscience.2014.12.021

[114] Ramsay RE, Rowan AJ, Pryor FM. Special considerations in treating the elderly patient with epilepsy. Neurology. 2004 Mar 9;**62**(5 Suppl 2):S24-S29. DOI: 10.1212/wnl.62.5_suppl_2.s24

[115] Tomari S, Tanaka T, Matsubara S, Fukuma K, Ihara M, Nagatsuka K, et al. Risk factors for nonconvulsive status epilepticus after stroke. European Neurology. 2018;**80**(5-6):256-260. DOI: 10.1159/000496512

[116] Bouma HK, Labos C, Gore GC, Wolfson C, Keezer MR. The diagnostic accuracy of routine electroencephalography after a first unprovoked seizure. European Journal of Neurology. 2016 Mar;**23**(3):455-463. DOI: 10.1111/ene.12739

[117] Yoshimura H, Matsumoto R, Ueda H, Ariyoshi K, Kawamoto M, Ishii J, et al. Status epilepticus in the elderly: Prognostic implications of rhythmic and periodic patterns in electroencephalography and hyperintensities on diffusion-weighted imaging. Journal of the Neurological Sciences. 2016 Nov 15;**370**:284-289. DOI: 10.1016/j.jns.2016.09.062

[118] Yoshimura H, Matsumoto R, Ueda H, Ariyoshi K, Ikeda A, Takahashi R, et al. Status epilepticus in the elderly: Comparison with younger adults in a comprehensive community hospital. Seizure. 2018 Oct;**61**:23-29. DOI: 10.1016/j.seizure.2018.07.013

[119] Hirsch LJ, LaRoche SM, Gaspard N, Gerard E, Svoronos A, Herman ST, et al. American Clinical Neurophysiology Society's Standardized Critical Care EEG Terminology: 2012 version. Journal of Clinical Neurophysiology. 2013 Feb;**30**(1):1-27. DOI: 10.1097/WNP.0b013e3182784729

[120] Leitinger M, Trinka E, Gardella E, Rohracher A, Kalss G, Qerama E, et al. Diagnostic accuracy of the Salzburg EEG criteria for non-convulsive status epilepticus: a retrospective study. Lancet Neurology. 2016 Sep;**15**(10):1054-1062. DOI: 10.1016/S1474-4422(16)30137-5

[121] Shimogawa T, Morioka T, Sayama T, Haga S, Kanazawa Y, Murao K, et al. The initial use of arterial spin labeling perfusion and diffusion-weighted magnetic resonance images in the diagnosis of nonconvulsive partial status epileptics. Epilepsy Research. 2017 Jan;**129**:162-173. DOI: 10.1016/j.eplepsyres.2016.12.008

[122] Takahara K, Morioka T, Shimogawa T, Haga S, Kameda K, Arihiro S, et al. Hemodynamic state of periictal hyperperfusion revealed by arterial spin-labeling perfusion MR images with dual postlabeling delay. eNeurologicalSci. 2018 Jun 26;**12**:5-18. DOI: 10.1016/j.ensci.2018.06.001

[123] Trinka E, Brigo F. Antiepileptogenesis in humans: disappointing clinical evidence and ways to move forward. Current Opinion in Neurology. 2014 Apr;**27**(2):227-235. DOI: 10.1097/WCO.0000000000000067

[124] Gilad R, Lampl Y, Eschel Y, Sadeh M. Antiepileptic treatment in patients with early postischemic stroke seizures: a retrospective study. Cerebrovascular Diseases. 2001;**12**(1):39-43. DOI: 10.1159/000047679

[125] Marson A, Jacoby A, Johnson A, Kim L, Gamble C, Chadwick D; Medical Research Council MESS Study Group. Immediate versus deferred antiepileptic drug treatment for early epilepsy and single seizures: a randomised controlled trial. Lancet. 2005 Jun 11-17;365(9476):2007-2013. doi: 10.1016/S0140-6736(05)66694-9.

[126] Youssef S, Stüve O, Patarroyo JC, Ruiz PJ, Radosevich JL, Hur EM, et al. The HMG-CoA reductase inhibitor, atorvastatin, promotes a Th2 bias and reverses paralysis in central nervous system autoimmune disease. Nature. 2002 Nov 7;**420**(6911):78-84. DOI: 10.1038/nature01158

[127] Guo J, Guo J, Li J, Zhou M, Qin F, Zhang S, et al. Statin treatment reduces the risk of poststroke seizures. Neurology. 2015 Aug 25;**85**(8):701-707. DOI: 10.1212/WNL.0000000000001814

[128] Vitturi BK, Gagliardi RJ. The influence of statins on the risk of post-stroke epilepsy. Neurological Sciences. 2020 Jul;**41**(7):1851-1857. DOI: 10.1007/s10072-020-04298-5

[129] Leone MA, Giussani G, Nolan SJ, Marson AG, Beghi E. Immediate antiepileptic drug treatment, versus placebo, deferred, or no treatment for first unprovoked seizure. Cochrane Database of Systematic Reviews. 2016 May 6;**2016**(5):CD007144. DOI: 10.1002/14651858.CD007144.pub2

[130] Jin J, Chen R, Xiao Z. Post-epilepsy stroke: A review. Expert Review of Neurotherapeutics. 2016;**16**(3):341-349. DOI: 10.1586/14737175.2016.1151355

[131] Brigo F, Lattanzi S, Zelano J, Bragazzi NL, Belcastro V, Nardone R, et al. Randomized controlled trials of antiepileptic drugs for the treatment of post-stroke seizures: A systematic review with network meta-analysis. Seizure. 2018 Oct;**61**:57-62. DOI: 10.1016/j.seizure.2018.08.001

[132] Katsiki N, Mikhailidis DP, Nair DR. The effects of antiepileptic drugs on vascular risk factors: a narrative review. Seizure. 2014 Oct;**23**(9):677-684. DOI: 10.1016/j.seizure.2014.05.011

[133] Isojärvi JI, Laatikainen TJ, Knip M, Pakarinen AJ, Juntunen KT, Myllylä VV. Obesity and endocrine disorders in women taking valproate for epilepsy. Annals of Neurology. 1996 May;**39**(5):579-584. DOI: 10.1002/ana.410390506

[134] Verrotti A, Manco R, Agostinelli S, Coppola G, Chiarelli F. The metabolic syndrome in overweight epileptic patients treated with valproic acid. Epilepsia. 2010 Feb;**51**(2):268-273. DOI: 10.1111/j.1528-1167.2009.02206.x

[135] Zeng K, Wang X, Xi Z, Yan Y. Adverse effects of carbamazepine, phenytoin, valproate and lamotrigine monotherapy in epileptic adult Chinese patients. Clinical Neurology and Neurosurgery. 2010 May;**112**(4):291-295. DOI: 10.1016/j.clineuro.2009.12.014

[136] Biton V. Effect of antiepileptic drugs on bodyweight: overview and clinical implications for the treatment of epilepsy. CNS Drugs. 2003;**17**(11):781-791. DOI: 10.2165/00023210-200317110-00002

[137] Apovian CM, Aronne LJ. Zonisamide for weight reduction in obese adults. Journal of the American Medical Association. 2013 Aug 14;**310**(6):637-638. DOI: 10.1001/jama.2013.101049

[138] Janousek J, Barber A, Goldman L, Klein P. Obesity in adults with epilepsy. Epilepsy & Behavior. 2013 Sep;**28**(3):391-394. DOI: 10.1016/j.yebeh.2013.05.012

[139] Talaat FM, Kamel T, Rabah AM, Ahmed SM, El-Jaafary SI, Abdelaziz GH. Epilepsy and antiepileptic drugs: risk factors for atherosclerosis. The International Journal of Neuroscience. 2015;**125**(7):507-511. DOI: 10.3109/00207454.2014.949704

[140] Chuang YC, Chuang HY, Lin TK, Chang CC, Lu CH, Chang WN, et al. Effects of long-term antiepileptic drug monotherapy on vascular risk factors and atherosclerosis. Epilepsia. 2012 Jan;**53**(1):120-128. DOI: 10.1111/j.1528-1167.2011.03316.x

[141] Yiş U, Doğan M. Effects of oxcarbazepine treatment on serum lipids and carotid intima media thickness in children. Brain & Development. 2012 Mar;**34**(3):185-188. DOI: 10.1016/j.braindev.2011.05.009

[142] Ashjazadeh N, Fathi M, Shariat A. Evaluation of homocysteine level as a risk factor among patients with ischemic stroke and its subtypes. Iranian Journal of Medical Sciences. 2013 Sep;**38**(3):233-239

[143] Belcastro V, Striano P, Gorgone G, Costa C, Ciampa C, Caccamo D, et al. Hyperhomocysteinemia in epileptic patients on new antiepileptic drugs. Epilepsia. 2010 Feb;**51**(2):274-279. DOI: 10.1111/j.1528-1167.2009.02303.x

[144] Marchi A, Pennaroli D, Lagarde S, McGonigal A, Bonini F, Carron R, et al. Epileptogenicity and surgical outcome in post stroke drug resistant epilepsy in children and adults. Epilepsy Research. 2019 Sep;**155**:106155. DOI: 10.1016/j.eplepsyres.2019.106155

[145] Lee CY, Yeh SJ, Tsai LK, Tang SC, Jeng JS. Dural arteriovenous fistula presenting with status epilepticus treated successfully with endovascular intervention. Acta Neurologica Taiwanica. 2015 Jun;**24**(2):52-56

Section 3

Neurophysiological Techniques to Study Epilepsy and Epileptic Seizures

Chapter 6

Clinical Applications of Brain Mapping in Epilepsy

Sandro Misciagna

Abstract

EEG brain mapping is a neurophysiological technique based on computer-assisted analysis of conventional EEG. This technique, generally consisting in quantitative analysis of EEG (QEEG), includes topographic displays of frequency or voltage, statistical comparison to normal values and discriminant analysis. QEEG assessment still remains controversy about its clinical role. QEEG topographic analysis could be useful in many neurological diseases: in cerebrovascular disease EEG analysis is useful since EEG parameters are highly correlates with regional blood and metabolism; in degenerative disease (as dementia or encephalopathies) quantitative EEG frequency analysis could suggest an organic base of the disorder even if it is not able to distinguish between the types of dementia. QEEG techniques are also potentially useful in identifying anomalies in patients with cerebral trauma or in children with cognitive disorders. In the field of epilepsy EEG brain mapping could help clinics to detect spikes, locate an epileptic focus and suggest the type of epilepsy. In this chapter author describes principles of EEG brain mapping and its potential applications in particular in the epileptic field.

Keywords: brain mapping, epilepsy, quantitative EEG, QEEG, brain maps, digital EEG, EEG spatial analysis, spike detection, spike analysis, seizure detection, epileptic focus, focus localization

1. Introduction

EEG was first described as a promise to provide a "window into the brain" in 1929 by Hans Berger [1]. In spite of recent advances, the analytic potential of EEG has not been fully employed. On the other hand, brain function studies and neuroimaging methods have been deeply improved, severely discrediting EEG use. However, it is important to insist that EEG can give relevant information about topography of cerebral activity, even if it is difficult to have topographic information with a conventional EEG recording.

EEG recording is based on two-dimensional representation of potential differences between two electrodes in function of time and topographic information is based on integration of information across different channels [2].

Introduction of digital EEG techniques not only displays the EEG tracing but can provide additional measurement with quantitative EEG (QEEG), also called "EEG brain mapping".

The use of EEG brain mapping is based on visualisation of coloured brain maps generated by digital analysis of cerebral electrical activity. These maps display many features that can be instantaneous of an averaged period of time. The cerebral maps include topographic displays of voltage, frequencies, power and statistical analysis with comparison with a normal reference population.

Still nowadays the clinical utility of QEEG techniques remains a controversial matter so that it could be considered as a useful tool, but also as a dangerous toy.

2. Short history of EEG spatial analysis

EEG is traditionally analysed in terms of temporal waveforms at different channels, looking at power of rhythms in terms of frequency, latency of peaks or presence of particular grapho-elements. This type of traditional EEG analysis provides important insights about brain functioning in health subjects and diseases that interfere with electric brain activity, even if it cannot be considered as an imaging method.

Numerical analysis of cerebral activity was started as early as the 1930s by Dietsch [3], followed by Grass and Gibbs [4] and Drohocki [5] who applied Fourier analysis to disassemble EEG signal. Successively, in 1943, Walter [6] described an automatic analogue frequency analyser and later in 1951 Walter and Shipton [7] developed an automated topographic display called "toposcope".

With the development of microcomputers with colour graphic Duffy [8, 9] and many other researchers improved techniques for brain electrical activity mapping, EEG quantification and topographic analysis. Researchers as Lehmann directed their studies to the analysis of specific EEG spike–wave patterns, analysis of topography of a particular EEG feature at an instant time or the average of a recurring event [10].

3. General principles of EEG brain maps

EEG brain maps are produced using from 16 to 32 electrodes arranged in a grid pattern of human scalp, giving a spatial resolution of about 6 cm [11] (see **Figure 1**).

Brain maps are sensitive to the quality of data acquisition of the EEG in terms of montages, references, control settings or biological factors (such as medications, clinical problems or level of awareness), which must be considered in every cases before interpreting the data.

In fact, as Duffy himself has written "brain map without the EEG is blind" [12].

Cerebral maps are produced by a process of interpolation between the electrode sites. There are several methods of interpolation and still nowadays it is an object of controversy.

The use of EEG quantification, for example by spectral analysis, gives the possibility to reduce data and describe a long record by few numerical data. These data may be subjected to statistical analyses including visual EEG interpretation or clinical decision-making.

Recent development in the quantitative analysis of complex networks by using computer graphics has increased the availability of brain mapping, contributing to a renewed interest in quantitative investigations of EEG and it has been rapidly translated to studies of brain network organisation [13]. This is a welcome development, but the problem of mapping lies not so much in the method itself, particularly by uninformed users who can see cerebral maps as a neuroimaging technique.

But, instead, mapping systems must be operated by EEG certified neurologist expertise in the use of brain mapping [14].

DOI: http://dx.doi.org/10.5772/intechopen.95121

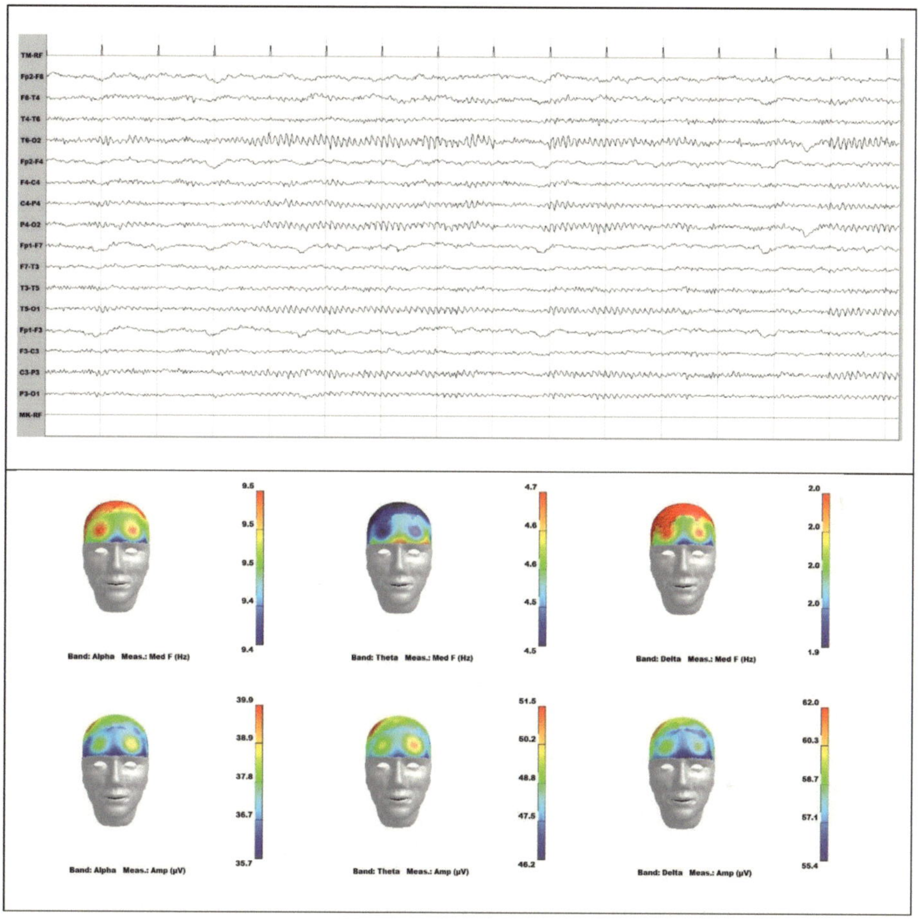

Figure 1.
Example of brain mapping in a traditional EEG showing absence of anomalies.

4. Problems related to use of EEG mapping

One of the major problems of the brain maps is that similarity of brain mapping to classical neuroimaging techniques (CT, MRI or PET scans) is illusory. In classical neuroimaging techniques there is a direct and close correspondence between the image and the affected structure. On the contrary, in the case of topographic changes in electrical activity, there is a more complex relationship to function and cerebral pathology.

Cerebral maps could be easily misinterpreted. In fact, the selection of what to map is at the discretion of the user, there aren't clear standards and interpretation is strongly subjective.

Maps do not distinguish between cerebral potentials and artefacts or between the feature of interest and a superimposed activity with different topography. Consequently, it is essential that users analyse with attention the trace recorded before plotting cerebral maps.

Another problem of quantitative EEG analysis is to determine the best method of deriving the signal to be analysed. Common reference derivation seems be the obvious choice. However asymmetrical activity involving ears reference is particularly open to misinterpretation so that asymmetries in alpha activity may be shown as reversed [15]. A paradox of EEG mapping is that when a focal activity occurs at or near the reference, the deflections produced are greatest on channels recording from the most distant electrodes [16]. This effect is particularly liable to misinterpretation in spectral maps: thus focal temporal delta activity may be misallocated to the contralateral central region [17].

5. General applications of EEG mapping

EEG topographic analysis could be useful in many neurological diseases as cerebrovascular diseases, degenerative encephalopathies, demyelinating diseases, head injuries, headache and study of different cognitive disorders (such as learning and attention disorders) or psychiatric pathologies.

In cerebrovascular disease EEG quantitative parameters are highly correlated with regional blood flow and regional cerebral metabolism. When used by neurologist expertise in EEG interpretation, EEG mapping could be used for detection of focal ischemia related to a cerebral impairment [18]. However, EEG anatomical localization is inferior to that found with conventional neuroradiological techniques as CT or MRI that remain the examinations of choice. Moreover, EEG quantitative changes are unable to differentiate a cerebral infarction from an haemorrhage, a tumour or another focal cerebral lesion [19]. Conventional EEG remains indicated in patients with cerebrovascular problems as possible seizures or coma. Intraoperative EEG quantitative analysis, as frequency analysis, could be used in patients who undergo carotid endarterectomy, during surgical procedure to identify or better measure changes in electrical brain activity [20].

In neurological degenerative pathologies as dementia, EEG quantitative analysis is useful in detecting focal or generalised slowing that strongly suggest an organic basis rather than a depressive condition [21]. EEG frequency analysis cannot distinguish between the types of dementias, but EEG waves patterns are highly suggestive of certain dementing disorders. The degree of EEG frequency analysis abnormality corresponds to the degree of dementia and disease progression so that it has been experimentally used to separate normal controls from patients with mild–moderate Alzheimer disease [22]. EEG spatial analysis conducted on patients with Alzheimer disease has showed decreased duration and increased number of microstates [23]. Quantitative EEG in expert hands could also be useful in evaluation of certain patients with dementia whose neuroimaging and routine EEG studies are not conclusive.

In patients with demyelinating disease as multiple sclerosis, studies of topographic analysis of multichannel recording of evoked potentials have been directly compared in sensitivity and specificity of values obtained from canonical analysis of individual evoked potentials waveforms [24].

Some studies, reports and retrospective observations have addressed EEG brain mapping techniques in patients with head injury [25]. In a small group of patients with post-concussion syndrome it has been reported an increase in 8 to 10 hz of alpha rhythm [26]. Other reports have confirmed alpha reduction in a much larger group of patients after head injury so that it has been proposed as a prognostic element [27]. In coma patients due to severe head injury, EEG monitoring, with or without frequency analysis, has been shown to predict outcome and able to detect non-convulsive seizures or other complications [28]. Even if EEG brain mapping techniques have reported interesting changes in some studies the results are not sufficient to support its use in diagnosis of patients with minor-moderate head trauma or post-concussive syndrome.

In a study of patients with headache Pechadre et al. [29] have demonstrated that migraineurs have specific findings upon EEG mapping during photo-stimulation, suggesting that neuronal excitability of visual cortex is altered in migraine patients [30].

EEG spatial analysis has been applied in the study of different cognitive disorders such as memory disorders, mechanism of memory formation and retrieval in human patients with amnesia [31] or language disorders such word production in stroke patients with aphasia [32]. EEG spatial analysis has also been applied to study the characteristics of brain function difficulties in children with Attention Deficits and Hyperactivity Disorders (ADHD) to evaluate time processing [33], to predict reading skills [34] or to evaluate treatment efficacy and predict changes in use of grammar in children with specific language disorders [35]. EEG specific patterns have been proposed in children with learning and attention disorders and researchers have proposed a relationship between EEG patterns and outcomes of therapy. EEG brain mapping have not been proven useful in establishing diagnosis or treatment for children with cognitive learning disabilities. Quantitative EEG is not recommended as an exam for diagnosing learning disabilities or attention disorders.

Finally, EEG spatial analysis, in the time as well as in the frequency domain, has been used to characterise different pathological states, particularly related to psychiatric pathologies. EEG analysis can identify slow wave or epileptiform abnormalities, which can occur in intoxication, delirium or other psychiatric disorders [36]. Frequency domain source localization has been used to identify brain regions with altered rhythms in patients with psychiatric disorders [37]. EEG microstate analysis has demonstrated that spatial characteristics of microstates are a sensitive measure of different mental states. For example, schizophrenic patients have a decreased duration and reduced number of some microstates [38] that could change and be normalised with medications [39]. Study of resting state in schizophrenic patients have showed that specific short microstates could be observed during auditory verbal hallucinations [40]. In depression microstates duration was also reduced or some microstates were repeated more frequently [41]. Anxiolytic or antipsychotic drugs as well as meditation or hypnosis can also alter the characteristics of cerebral microstates [42].

6. Applications of brain mapping in epilepsy

The most studied application of spatial EEG analysis is in the study of epilepsy in particular as a method to locate an epileptic focus (see **Figure 2**) and determine the type of epileptic syndrome [43].

Digital spike and seizure detection can help to identify electric cerebral events that might be epileptic spikes even if are frequent false-positive detections. In long-term EEG monitoring records, candidate spikes or seizure events are automatically selected and saved but there is need of a professional visual review and confirmation, especially in recording lasting several days [44].

Automated seizure detection can also identify non-convulsive seizure occurring in intensive care unit patients at risk for such complication [45] or to monitory convulsive status epilepticus in patients requiring neuromuscular blockade [46].

Quantitative analysis of spikes characteristic (as spike dipole analysis) can suggest location of cortical generators, existence of multiple separate spike generators and direction of propagation of spikes especially if this information is combined with visual review of voltage mapping.

These techniques might be useful in non-invasive evaluation of epileptic patient candidate for epilepsy surgery, even if the information obtained with dipole analysis is not mathematically and anatomically precise.

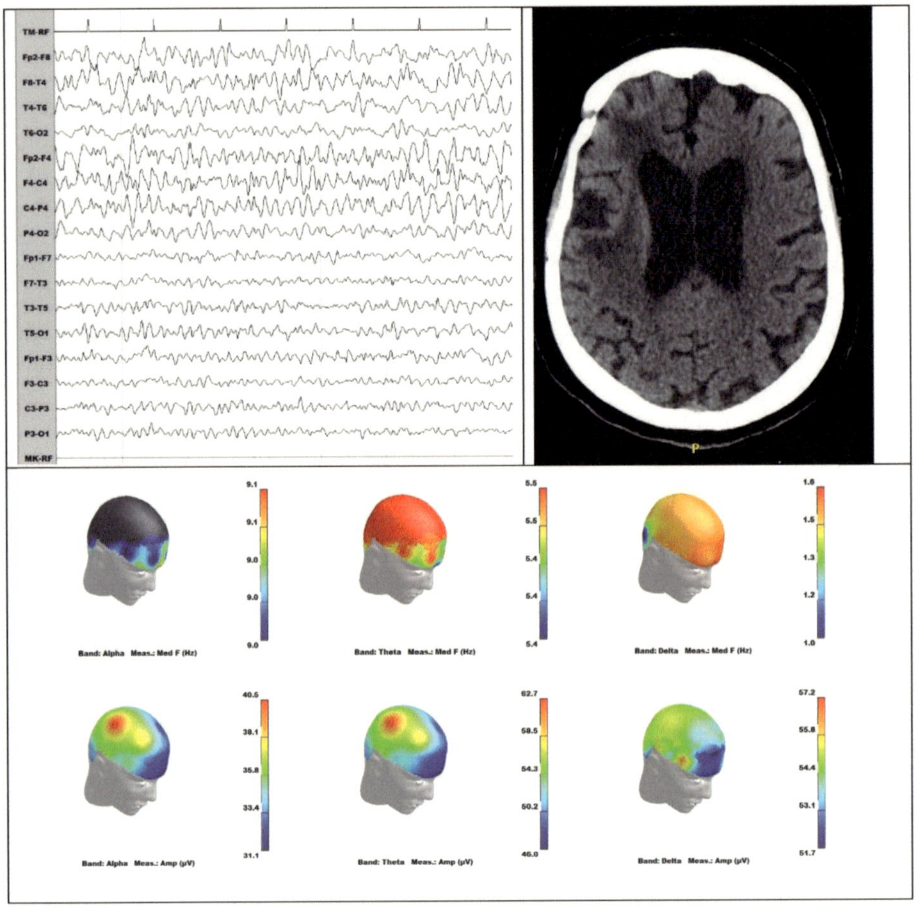

Figure 2.
Example of patient in which traditional electroencephalograms shows a right temporo-parietal epileptiform grapho-elements. TC brain scan shows ipodensity area in right hemisphere, where a cerebral glioma was surgically removed. EEG brain mapping confirms topography of discharges in right hemisphere with prevalence of rhythms in theta band.

A large number of studies have demonstrated that EEG mapping is a powerful tool to non-invasively localise an epileptic focus. The major advantage in the study of an epileptic focus localization compared to other neuro-functional conventional studies (such as fMRI or PET) is the high temporal resolution that allows for separating initiation from rapid propagation of epileptic activity.

The localization of epileptogenic foci with EEG mapping has been found in particular in mesial temporal lesions [47].

Sperli et al. [48], after EEG imaging analysis on 30 operated and seizure free children, reported correct localization of epileptic focus on a lobar level in 90% of cases. In another study, Michel et al. [49] showed 79% localization precision on a sublobar level. In a study conducted by Brodbeck et al. [50] were analysed 10 operated patients with normal MRI in which EEG spatial analysis showed in 8 of them correct localization within the resect margin. In a study conducted by Zumsteg et al. [51] in 2005, based on the analysis in 15 patients with mesial temporal lobe epilepsy the authors compared EEG imaging obtained by cortical electrodes with simultaneously recorded data from foramen ovale electrodes. They showed that 14 of the 19 patterns seen by foramen ovale electrodes could be correctly identified with source imaging, indicating that even mesial temporal sources can be recorded by scalp EEG as also previously demonstrated by Lantz et al. [52] in simultaneous cortical and intracranial EEG recording. Brodbeck et al. [53] were also able to localise correctly spike activity within the resected zone in 12 of 14 patients with large cerebral lesions.

Regional or focal EEG slowing has long been valued to help to lateralize an epileptic focus that might be overlooked by a routine visual evaluation [54].

Brain mapping techniques may highlight to characteristics not obvious to the observer, drawing attention to particular features of a transient event. Clinical examples of applications in epilepsy include the mid-frontal positivity of typical Rolandic spike in benign childhood epilepsy [55]. In Benign Rolandic Epilepsy in Childhood (BREC) quantitative spike voltage analysis has been demonstrated to be useful in determining field complexity and dipole model stability and differentiating "typical" from "atypical" forms, a distinction with prognostic and therapeutic significance [56].

Some quantitative EEG techniques are useful to differentiate primary generalised discharges from secondary bilateral synchrony by looking for interhemispheric small time differences during spike–wave activity and the characteristic distribution of maximal activity [57]. This analysis could be useful to choose the best antiepileptic drug as well as pre-surgical localization of epileptic focus. This potential application has not been clearly demonstrated to be used in general clinical use.

Data manipulations used to enhance isopotential maps and mapping of averages have been used to show subtle features and pattern of propagations [55].

In a retrospective study conducted on 152 operated patients Brodbeck et al. [58] showed that EEG source imaging has a sensitivity of 84% and a specificity of 88% if the EEG is recorded with a large number of electrodes, 128–256 channels and the individual MRI is used as head model. The obtained values resulted comparable to those of structural MRI, PET and ictal-interictal PET. Specificity and sensitivity of EEG mapping and source imaging decreased significantly with use of a low number of electrodes (<32) and a template of head model. On the bases of this study authors concluded that EEG source imaging analysis should be used as standard tool in pre-surgical evaluation of epileptic patients, especially in consideration of its low costs and high flexibility if compared to other imaging methods. However, caution must be exercised since erroneous localizations could occur even for experienced users for the simplified spherical head model commonly used [59].

On the bases of the promising studies above illustrated, Plummer et al. [60] realised a comprehensive review proposing EEG source imaging as a routine work-up of patients with localization-related epilepsy, but concluded that a prospective validation study conducted on larger patients is still required.

EEG imaging has also been demonstrated to be useful in epileptic focus localization in combination with functional MRI. A series of studies conducted to evaluate spike-related analysis have revealed that the temporal resolution of EEG source imaging helps to identify spike-related BOLD responses that correspond to start of epileptic discharge [61–63].

Grouiller et al. [64] conducted a study in which they used EEG topographic analysis to help to analyse fMRI data of epileptic patients that had no spike in the scanner or no-related BOLD responses. In this study they used the average spike-map of EEG recorded during a long-term monitoring and demonstrated that 78% of the otherwise inconclusive fMRI studies could nonetheless be interpreted.

7. Conclusions

EEG analysis in recent times has moved from the traditional analysis of graphoelements to a comprehensive study of brain's electric fields at the scalp.

Quantitative EEG provides more information than visual inspection of traditional EEG used for routine in neurology practice.

Quantitative EEG or other EEG brain mapping techniques cannot diagnose whether a patient has epilepsy but is useful to give additional information in epileptic patients for screening of spikes or possible epileptic spikes in long term EEG monitoring.

EEG spatial analysis is not only a synonymous of source localization but a new insight in brain functioning obtained just analysing the spatial changes of the scalp potential maps over time principally based on the quantitative analysis of EEG waveforms in terms of frequency and amplitude.

Given to the flexibility, non-invasively, easy use and cost-effectiveness EEG mapping is a powerful and interesting brain imaging device that can be easily combined with other traditional imaging techniques.

The potential use of this technique has limitations since quality of EEG mapping depends on the raw data inputs and lack of universally valid normative data due to inter-individual variability of EEG.

The problem of inter-individual variability is reduced with computer-assisted analysis of EEG even if more engineering and analysis tools are still needed to better develop this technique that can be actually used only by physicians highly skilled in clinical EEG and in conjunction with traditional EEG.

Author details

Sandro Misciagna
Neurology Department, Belcolle Hospital, Viterbo, Italy

*Address all correspondence to: sandromisciagna@yahoo.it

References

[1] Berger H. Uber das Elektrenkephalogramm des Menschen. Archiv für Psychiatrie und Nervenkrankheiten. 1929;**87**:527-570

[2] Acharya JN, Acharya VJ. Overview of EEG montages and principles of localization. Journal of Clinical Neurophysiology. 2019 Sep;**36**(5):325-329

[3] Dietsch G. Fourier-analyser von Elektencephalogrammen des Menschen. Arch ges Physiol. 1932;**230**:106-112

[4] Grass AM, Gibbs FA. Fourier bandform of the electroencephalogram. Journal of Neurophysiology. 1937;**1**:521-526

[5] Drohocki Z. L'electrospectrographie du cerveau. CR Soc Biol. 1938;**129**: 889-893

[6] Walter WG. An automatic low frequency analyser. Electronic Engineering. 1943;**11**:237

[7] Walter WG, Shipton HW. A toposcopic display system applied to neurophysiology. J Br Inst Radio Eng. 1951;**3**:260-273

[8] Duffy FH, Burchfiel JL, Lombroso CT. Brain electrical activity mapping (BEAM): A method for extending the clinical utility of EEG and evoked potential data. Annals of Neurology. 1979;**5**:309-321

[9] Duffy FH, Bartels PH, Burchfiel JL. Significance probability mapping: An aid in the topographic analysis of brain electrical activity. Electroencephalography and Clinical Neurophysiology. 1981;**51**:455-462

[10] Lehmann D. Human scalp EEG fields: Evoked, alpha, sleep and spike-wave patterns. In: Petsche H, Brazier MAB, editors. Synchronization of EEG Activity in the Epilepsies. NewYork: Springer; 1972. pp. 307-326

[11] Spitzer AR, Cohen LG, Fabrikant J, Hallett M. A method for determining optimal interelectrode spacing for cerebral topographic mapping. Electroencephalography and Clinical Neurophysiology. 1989;**72**:355-361

[12] Duffy FH. Brain electrical activity mapping: ideas and answers. Topographic mapping of brain electrical activity. Boston: Butterworths. 1986;401-98.

[13] Bullmore E, Sporns O. Complex brain networks: Graph theoretical analysis of structural and functional systems. Nature Reviews. Neuroscience. 2009 Mar;**10**(3):186-198

[14] John ER. The role of quantitative EEG topographic mapping or "neurometrics" in the diagnosis of psychiatric and neurological disorders: The pros. Electroencephalography and Clinical Neurophysiology. 1989;**73**:2-4

[15] Fisch BJ, Hauser WA, Keller DL, Pedley TA. EEG topography: A comparison of bipolar and linked ear reference recordings. Electroencephalography and Clinical Neurophysiology. 1989;**73**:13P

[16] Macgillivray BB, Sawyers FJP. A comparison of common reference, average and source derivations in mapping. In: Sampson-Dollfus D, editor. Statistics and Topography in Quantitative EEG. Amsterdam: Elsevier; 1988. pp. 72-87

[17] Binnie CD. Pathological EEG phenomena. In: Osselton JW, Binnie CD, Cooper R, Fowler CJ, Maugiere F, Prior PM, eds. A Manual of Clinical Neurophysiology. London: di LF Haas. 1992.

[18] Nagata K, Mizukami M, Araki G, Kawase T, Hirano M. Topographic electroencephalographic study of cerebral infarction using computed mapping of the EEG. Journal of Cerebral Blood Flow and Metabolism. 1982;**2**:79-88

[19] Mies G, Hoppe G, Hossmann K-A. Limitations of EEG frequency analysis in the diagnosis of intracerebral diseases. In: Pfurtscheller G, Jonkman EJ, Lopes da Silva FH, Eds Brain Ischemia: Quantitative EEG and Imaging Techniques, vol62. Amsterdam: Elsevier; 1984. pp. 85-103

[20] Redekop G, Ferguson G. Correlation of contralateral stenosis and intraoperative electroencephalogram change with risk of stroke during carotid endarterectomy. Neurosurgery. 1992;**30**:191-194

[21] Brenner RP, Ulrich RF, Spiker DG, et al. Computerized EEG spectral analysis in elderly normal, demented and depressed subjects. Electroencephalography and Clinical Neurophysiology. 1986;**64**:483-492

[22] Pritchard WS, Duke DW, Coburn KL, et al. EEG-based, neural-net predictive classification of Alzheimer's disease versus control subjects is augmented by non-linear EEG measures. Electroencephalography and Clinical Neurophysiology. 1994;**91**:118-130

[23] Dierks T, Jelic V, Julin P, Maurer K, Wahlund LO, Aimkvist O, et al. EEG-microstates in mild memory impairment and Alzheimer's disease. Possible association with disturbed information processing. Journal of Neural Transmission. 1997;**104**:483-495

[24] Lascano AM, Brodbeck V, Lalive PH, Chofflon M, Seek M, Michel CM. Increasing the diagnostic value of evoked potentials in multiple sclerosis by quantitative topographic analysis of multichannel recordings. Journal of Clinical Neurophysiology. 2009;**26**:316-325

[25] Johnstone J, Thatcher RW. Quantitative EEG analysis and rehabilitation issues in mild traumatic brain injury. Journal of Insurance Medicine. 1991;**23**:228-232

[26] Tebano MT, Cameroni M, Gallozzi G, et al. EEG spectral analysis after minor head injury in man. Electroencephalography and Clinical Neurophysiology. 1988;**70**:185-189

[27] Thatcher RW, Cantor DS, McAlaster R, Geisler F, Krause P. Comprehensive predictions of outcome in closed head-injured patients. The development of prognostic equations. Ann NY Acad Sci. 1991;**620**:82-101

[28] Karnaze DS, Marshall LF, Bickford RG. EEG monitoring of clinical coma: Spectral array. Neurology. 1982;**32**:289-292

[29] Pechadre JC, Beudin P, Lauxerois M, Gibert J, Beorchia S, Loisy C. Specific EEG brain mapping reactivity to photic stimulation in migraneurs. In: Rose FC, editor. New Advances in Headache Eserch. London: Smith-Gordon; 1989. pp. 51-56

[30] Klotz JM, Heils A, Langohr HD. Quantitative und topographische analyse des photic driving Effektes (PDE) bei patienten mit migrane. Nervenheikunde. 1992;**11**:316-322

[31] Barcellona-Lehmann S, Morand S, Bindschedler C, Nahum L, Gabrel D, Schnider A. Abnormal cortical network activation in human amnesia: A high-resolution evoked potential study. Brain Topography. 2010;**23**:72-81

[32] Laganaro M, Morand S, Michel CM, Spinelli L, Schnider A. ERP correlates of word production before and after stroke in aphasic patients. Journal of Cognitive Neuroscience. 2011;**23**:374-381

[33] Valko L, Schneider G, Doehnert M, Muller U, Brandeis D, Steinhausen HC, et al. Time processing in children and adults with ADHD. Journal of Neural Transmission. 2010;**117**:1213-1228

[34] Bach S, Richardson U, Brandeis D, Martin E, Brem S. Print-specific multimodal brain activation in kindergarten improves prediction of reading skills in second grade. Neuroimage. 2013;Nov 15;82:605-15

[35] Yoder PJ, Molfese D, Murray M. Key APF. Normative topographic ERP analyses of speed of speech processing and grammar before and after grammatical treatment Dev Neuropsychol. 2013;**38**(8):514-533

[36] American Psychiatric Association. Quantitative electroencephalography: a report on the present state of computerized EEG techniques. American Psychiatric Association Task Force on Quantitative Electrophysiological Assessment. Am J Psychiatry. 1991;148:961-964.

[37] Saletu B, Anderer P, Saletu-Zyhlarz GM, Pascual-Marqui RD. EEG mapping and low-resolution brain electromagnetic tomography (LORETA) in diagnosing and therapy of psychiatric disorders: Evidence for a key-lock principle. Clinical EEG and Neuroscience. 2005;**36**:108-115

[38] Lehmann D, Faber PL, Galderisi S, Herrmann WM, Kinoshita T, Koukkou M, et al. EEG microstate duration and sintax in acute, medication naïve, first-episode schizophrenia: A multi-Centre study. Psychiatry Research. 2005;**138**:141-156

[39] Kikuchi M, Koenig T, Wada Y, Higashima M, Koshino Y, Strik W, et al. Native EEG and treatment effects in neuroleptic-naïve schizophrenic patients: Time and frequency domain approaches. Schizophrenia Research. 2007;**97**:163-172

[40] Kindler J, Hubl D, Strik WK, Dierks T, Koenig T. Resting-state EEG in schizophrenia: Auditory verbal allucinations are related to shortening of specific microstates. Clinical Neurophysiology. 2011;**122**:1179-1182

[41] Strik W, Dierks T, Becker T, Lehmann D. Larger topographical variance and decreased duration of brain electric microstates in depression. Journal of Neural Transmission. General Section. 1995;**99**:213-222

[42] Katayama H, Giannotti LR, Isotani T, Faber PL, Sasada K, Kinoshita T, et al. Classes of microchannel EEG microstates in light and deep hypnotic conditions. Brain Topography. 2007;**20**:7-14

[43] Michel CM & Murray MM. Towards the utilization of EEG as a brain imaging tool. 2012;Jun;61(2):371-85.

[44] Whisler JW, ReMine WJ, Leppik IE, McLain LW Jr, Gumnit RJ. Machine detection of spike-wave activity in the EEG and its accuracy compared with visual interpretation. Electroencephalogr Clin Neurophysiol. 1982;**54**:541-551

[45] Jordan KG. Continuous EEG and evoked potential monitor- ing in the neuroscience intensive care unit. J Clin Neuro- physiol. 1993;10:445-475

[46] Michelucci R, Tassinari CA, Zapoli R. Status epilepticus. In: Gotman J, Ives JR, Gloor P, editors. Long-Term Monitoring in Epilepsy. Amsterdam: Elsevier; 1985. pp. 241-265

[47] Ebersole JS. Equivalent dipole modelling-a new EEG method for localisation of epileptogenic foci. In: Pedley TA, Meldrum BS, editors. Current problems in epilepsy. Edinburgh: Churchill Livingstone; 1992. pp. 51-71

[48] Sperli F, Spinelli L, Seeck M, Kurian M, Michel CM, Lantz G. EEG source imaging in paediatric epilepsy surgery. A new perspective in presurgical workup. Epilepsia. 2006;**47**:981-990

[49] Michel CM, Lantz G, Spinelli L, De Peralta RG, Landis T, Seek M. 128-channel EEG source imaging in epilepsy. Clinical yield and localization precision. Journal of Clinical Neurophysiology. 2004;**21**:71-83

[50] Brodbeck V, Spinelli L, Lascano AM, Pollo C, Schaller K, Vargas MI, et al. Electrical source imaging for presurgical focus localization in epilepsy patients with normal MRI. Epilepsia. 2010;**51**:583-591

[51] Zumsteg D, Friedman A, Wennberg RA, Wieser HG. Source localization of mesial temporal interictal epileptiform discharges: Correlation with intracranial foramen ovale epectrode recording. Clinical Neurophysiology. 2005;**116**:2810-2818

[52] Lantz G, de Peralta, Grave, Menendez R, Gonzalez Andino S, Michel CM. 2001. Non-invasive localization of electromagnetic epileptic activity. Demonstration of sublobar accuracy in patients with simultaneous surface and depth recording. Brain Topography;14:139-147.

[53] Brodbeck V, Lascano AM, Spinelli L, Seeck M, Michel CM. Accuracy of EEG source imaging of epileptic spikes in patients with large brain lesions. Clinical Neurophysiology. 2009;**120**:679-685

[54] Lieb JP, Sperling MR, Mendius JR, Skomer CE, Engel J Jr. Visual versus computer evaluation of thiopental-induced EEG changes in temporal lobe epilepsy. Electroencephalography and Clinical Neurophysiology. 1986;**63**:395-407

[55] Gregory DL, Wong PK. Topographical analysis of the centrotemporal discharges in benign Rolandic epilepsy of childhood. Epilepsia. 1984;25:705-1 1.

[56] Van der Meij W, Van Huffelen AC, Wieneke GH, Willemse J. Sequential EEG mapping may differentiate “epileptic” from “non-epileptic” rolandic spikes. Electroencephalogr Clin Neu- rophysiol. 1992;**82**:408-414

[57] Kobayashi K, Ohtsuka Y, Oka E, Ohtahara S. Primary and secondary bilateral synchrony in epilepsy: Differentiation by estimation of interhemispheric small time differences during short spike-wave activity. Electroencephalogr Clin Neuro- physiol. 1992;**83**:93-103

[58] Brodbeck V, Spinelli L, Lascano AM, Wissmeyer M, Vargas MI, Vulliemoz S, et al. Electroencephalographic source imaging: A prospective study of 152 operated epileptic patients. Brain. 2011;**134**:2887-2897

[59] Nakasato N, Levesque MF, Barth DS, Baumgartner C, Rogers RL, Sutherling WW. Comparisons of MEG, EEG, and ECoG source localization in neocortical partial epilepsy in humans. Electroencephalography and Clinical Neurophysiology. 1994;**91**:171-117

[60] Plummer C, Harvey AS, Cook M. EEG source localization in focal epilepsy: Where are we now? Epilepsia. 2008;**49**:201-218

[61] Groening K, Brodbeck V, Moeller F, Wolff S, van Baalen A, Michel CM, et al. Combination of EEG-fMRI and EEG source analysis improves interpretation of spike-associated activation networks in paediatric pharmacoresistent focal epilepsies. NeuroImage. 2009;**46**:827-833

[62] Siniatchkin M, Groening K, Moehring J, Moeller F, Boor R,

Brodbeck V, et al. Lemieux l, Stephani U. neuronal networks in children with continuous spikes and waves during slow sleep. Brain. 2010;**133**:2798-2813

[63] Vulliemoz S, Lemieux L, Daunizeau J, Michel CM, Duncan JS. The combination of EEG source imaging and EEG-correlated functional MRI to map epileptic networks. Epilepsia. 2010;**51**:491-505

[64] Grouiller F, Thornton RC, Groening K, Spinelli L, Duncan JS, Schaller K, et al. With or without spikes. Localization of focal epileptic activity by simultaneous electroencephalography and functional magnetic resonance imaging. Brain. 2011;**134**:2867-2866

Chapter 7

Is EEG a Useful Examination Tool for Diagnosis of Epilepsy and Comorbid Psychiatric Disorders?

Hideki Azuma

Abstract

Diagnosis of epilepsy usually involves interviewing the patients and the individuals who witnessed the seizure. An electroencephalogram (EEG) adds useful information for the diagnosis of epilepsy when epileptic abnormalities emerge. EEG exhibits nonlinearity and weak stationarity. Thus, nonlinear EEG analysis may be useful for clinical application. We examined only about English language studies of nonlinear EEG analysis that compared normal EEG and interictal EEG and reported the accuracy. We identified 60 studies from the public data of Andrzejak 2001 and two studies that did not use the data of Andrzejak 2001. Comorbid psychiatric disorders in patients with epilepsy were not reported in nonlinear EEG analysis except for one case series of comorbid psychotic disorders. Using a variety of feature extraction methods and classifier methods, we concluded that the studies that used the data of Andrzejak 2001 played a valuable role in EEG diagnosis of epilepsy. In the future, according to the evolution of artificial intelligence, deep learning, new nonlinear analysis methods, and the EEG association with the rating scale of the quality of life and psychiatric symptoms, we anticipate that EEG diagnosis of epilepsy, seizures, and comorbid psychiatric disorders in patients with epilepsy will be possible.

Keywords: epilepsy, EEG, diagnosis, nonlinear analysis, comorbid psychiatric disorders

1. Introduction

1.1 EEG and epilepsy

Epileptic seizures usually do not emerge during the consultation. The diagnosis of epilepsy begins with a conversation with the individual and those who witnessed the seizures. [1] An electroencephalogram (EEG) is also used for the diagnosis of epilepsy. The gold standard for diagnosis of epilepsy is simultaneous ictal EEG recording with video, but this method is not applicable for many patients. The presence of epileptic paroxysmal abnormalities can help with the diagnosis. If a non-expert makes the diagnosis based on EEG findings alone rather than seizure symptoms, misinterpretation of the EEG findings may increase the false-positive diagnosis of epilepsy. Many physicians anticipate that EEG diagnosis for epilepsy will become possible with technological advances, even when no EEG abnormalities are present. EEG is useful not only for diagnosis, but also for monitoring during the course of treatment. [2] Psychiatric disorders occur more frequently as comorbidities in patients with epilepsy [3], and they can affect quality of life. [4]

1.2 EEG and nonlinearity

EEG is characterized by its nonlinearity. [5] Nonlinear dynamics is a concept that includes chaos. Therefore, the adaptation of nonlinear EEG analysis is more useful than that of linear EEG analysis. [6] In nonlinear dynamics, the time series data of EEG can be transformed into a reconstructed state space, which is calculated according to the embedded theorem [7, 8], and the dynamic attractors can be reconstructed. The reconstruction enables us to estimate nonlinear statistics such as fractal dimension and bifurcation structure. The attractor here is a set of trajectories where all of the nearest trajectories converge. [9] CD [9–11], which is a kind of fractal dimension, is a dimension that is occupied by the attractor in phase space. The method of Grassberger et al. is often used. [10] The lyapunov exponent is the degree of exponential separation between orbits, and measures the extent by which nearby points on an attractor diverge or converge with respect to each other while moving along any trajectory of the attractor. [9, 12] If the largest lyapunov exponent is greater than zero, this shows the presence of deterministic chaos. If the lyapunov exponent is less than or equal to zero, this shows a periodic or quasiperiodic motion, respectively. Furthermore, to show the nonlinearity of EEG, generation of surrogate data with linear characteristics and demonstration of a significant difference between them are necessary. In addition, nonlinear analysis is possible with the assumption that EEG exhibits weak stationarity, that the mean and the variance are normally distributed in the evaluated interval, and that no noise is present. [13]

1.3 Epilepsy and nonlinear EEG analysis

Many studies on the nonlinear analysis of EEG and epilepsy have been reported, including reviews concerning ictal EEG detection and machine leaning approaches. [14–16] Ideally, interictal EEG with no paroxysmal abnormalities should be used to diagnose epilepsy and comorbid psychiatric disorders by using computerized analysis rather than expert observation and interpretation.

1.4 Objectives in this review

Therefore, in the present review, we investigated the reports on the nonlinear analysis of EEG between normal and epileptic groups, focusing on the diagnosis of epilepsy and comorbid psychiatric disorders.

2. Methods

2.1 Public data set in Andrzejak 2001

A literature search of Scopus and PubMed was performed. In addition, we identified other relevant literature. We selected only about English language reports that compared normal and epilepsy groups. Many reports used data from Andrzejak 2001. [17] They prepared and used five different data sets, A-E, which each contain 100 single channels from EEG segments of 23.6-sec duration. These segments were selected and extracted from continuous multichannel EEG recordings after visual inspection for artifacts, e.g., due to muscle activity or eye movements. Set A and set B consisted of EEGs from five healthy volunteers with eyes open and closed, respectively. Set C and set D consisted of EEGs from five patients in the epileptogenic zone (set D) and from the hippocampal formation of the opposite hemisphere of set D (set C). Set E contains ictal activity. Set A and set B were recorded extracranially, whereas set C, set D, and set E were recorded intracranially.

2.2 Nonlinearity of the data set

The objective of the study by Andrzejak 2001 was examination of nonlinearity. They generated 39 surrogate data points from all EEG segments for nonlinear prediction error and CD according to the weak stationarity assumption. Nonlinearity was found except in set A for nonlinear prediction error, but only in set D and set E for CD. They discussed that they cannot rule out the possibility that the surrogate test compared to the surrogate data with linear properties including the weak stationarity may result in a false-positive rejection of nonstationarity, and that the surrogate test has neither high sensitivity nor specificity for nonstationarity in nonlinear dynamics systems. [17] Thuraisingham reexamined the data using MPR complexity and normalized shanon spectral entropy, taking into account the probability distribution function. [18] He carried out a surrogate test using the Amplitude Adjusted Fourier Transform method to generate 1000 surrogate data points for evaluation of entropy and complexity. The degree of nonlinearity was set E > set D > set C > set B > set A. However, when adjusted for the effect of noise, all data showed the same degree of nonlinearity by the above method. Set A showed more nonlinearity than set B, and Thuraisingham concluded that denoising with a wavelet was effective for nonlinearity. In light of these results, we considered all five EEG sets as nonlinear and examined the difference between the normal EEG and interictal EEG among the five EEG sets. There were many studies on the comparison between other sets vs. set E. However, an expert can easily interpret set E as ictal. The diagnosis of epilepsy from interictal EEG with no paroxysmal abnormalities is meaningful for both specialists and non-specialists. Therefore, in this review, in the studies with explicit comparisons with the data set of Andrzejak 2001, A vs. C, A vs. D, AB vs. CD vs. E, A vs. B vs. C vs. D vs. E, B vs. C, B vs. D, A vs. D vs. E, A vs. C vs. E, and AB vs. CD, were examined.

3. Results

3.1 Normal vs. epilepsy

The development of feature extraction with nonlinear analysis methods and machine learning has been reported in studies of various combinations of classifications on EEG diagnosis of epilepsy. (**Table 1**). [19–79] **Table 2** shows the details of the classification. Sixty studies using the Andrzejak 2001 data set were selected, and two studies between normal and epileptic groups were selected. Although set C (the opposite site of the epileptogenic zone) and set D (the site of the epileptogenic zone) were interictal and intracranial EEG, the results for B vs. C (99.3% accuracy) and B vs. D (99.5% accuracy) by Gupta 2018 [29] and the results for A vs. D (100% accuracy) by Kaya 2015 [45] and 2018 [30] and for A vs. C (99.7% and 99.6% accuracy) by Raghu 2017 [36] and Liu 2020 [21] were reported. The feature extraction methods and the classifiers were different in each study. Nevertheless,

Author (year) [reference number]	Feature extraction	Classifiers	Comparisons [accuracy%]
Gao (2020) [19]	ApEn, RQA	CNN, BRBP	AB vs. CDE [99.2]
Goshvarpour (2020) [20]	PP	KNN, PNN	A vs. D vs. E [98.3]
Liu (2020) [21]	WPE, WEE, TEE, PSD, 1D-LBP, LNDP, 1D-LGP, LSP, SampEn, LSPA, NEO, HSFV*	AB*, NB, DA, KNN, SVM	A vs. D vs. E [99.0], AB vs. CD vs. E [98.1], AB vs. CD [99], A vs. D [99.5], A vs. C [98.6], B vs. C [99.6], B vs. D [99.6], A vs. CD [98.8], B vs. CD [99.1]
Abedin (2019) [22]	Multilevel DWT	Nonlinear ANN	A vs. D vs. E [97.3]
Fasil (2019) [23]	ExpEn	SVM	A vs. D vs. E [89], A vs. C vs. E [91.6]
Ghayab (2019) [24]	TQWT	KNN*, SVM, BT	AB vs. CD vs. E [100], A vs. B vs. C vs. D vs. E [100]
Kaur (2019) [25]	DWT	BSVM	A vs. C [76], B vs. C [81.6], A vs. D [72.8], B vs. D [71.1]
Sun (2019) [26]	ESN, AR	ELM	A vs. D vs. E [98.3]
Torse (2019) [27]	RP, RQA	SVM*, ANN, PNN	AB vs. CD vs. E [91.2]
Tuncer (2019) [28]	LSP	LDA-SVM*, QDA, KNN	A vs. D vs. E [98.6], A vs. B vs. C vs. D vs. E [93], A vs. D [99.5]
Gupta (2018) [29]	DCT, HE, ARMA	SVM	A vs. C [96.5], A vs. D [98.4], B vs. C [99.3], B vs. D [99.5], AB vs. CD [97.7]
Kaya (2018) [30]	1D-TP (1; lower features, 2; upper features)	ANN*, RF†, FT‡, SVM, BayesNet	1; A vs. D vs. E [95.7]†, A vs. D [99]*, 2; A vs. D vs. E [94] †, A vs. D [100]†,‡,
Sairamya (2018) [31]	LNGP†, SWLNGP‡	ANN*, KNN, QLDA, SVM	A vs. D vs. E [99.7] † [99.6] ‡, AB vs. CD vs. E [99.5] † [99.3] ‡, A vs. D [99.9] †, [99.9] ‡
Zhang (2018) [32]	fDistEn, WPD	KNN*, Kruskal-Wallis, nonparametric ANOVA	A vs. D vs. E [99.3], A vs. B vs. C vs. D vs. E [76]
Abdulhay (2017) [33]	ApEn, SampEn, PE, HE, HFD, HOS	KNN, SVM, NB	A vs. D vs. E [98.5]
Jaiswal (2017) [34]	1D-LBP†, LNDP‡, 1D-LGP	ANN*, NN, SVM, DT	A vs. D vs. E [97.0] † [98.2] ‡, A vs. D [99.3] †[99.9] ‡
Kalbkhani (2017) [35]	ST, KPCA	NN	A vs. D vs. E [99.3], AB vs. CD vs. E [99.5], A vs. C vs. E [99.9]
Raghu (2017) [36]	WPD, LEEn*, NE†	REN	A vs. C [99.7]*, [99.3] †
Tiwari (2017) [37]	LBP	SVM	AB vs. CD vs. E [98.8]
Wang (2017) [38]	LDWT	NSVM	A vs. D vs. E [98.4]
Wen (2017) [39]	GAFDS, SampEn, HE, LE, MFDFA	KNN*, LDA, DT, AB, MLP, NB	A vs. D vs. E [97.3]
Zhang (2017) [40]	LMD, RE, HE	GASVM*, BPNN, KNN, LDA, SVM	AB s CD vs. E [98.4]
Hekim (2016) [41]	DWT, EWD, EFD, SE	ANFIS	AB vs. CD [96.5]

Author (year) [reference number]	Feature extraction	Classifiers	Comparisons [accuracy%]
Murugavel (2016) [42]	LLE, ApEn, DWT	H-MSVM*, ANN	A vs. D vs. E [96], AB vs. CD vs. E [95], A vs. B vs. C vs. D vs. E [94]
Peker (2016) [43]	DTCWT	CVANN	A vs. D vs. E [99.3], AB vs. CD vs. E [98.2]
Abalsaud (2015) [44]	DCT, DWT	NSC*, ANN, NB, KNN, SVM	A vs. C vs. E [90]
Kaya (2015) [45]	1D-LBP	GRA	A vs. D [100]
Martis (2015) [46]	DWT, LLE, HFD, HE, SampEn	RBFSVM*, LSVM, PSVM, QSVM, DT, KNN	A vs. D vs. E [98]*
Riaz (2015) [47]	EMD	SVM*, DT, KNN, ANN	A vs. D vs. E [91], A vs. B vs. C vs. D vs. E [94]
Tawfik (2015) [48]	WPE, DWT	LSVM*, NSVM†, ANN	A vs. D vs. E [97.2]* [97.5] †, A vs. B vs. C vs. D vs. E [91.6]* [93.7] †
Kaya (2014) [49]	LBP, 1DLBP	BayesNet*, SVM, ANN, LR, FT	A vs. D vs. E [95.6], A vs. D [95.5]
Sivasankari (2014) [50]	ICA, STFT, CD, LE	FFBPNN*, ANFIS	A vs. D vs. E [100], A vs. B vs. C vs. D vs. E [96.2]
Acharya (2013) [51]	CWT, HOS, CM, RLM, LBP, LME	SVM*, ANOVA, DT, KNN, PNN	AB vs. CD vs. E [96]
Alam (2013) [52]	EMD	ANN	A vs. D vs. E [100], AB vs. CD vs. E [80]
Fernández-Blanco (2013) [53]	GP		A vs. D vs. E [98.5], AB vs. CD vs. E [97.8]
Hosseini (2013) [54]	HE, LLE	ANFIS	AB vs. CD [97.4]
Niknazar (2013) [55]	RQA, DWT	ECOC	AB vs. CD vs. E [98.6]
Peker (2013) [56]	FCBFA	CVANN	A vs. D vs. E [97]
Seng (2013) [57]	HE, FD, ApEn, LLE, CD	RBFSVM	AB vs. CD vs. E [97.1]
Wang (2013) [58]	BD, FI	SVM	A vs. D vs. E [97.1]
Zhu (2013) [59]	SampEn	MKM*, KMA, SVM	A vs. C [95], A vs. D [96]
Acharya (2012) [60]	ApEn, SampEn, FD, HOS, HE	FSC*, DT, GMM, KNN, RBFSVM, PNN	A vs. D vs. E [99.7]
Acharya (2012–2) [61]	DWT(23.6 sec), ICA	RBFSVM*, DT, KNN, PNN, FSC, GMM	A vs. D vs. E [96]
Martis (2012) [62]	EMD	DT*, ANOVA	A vs. D vs. E [95.3]
Acharya (2011) [63]	RP, RQA	SVM*, GMM, FSC, KNN, NB, DT, PNN	A vs. D vs. E [94.4]
Guo (2011) [64]	DWT, GP	KNN	A vs. D vs. E [93.5]
Mhandoost (2011) [65]	DWT	GARCH*, MRF	A vs. D vs. E [98.8], A vs. C vs. E [98]
Orhan (2011) [66]	DWT	MLP-NN*, KMC	A vs. D vs. E [96.6]

Author (year) [reference number]	Feature extraction	Classifiers	Comparisons [accuracy%]
Ballli (2010) [67]	HOA, TRA, ApEn, LLE, CD, NPE, HE, AR	SFFS-LDA	A vs. B vs. C vs. D vs. E [81.4]
Liang (2010) [68]	ApEn, AR, GA, PCA	RBFSVM*, LLS, LDA, BPNN, LISVM	A vs. D vs. E [98.6], A vs. B vs. C vs. D vs. E [85.9]
Song (2010) [69]	SmpEn	ELM*, BPNN	A vs. D vs. E [95.6]
Acharya (2009) [70]	CD, HE, ApEn, LLE	GMM*, SVM	AB vs. CD vs. E [95]
Übeyli (2009) [71]	DWT	MLP + LMA NN	A vs. D vs. E [94.8]
Übeyli (2008) [72]	DWT	ME*, EMA, MLP-NN	A vs. D vs. E [93.1]
Güler (2007) [73]	DWT, LE	RBFSVM*, MLP-NN, PNN, MSVM	A vs. B vs. C vs. D vs. E [99.2]
Tzallas (2007) [74]	STFT, PSD	FFANN	A vs. D vs. E [100], A vs. B vs. C vs. D vs. E [89]
Tzallas (2007–2) [75]	SPWVD	FFANN, PCA	A vs. D vs. E [99.2], AB vs. CD vs. E [97.7]
Übeyli (2007) [76]	PM, MUSIC, MN, PSD	MME *, ME	A vs. B vs. C vs. D vs. E [98.6]
Sadati (2006) [77]	DWT	ANFN*, ANFIS, RBFSVM, FFBPNN	A vs. D vs. E [85.9]
Güler (2005) [78]	LE, LMA	RNN	A vs. D vs. E [96.7]
Güler (2005–2) [79]	DWT	ANFIS*, BP, GDM, LLS	A vs. B vs. C vs. D vs. E [98.6]

Accuracy = (TP+ TN)/(TP + FP+ TN+ FN); TP, TN, FP and FN mean true positive, true negative, false positive and false negative, respectively.
*, †, ‡ *The accuracy corresponds to each feature extraction and classifier with the symbol.*

Table 1.
Results for the data of Andrzejak 2001.

Comparisons	Mean(SD) [range]	Number of results
A vs. D vs. E	96.8(2.9) [85.9–100]	44 results in 40 studies
A vs. B vs. C vs. D vs. E	92.2(6.7) [76–100]	14 results in 13 studies
AB vs. CD vs. E	96.3(4.9) [80–100]	15 results in 14 studies
A vs. C vs. E	94.8(4.1) [90–99.9]	4 results in 4 studies
AB vs. CD	97.6(0.8) [96.5–99]	4 results in 4 studies
A vs. D	96.7(7.3) [72.8–100]	12 results in 10 studies
A vs. C	94.1(8.2) [76–99.7]	6 results in 5 studies
B vs. D	90.0(13.4) [71.1–99.6]	3 results in 3 studies
B vs. C	93.5(8.4) [81.6–99.6]	3 results in 3 studies

Table 2.
The mean (standard deviation) and number of results for each comparison.

these results were clinically interesting and reasonable. Gruszczyńska 2019 (86.8% accuracy) reported that interictal Fp1 EEG and normal Fp1 EEG using the feature extraction of RQA and RP were classified by SVM. [80] No detailed descriptions were provided for the focal side. Jacob 2016 (100% accuracy) reported the classification of interictal EEG and normal EEG. [81] However, no detailed description was provided of EEGs that were artifact free or with no paroxysmal abnormalities.

3.2 Comorbid psychiatric disorders

No literature on nonlinear EEG analysis for the diagnosis of comorbid psychiatric disorders with epilepsy has been published, and we only found a case series with nonlinear analysis of comorbid psychiatric symptoms with epilepsy. [82] Azuma reported that EEG was artifact free and had no paroxysmal abnormalities and that patients including controls had uncontrolled seizures before and after psychosis. SampEn may not only decrease in the right frontal and frontal-anterior temporal regions before psychosis, but it may also increase in the frontal and frontal-temporal regions during psychosis. Further reports about prodromal periods are needed. Several studies and reviews about forced normalization have been published [83, 84], but none have reported nonlinear analysis as well.

4. Discussion

4.1 Normal vs. epilepsy

In studies on Andrzejak 2001 data, comparisons of A or B vs. C and A or B vs. D have increased in recent years (**Table 1**). Set C and set D consist of intracranial EEG. Usually, intracranial EEG is less noisy, but it provides more localized EEG information. [85, 86] Thus, in the future, comparisons using interictal surface EEG data are needed. This review revealed that the studies in **Table 1** using nonlinear feature extraction methods and classifier methods play a valuable role on EEG diagnosis for epilepsy (A or B vs. C (93.8% accuracy) and A or B vs. D (93.4% accuracy). These results can be further examined in future studies. Thus, consideration and examination with denoising with wavelets [18] and the date of EEG and seizures [87] in nonlinear EEG analysis may be needed in future studies.

4.2 Comorbid psychiatric disorders

In many studies on the diagnosis of depression and schizophrenia [88–97], the nonlinear EEG analysis have been reported, but no nonlinear EEG analysis with accuracy has been reported for comorbid psychotic disorders and depression in patients with epilepsy. Psychiatric comorbidities are common in patients with epilepsy [3], and associations for psychosis with the age at onset, duration of epilepsy, and seizure frequency have been reported. [98, 99] Prodromal symptoms should also be considered when evaluating the onset of psychiatric symptoms. [100] Nonlinear EEG analysis of patients with schizophrenia and depression have been reported, but no nonlinear EEG analysis with accuracy has been reported for comorbid psychotic disorders and depression in patients with epilepsy. No study on forced normalization has been reported using nonlinear EEG analysis. Because psychiatric symptoms affect quality of life in patients with epilepsy [4], we expect that the studies of the association between nonlinear EEG analysis, cognitive function [101–103] and the psychiatric rating scales [104, 105] in the future.

5. Conclusion

EEG exhibits nonlinearity and weak stationarity. Thus, nonlinear EEG analysis is useful to investigate the clinical application for epilepsy, as shown in studies using the public record of Andrzejak 2001. We reviewed the studies using this data set. Using a variety of feature extraction methods and classifier methods, we conclude that these studies played a valuable role in EEG diagnosis for epilepsy. Comorbid psychiatric disorders in patients with epilepsy have not been reported in nonlinear EEG analysis except for one case series of comorbid psychotic disorders. In the future, according to the evolution of artificial intelligence, deep learning, new nonlinear analysis, and the association with the rating scale of the quality of life and psychiatric symptoms, we anticipate that EEG diagnosis for epilepsy, seizures, and comorbid psychiatric disorders in patients with epilepsy will become possible.

Acknowledgements

The authors would like to thank all of the authors for participating in this review.

Conflict of interest

None of the authors has any conflict of interest to disclose.

Abbreviations

A

AB; AdaBoost, ANFIS; Adaptive neuro-fuzzy inference system, ANFN; Adaptive neural fuzzy network, ANN; Artificial Neural Network, ApEn; Approximate entropy, AR; Autoregressive model, ARMA; Autoregressive moving average model.

B

BayesNet; Bayes networks; BD; Blancket dimension, BP; Backpropagation, BPNN; Back propagation neural network, BRBP; Bayesian regularization back-propagation, BSVM; Bagged support vector machine, BT; Bagging tree.

C

CD; Correlation dimension, CM; Co-occurrence matrix, CNN; Convolutional neural network, CVANN; Complex-valued neural networks, CWPS; Continuous wavelet power spectra, CWT; Continuous wavelet transform.

D

DA; Discriminant analysis, DCT; Discrete cosine transform, DT; Decision tree, DTCWT; Dual-tree complex wavelet transformation, DWPS; Discrete wavelet power spectra, DWT; Discrete wavelet transform.

E

ECOC; Error-correction output codes, EFD; Equal frequency discretization, ELM; Extreme learning machine, EMA; Expectation–maximization algorithm, EMD; Empirical Mode Decomposition, ENSC; Ensemble noise-aware signal combination; ESN; Echo state network, EWD; Equal width discretization, ExpEn; Exponential energy.

F

FCBFA; Fast Correlation Based Filter algorithm, FD; Fractal dimension, fDistEn; Fuzzy distribution entropy, FE; Fuzzy entropy, FFANN; Feed-forward artificial neural network, FFBPNN; Feed forward back-propagation neural network, FI; Fractal intercept, FPCA; Functional principal component analysis, FSC; Fuzzy Sugeno Classifier, FT; Functional trees.

G

GA; Genetic algorithm, GAFDS; Genetic algorithm-based frequency-domain feature search, GASVM; Genetic algorithm support vector machine, GARCH; Generalized autoregressive conditional heteroscedasticity, GDM; Gradient descent method, GEO; Gradient energy operator, GMM; Gaussian mixture model, GP; Genetic programming, GRA; Gray relational analysis.

H

HE; Hurst exponent, HFD; Higuchi fractal dimension, H-MSVM; Hierarchical multi-class support vector machine, HOA; Higher order autocovariance, HOS; Higher order spectra, HSFV; Hybrid-selection-feature vector.

I

ICA; Independent component analysis, ICNC; Inverse correlation network coupling, IShE; Indirect shannon entropy.

K

KMA; K-means algorithm, KMC; K-means clustering, KNN; K-nearest neighbor, KPCA; Kernel principal component analysis, KSE; Kolmogorov Sinai entropy.

L

LE; Lyapunov exponent, LBP; Local binary pattern, LEEn; Log energy entropy, LDA; Linear discriminant analysis, LLS; Linear least squares, LMA; Levenberg–marquardt algorithm, LMD; Local mean decomposition, LME; Laws mask energy, LNDP; Local neighbor descriptive pattern, LNGP; Local neighbor gradient pattern, LR; Logistic regression, LSP; Local speed pattern, LSP; Local senary pattern, LSPA; Lorenz scatter plot area, LS-SVM; Last squares support vector machine, LSVM; Linear support vector machine.

M

ME; Mixture of experts, MFDFA; MKM; Multi-scale K-means algorithm, Multifractal detrended fluctuation analysis, MLP; Multilayer perceptron, MME; Modified mixture of experts, MN; Minimum-Norm, MPE; Multiscale permutation entropy, MPEr; Multiscale permutation renyi entropy, MRF; Markov random field, MSVM; Multiclass support vector machine, MUSIC; Multiple signal classification.

N

NB; Naive Bayes, NE; Norm entropy, NEO; Nonlinear energy operator, NN; Nearest neighbor, NN; Neural network, NPE; Nonlinear prediction error, NSVM; Nonlinear support vector machine.

O

OC; Omega complexity, 1D-LBP; One-dimensional local binary pattern, 1D-LGP; One-dimensional local gradient pattern, 1D-TP; One-dimensional ternary patterns.

P

PCA; Principal component analysis, PE; Permutation entropy, PM; Pisarenko method, PNN; Probabilistic neural network, PP; Poincare plot, PS; Phase synchrony; PSD; Power spectral density, PSVM; Polynominal support vector machine.

Q

QDA; Quadratic discriminant analysis, QLDA; Quadratic linear discriminant analysis, QSVM; Quadratic support vector machine.

R

RBFSVM; Radial basis function support vector machine, RE; Renyi entropy, REN; Recurrent elman neural network, RF; Random trees, RLM; Run length matrix, RNN; Recurrent neural network, RP; Recurrence plots, RQA; Recurrence quantification analysis.

S

SampEn; Sample entropy, SE; Shannon entropy, SELM; Sparse extreme learning machine, SFFS-LDA; Sequential floating forward search with linear discriminant analysis method, SLMC; Spatial linear mode complexity, SSE; Shannon spectral entropy, ST; Stockwell transform, STFT; Short time fourier transform, SPWVD; Smoothed pseudo-wigner-ville distribution, SVM; Support vector machine, SWLNGP; Symmetrically weighted local neighbor gradient pattern.

T

TEE; Temporal energy entropy, TQWT; Tunable Q-factor wavelet transform, TRA; Time reversal asymmetry.

V

VGA; Visibility graph algorithm.

W

WEE; Wavelet energy entropy, WPE; Wavelet packet energy, WPE; Weighted permutation Entropy, WPD; Wavelet packet decomposition.

Author details

Hideki Azuma
Department of Psychiatry and Cognitive-Behavioral Medicine, Nagoya City University Graduate School of Medical Sciences, Mizuho-Cho, Mizuho-Ku, Nagoya, Japan

*Address all correspondence to: azma@med.nagoya-cu.ac.jp

References

[1] NICE Guidelines. Epilepsy: Diagnosis and management. 2012.

[2] Krumholz A, Wiebe S, Gronseth G, Shinnar S, Levisohn P, Ting T, et al. Practice Parameter: evaluating an apparent unprovoked first seizure in adults (an evidence-based review): report of the Quality Standards Subcommittee of the American Academy of Neurology and the American Epilepsy Society. Neurology. 2007 Nov;69(21):1996-2007.

[3] Clancy MJ, Clarke MC, Connor DJ, Cannon M, Cotter DR. The prevalence of psychosis in epilepsy; a systematic review and meta-analysis. BMC Psychiatry. 2014 Mar;14:75.

[4] Azuma H, Akechi T. Effects of psychosocial functioning, depression, seizure frequency, and employment on quality of life in patients with epilepsy. Epilepsy Behav. 2014;41.

[5] Stam CJ. Nonlinear dynamical analysis of EEG and MEG: review of an emerging field. Clin Neurophysiol. 2005 Oct;116(10):2266-2301.

[6] Holger Kantz TS. Nonlinear Time Series Analysis. 2nd ed. Cambridge: Cambridge University Press; 2003.

[7] Roux J-C, Simoyi RH, Swinney HL. Observation of a strange attractor. Phys D Nonlinear Phenom. 1983;8(1):257-266.

[8] Takens F. Detecting strange attractors in turbulence BT - Dynamical Systems and Turbulence, Warwick 1980. In: Rand D, Young L-S, editors. Berlin, Heidelberg: Springer Berlin Heidelberg; 1981. p.366-381.

[9] Strogatz SH. Nonlinear Dynamics And Chaos: With Applications To Physics, Biology, Chemistry, And Engineering. Perseus Books Publishing, LLC, Westview: 1994.

[10] Grassberger P, Procaccia I. Characterization of Strange Attractors. Physical review letters. 1983; 50: 346-349.

[11] Grassberger P, Procaccia I. Measuring the Strangeness of Strange Attractors. Physica 9D. 1983; 189-208.

[12] Wolf A, Swift J, Swinney H, Vastano JA. Determining lyapnov exponents from a time series. Phys D Nonlinear Phenom. 1985;16:285-317.

[13] Blanco S, Garcia H, Quiroga R, Romanelli L, Rosso O. Stationarity of the EEG series. IEEE Eng Med Biol Mag. 1995;14:395-399.

[14] Beniczky S, Karoly P, Nurse E, Ryvlin P, Cook M. Machine learning and wearable devices of the future. Epilepsia. 2020 Jul;1-9.

[15] Siddiqui MK, Morales-Menendez R, Huang X, Hussain N. A review of epileptic seizure detection using machine learning classifiers. Brain informatics. 2020 May;7(1):5.

[16] Abbasi B, Goldenholz DM. Machine learning applications in epilepsy. Epilepsia. 2019 Oct;60(10):2037-2047.

[17] Andrzejak RG, Lehnertz K, Mormann F, Rieke C, David P, Elger CE. Indications of nonlinear deterministic and finite-dimensional structures in time series of brain electrical activity: dependence on recording region and brain state. Phys Rev E Stat Nonlin Soft Matter Phys. 2001 Dec;64(6 Pt 1):61907.

[18] Thuraisingham RA. Examining nonlinearity using complexity and entropy. Chaos. 2019 Jun;29(6):63109.

[19] Gao X, Yan X, Gao P, Gao X, Zhang S. Automatic detection of epileptic seizure based on approximate entropy, recurrence quantification

analysis and convolutional neural networks. Artif Intell Med. 2020;102:101711

[20] Goshvarpour A, Goshvarpour A. Diagnosis of epileptic EEG using a lagged Poincare plot in combination with the autocorrelation. Signal, Image Video Process. 2020;14(7):1309-1317.

[21] Liu X, Shen J, Zhao W. Epileptic EEG identification based on hybrid feature extraction. J Mech Med Biol. 2020; 2050025.

[22] Abedin MZ, Akther S, Hossain MS. An artificial neural network model for epilepsy seizure detection. In: 2019 5th International Conference on Advances in Electrical Engineering, ICAEE 2019. 2019. p. 860-865.

[23] Fasil OK, Rajesh R. Time-domain exponential energy for epileptic EEG signal classification. Neurosci Lett. 2019;694:1-8.

[24] Al Ghayab HR, Li Y, Siuly S, Abdulla S. A feature extraction technique based on tunable Q-factor wavelet transform for brain signal classification. J Neurosci Methods. 2019;312:43-52.

[25] Kaur A, Verma K, Bhondekar AP, Shashvat K.Implementation of Bagged SVM Ensemble Model for Classification of Epileptic States Using EEG. Curr Pharm Biotechnol. 2019;20(9):755-765.

[26] Sun L, Jin B, Yang H, Tong J, Liu C, Xiong H. Unsupervised EEG feature extraction based on echo state network. Inf Sci (Ny). 2019;475(January):1-17.

[27] Torse DA, Khanai R, Desai VV. Classification of epileptic seizures using recurrence plots and machine learning techniques. In: Proceedings of the 2019 IEEE International Conference on Communication and Signal Processing, ICCSP 2019. 2019. p. 611-615.

[28] Tuncer T, Dogan S, Akbal E. A novel local senary pattern based epilepsy diagnosis system using EEG signals. Australas Phys Eng Sci Med. 2019;42(4):939-948.

[29] Gupta A, Singh P, Karlekar M. A Novel Signal Modeling Approach for Classification of Seizure and Seizure-Free EEG Signals. IEEE Trans Neural Syst Rehabil Eng. 2018;26(5):925-935.

[30] Kaya Y, Ertuğrul ÖF. A stable feature extraction method in classification epileptic EEG signals. Australas Phys Eng Sci Med. 2018;41(3):721-730.

[31] Sairamya NJ, Thomas George S, Balakrishnan R, Subathra MSP. An effective approach to classify epileptic EEG signal using local neighbor gradient pattern transformation methods. Australas Phys Eng Sci Med. 2018;41(4):1029-1046.

[32] Zhang T, Chen W, Li M. Fuzzy distribution entropy and its application in automated seizure detection technique. Biomed Signal Process Control. 2018;39:360-377.

[33] Abdulhay E, Elamaran V, Chandrasekar M, Balaji VS, Narasimhan K. Automated diagnosis of epilepsy from EEG signals using ensemble learning approach. Pattern Recognit Lett. 2017; https://doi.org/10.1016/j.patrec.2017.05.021.

[34] Jaiswal AK, Banka H. Local pattern transformation based feature extraction techniques for classification of epileptic EEG signals. Biomed Signal Process Control. 2017;34:81-92.

[35] Kalbkhani H, Shayesteh MG. Stockwell transform for epileptic seizure detection from EEG signals. Biomed Signal Process Control. 2017;38:108-118.

[36] Raghu S, Sriraam N, Kumar GP. Classification of epileptic seizures using

wavelet packet log energy and norm entropies with recurrent Elman neural network classifier. Cogn Neurodyn. 2017;11(1):51-66.

[37] Tiwari AK, Pachori RB, Kanhangad V, Panigrahi BK. Automated Diagnosis of Epilepsy Using Key-Point-Based Local Binary Pattern of EEG Signals. IEEE J Biomed Heal informatics. 2017 Jul;21(4):888-896.

[38] Wang Y, Li Z, Feng L, Bai H, Wang C. Hardware design of multiclass SVM classification for epilepsy and epileptic seizure detection. IET Circuits, Devices Syst. 2018;12(1):108-115.

[39] Wen T, Zhang Z. Effective and extensible feature extraction method using genetic algorithm-based frequency-domain feature search for epileptic EEG multiclassification. Med (United States). 2017;96(19):1-11.

[40] Zhang T, Chen W. LMD Based Features for the Automatic Seizure Detection of EEG Signals Using SVM. IEEE Trans Neural Syst Rehabil Eng. 2017;25(8):1100-1108.

[41] Hekim M. The classification of EEG signals using discretization-based entropy and the adaptive neuro-fuzzy inference system. Turkish J Electr Eng Comput Sci. 2016;24(1):285-297.

[42] Murugavel ASM, Ramakrishnan S. Hierarchical multi-class SVM with ELM kernel for epileptic EEG signal classification. Med Biol Eng Comput. 2016;54(1):149-161.

[43] Peker M, Sen B, Delen D. A novel method for automated diagnosis of epilepsy using complex-valued classifiers. IEEE J Biomed Heal Informatics. 2016;20(1):108-118.

[44] Abualsaud K, Mahmuddin M, Saleh M, Mohamed A. Ensemble classifier for epileptic seizure detection for imperfect EEG data. Sci World J. 2015; http://dx.doi.org/10.1155/2015/945689.

[45] Kaya Y. Hidden pattern discovery on epileptic EEG with 1-D local binary patterns and epileptic seizures detection by grey relational analysis. Australas Phys Eng Sci Med. 2015;38(3):435-446.

[46] Martis RJ, Tan JH, Chua CK, Loon TC, Yeo SWJ, Tong L. Epileptic EEG classification using nonlinear parameters on different frequency bands. J Mech Med Biol. 2015;15(3). 1550040.

[47] Riaz F, Hassan A, Rehman S, Niazi IK, Dremstrup K. EMD-based temporal and spectral features for the classification of EEG signals using supervised learning. IEEE Trans Neural Syst Rehabil Eng. 2016;24(1):28-35.

[48] Tawfik NS, Youssef SM, Kholief M. A hybrid automated detection of epileptic seizures in EEG records. Comput Electr Eng. 2016;53(February 2019):177-190.

[49] Kaya Y, Uyar M, Tekin R, Yildirim S. 1D-local binary pattern based feature extraction for classification of epileptic EEG signals. Appl Math Comput. 2014;243:209-219.

[50] Sivasankari K, Thanushkodi K. An improved EEG signal classification using Neural Network with the consequence of ICA and STFT. J Electr Eng Technol. 2014;9(3):1060-1071.

[51] Acharya UR, Yanti R, Zheng JW, Krishnan MMR, Tan JH, Martis RJ, et al. Automated diagnosis of epilepsy using CWT, HOS and texture parameters. Int J Neural Syst. 2013;23(3).

[52] Alam SMS, Bhuiyan MIH. Detection of seizure and epilepsy using higher order statistics in the EMD domain. IEEE J Biomed Heal Informatics. 2013;17(2):312-318.

[53] Fernández-Blanco E, Rivero D, Gestal M, Dorado J. Classification of signals by means of Genetic Programming. Soft Comput. 2013;17(10):1929-1937.

[54] Hosseini SA, Akbarzadeh-T M-R, Naghibi-Sistani M-B. Qualitative and Quantitative Evaluation of EEG Signals in Epileptic Seizure Recognition. Int J Intell Syst Appl. 2013;5(6):41-46.

[55] Niknazar M, Mousavi SR, Vosoughi Vahdat B, Sayyah M. A new framework based on recurrence quantification analysis for epileptic seizure detection. IEEE J Biomed Heal Informatics. 2013;17(3):572-578.

[56] Peker M. AWERProcedia Information Technology & Computer Science A new complex-valued intelligent system for automated epilepsy diagnosis using EEG signals. 2013;03:1121-1128.

[57] Seng KC. Epilepsy risk index (ERI) for diagnosis of epilepsy: A new paradigm features. J Med Imaging Heal Informatics. 2013;3(2):314-320.

[58] Wang Y, Zhou W, Yuan Q, Li X, Meng Q, Zhao X, et al. Comparison of ictal and interictal eeg signals using fractal features. Int J Neural Syst. 2013;23(6).

[59] Zhu G, Li Y, Wen P (Paul), Wang S, Zhong N. Unsupervised Classification of Epileptic EEG Signals with Multi Scale K-Means Algorithm BT - Brain and Health Informatics. In: Imamura K, Usui S, Shirao T, Kasamatsu T, Schwabe L, Zhong N, editors. Cham: Springer International Publishing; 2013. p. 158-167.

[60] Acharya UR, Sree SV, Ang PCA, Yanti R, Suri JS. Application of non-linear and wavelet based features for the automated identification of epileptic EEG signals. Int J Neural Syst. 2012;22(2).

[61] Acharya UR, Yanti R, Swapna G, Sree VS, Martis RJ, Suri JS. Automated diagnosis of epileptic electroencephalogram using independent component analysis and discrete wavelet transform for different electroencephalogram durations. Proc Inst Mech Eng Part H, J Eng Med. 2013 Mar;227(3):234-244.

[62] Martis RJ, Acharya UR, Tan JH, Petznick A, Yanti R, Chua CK, et al. Application of empirical mode decomposition (EMD) for automated detection of epilepsy using EEG signals. Int J Neural Syst. 2012;22(6): 1250027.

[63] Acharya UR, Sree SV, Chattopadhyay S, Yu W, Ang PCA. Application of recurrence quantification analysis for the automated identification of epileptic EEG signals. Int J Neural Syst. 2011;21(3):199-211.

[64] Guo L, Rivero D, Dorado J, Munteanu CR, Pazos A. Automatic feature extraction using genetic programming: An application to epileptic EEG classification. Expert Syst Appl. 2011;38(8):10425-10436.

[65] Mihandoost A. Automatic feature extraction using generalised autoregressive conditional heteroscedasticity model: an application to electroencephalogram classification. IET Signal Process. 2012;6(9):829-838.

[66] Orhan U, Hekim M, Ozer M. EEG signals classification using the K-means clustering and a multilayer perceptron neural network model. Expert Syst Appl [Internet]. 2011;38(10):13475-13481.

[67] Balli T, Palaniappan R. Classification of biological signals using linear and nonlinear features. Physiol Meas. 2010 Jul;31(7):903-920.

[68] Liang SF, Wang HC, Chang WL. Combination of EEG complexity and spectral analysis for epilepsy diagnosis and seizure detection. EURASIP J Adv Signal Process. 2010;2010:17-20.

[69] Song Y, Liò P. A new approach for epileptic seizure detection: sample entropy based feature extraction and extreme learning machine. J Biomed Sci Eng. 2010;03(06):556-567.

[70] Acharya UR, Chua CK, Lim T-C, Dorithy, Suri JS. Automatic identification of epileptic EEG signals using nonlinear parameters. J Mech Med Biol. 2009;9(4):539-553.

[71] Übeyli ED. Combined neural network model employing wavelet coefficients for EEG signals classification. Digit Signal Process A Rev J. 2009;19(2):297-308.

[72] Übeyli ED. Wavelet/mixture of experts network structure for EEG signals classification. Expert Syst Appl. 2008;34(3):1954-1962.

[73] Güler I, Übeyli ED. Multiclass support vector machines for EEG-signals classification. IEEE Trans Inf Technol Biomed. 2007;11(2):117-126.

[74] Tzallas AT, Tsipouras MG, Fotiadis DI. Automatic seizure detection based on time-frequency analysis and artificial neural networks. Comput Intell Neurosci. 2007; doi:10.1155/2007/80510.

[75] Tzallas AT, Tsipouras MG, Fotiadis DI. The use of time-frequency distributions for epileptic seizure detection in EEG recordings. Annu Int Conf IEEE Eng Med Biol - Proc. 2007;3-6.

[76] Übeyli ED, Güler I. Features extracted by eigenvector methods for detecting variability of EEG signals. Pattern Recognit Lett. 2007;28(5):592-603.

[77] Sadati N, Mohseni HR, Maghsoudi A. Epileptic seizure detection using neural fuzzy networks. IEEE Int Conf Fuzzy Syst. 2006;(July 2014):596-600.

[78] Güler NF, Übeyli ED, Güler I. Recurrent neural networks employing Lyapunov exponents for EEG signals classification. Expert Syst Appl. 2005;29(3):506-514.

[79] Güler I, Übeyli ED. Adaptive neuro-fuzzy inference system for classification of EEG signals using wavelet coefficients. J Neurosci Methods. 2005;148(2):113-121.

[80] Gruszczyńska I, Mosdorf R, Sobaniec P, Żochowska-Sobaniec M, Borowska M. Epilepsy identification based on EEG signal using RQA method. Adv Med Sci. 2019;64(1):58-64.

[81] Jacob JE, Sreelatha VV, Iype T, Nair GK, Yohannan DG. Diagnosis of epilepsy from interictal EEGs based on chaotic and wavelet transformation. Analog Integr Circuits Signal Process. 2016;89(1):131-138.

[82] Azuma H, Nagata H, Akechi T. Linear and non-linear EEG analyses before and after psychosis in patients with epilepsy. Epilepsy & Seizure. 2019;11:20-29.

[83] Kawakami Y, Itoh Y. Forced Normalization: Antagonism Between Epilepsy and Psychosis. Pediatr Neurol. 2017 May;70:16-19.

[84] Flor-Henry P. Determinants of psychosis in epilepsy: laterality and forced normalization. Biol Psychiatry. 1983 Sep;18(9):1045-1057.

[85] Casale M, Marcuse L, Young JJ, Jetté N, Panov FE, Bender H, et al. The Sensitivity of Scalp EEG at Detecting Seizures-A Simultaneous Scalp and Stereo EEG Study. J Clin Neurophysiol. 2020;

[86] Dubey A, Ray S. Cortical Electrocorticogram (ECoG) Is a Local Signal. J Neurosci. 2019 May;39(22):4299-4311.

[87] Yin Y, Sun K, He S. Multiscale permutation Rényi entropy and its application for EEG signals. PLoS One. 2018;13(9):e0202558.

[88] Čukić M, Stokić M, Simić S, Pokrajac D. The successful discrimination of depression from EEG could be attributed to proper feature extraction and not to a particular classification method. Cogn Neurodyn. 2020 Aug;14(4):443-455.

[89] Li X, Hu B, Sun S, Cai H. EEG-based mild depressive detection using feature selection methods and classifiers. Comput Methods Programs Biomed. 2016 Nov;136:151-161.

[90] Akdemir Akar S, Kara S, Agambayev S, Bilgic V. Nonlinear analysis of EEGs of patients with major depression during different emotional states. Comput Biol Med. 2015 Dec;67:49-60.

[91] Akar SA, Kara S, Agambayev S, Bilgic V. Nonlinear analysis of EEG in major depression with fractal dimensions. Annu Int Conf IEEE Eng Med Biol Soc IEEE Eng Med Biol Soc Annu Int Conf. 2015;2015:7410-7413.

[92] Kalev K, Bachmann M, Orgo L, Lass J, Hinrikus H. Lempel-Ziv and multiscale Lempel-Ziv complexity in depression. Annu Int Conf IEEE Eng Med Biol Soc IEEE Eng Med Biol Soc Annu Int Conf. 2015;2015:4158-4161.

[93] Siuly S, Khare SK, Bajaj V, Wang H, Zhang Y. A Computerized Method for Automatic Detection of Schizophrenia Using EEG Signals. IEEE Trans neural Syst Rehabil Eng a Publ IEEE Eng Med Biol Soc. 2020 Sep;PP.

[94] Goshvarpour A, Goshvarpour A. Schizophrenia diagnosis using innovative EEG feature-level fusion schemes. Australas Phys Eng Sci Med. 2020 Jan;

[95] Jahmunah V, Lih Oh S, Rajinikanth V, Ciaccio EJ, Hao Cheong K, Arunkumar N, et al. Automated detection of schizophrenia using nonlinear signal processing methods. Artif Intell Med. 2019 Sep;100:101698.

[96] Cerquera A, Gjini K, Bowyer SM, Boutros N. Comparing EEG Nonlinearity in Deficit and Nondeficit Schizophrenia Patients: Preliminary Data. Clin EEG Neurosci. 2017 Nov;48(6):376-382.

[97] Takahashi T, Cho RY, Mizuno T, Kikuchi M, Murata T, Takahashi K, et al. Antipsychotics reverse abnormal EEG complexity in drug-naive schizophrenia: a multiscale entropy analysis. Neuroimage. 2010 May;51(1):173-182.

[98] Adachi N, Matsuura M, Okubo Y, Oana Y, Takei N, Kato M, et al. Predictive variables of interictal psychosis in epilepsy. Neurology. 2000 Nov;55(9):1310-1314.

[99] Adachi N, Akanuma N, Fenwick P, Ito M, Okazaki M, Ishida S, et al. Seizure activity and individual vulnerability on first-episode interictal psychosis in epilepsy. Epilepsy Behav. 2018 Feb;79:234-238.

[100] Adachi N, Akanuma N, Ito M, Kato M, Hara T, Oana Y, et al. Epileptic, organic and genetic vulnerabilities for timing of the development of interictal psychosis. Br J Psychiatry. 2010 Mar;196(3):212-216.

[101] Prevey ML, Delaney RC, Cramer JA, Mattson RH. Complex partial and secondarily generalized seizure patients: cognitive functioning prior to treatment with antiepileptic medication. VA Epilepsy Cooperative Study 264 Group. Epilepsy Res. 1998 Mar;30(1):1-9.

[102] Pulliainen V, Kuikka P, Jokelainen M. Motor and cognitive

functions in newly diagnosed adult seizure patients before antiepileptic medication. Acta Neurol Scand. 2000 Feb;101(2):73-78.

[103] Mathon B, Bordes A, Amelot A, Carpentier A, Méré M, Dupont S, et al. Evaluation of psychomotor functions in patients with drug-resistant epilepsy. Epilepsy Behav. 2020 May;106:106985.

[104] Tadokoro Y, Oshima T, Fukuchi T, Kanner AM, Kanemoto K. Screening for major depressive episodes in Japanese patients with epilepsy: validation and translation of the Japanese version of Neurological Disorders Depression Inventory for Epilepsy (NDDI-E). Epilepsy Behav. 2012 Sep;25(1):18-22.

[105] Gillham R, Bryant-Comstock L, Kane K. Validation of the side effect and life satisfaction (SEALS) inventory. Seizure. 2000 Oct;9(7):458-463.

Chapter 8

EEG Signal Denoising Using Haar Transform and Maximal Overlap Discrete Wavelet Transform (MODWT) for the Finding of Epilepsy

Sasikumar Gurumoorthy, Naresh Babu Muppalaneni and G. Sandhya Kumari

Abstract

Wavelet transform filters the signal without changing the pattern of the signal. The transformation techniques have been applied to the continuous time domain signals. The chapter is devoted to the study of the EEG (ElectroEncephaloGram) Signal processing using Haar wavelet transform and Maximal overlap discrete wavelet transform (MODWT) for the analyzing of Epilepsy. Haar transform returns the approximation coefficients and detail coefficients. Detail coefficients are generally referred to as the wavelet coefficients and are a highpass representation of the input. In this chapter, with the help of Haar transform, the detailed coefficients of the input signal have been analyzed for the detection of Epilepsy. Maximal overlap discrete wavelet transform filters the noise coefficients of the input signal in each and every level, and it has displayed the filtered output signal.

Keywords: EEG, Haar, MODWT, wavelet transform, epilepsy

1. Introduction

EEG Signal processing is essential for the diagnosis of brain disorders. The brain EEG signal that has been acquired from the EEG equipment consists of noise disturbances such as eye ball movement, muscle contractions etc., where the particular brain signal cannot be analyzed without any filtration techniques. Due to the presence of noise coefficients in the input signal, the transformation techniques have been applied to the input signal. Haar transform and maximal overlap discrete wavelet transform are the transformation techniques that supported for the filtration of the noisy coefficients from the input EEG signal.

The transformation techniques that have been applied to the brain signal filtered the noise coefficients without disturbing the peak values of the input signal. With the help of peak points, it is possible to represent the presence of Epileptic seizure. Epileptic seizure is the brain disorder and it can be analyzed based on the sudden increase of the sudden increase in the input signal. For the analyzation of actual input signal, the transformations such as Haar transform and Maximal

Overlap Discrete Wavelet Transform (MODWT) has not been disturbed the peak points of the actual brain signal and filtered the noise coefficients efficiently.

2. Literature survey

Ozaydin and Alak have explained speech enhancement using maximal overlap discrete wavelet transform where they demonstrated the application of the Maximal overlap discrete wavelet transform in speech signal processing [1]. The analyzation algorithm was performed using Matlab platform. Rahul Kher et al. have presented a paper on signal processing techniques for removing high frequency noise from ECG signals with matlab platform.

Kumar and Joshi describe MODWT Based Time Scale Decomposition Analysis of BSE and NSE Indexes Financial Time Series, Where they concluded that MODWT based time scale decomposition analysis gives better results than the Fourier transform based spectral analysis [2]. Hostalkova et al. have been analyzed the multi-dimensional biomedical image de-noising using Haar transform, where the results are represented in numerical and graphical forms using three-dimensional visualization tools [3]. Ali Hajjaji et al. have published a paper regarding the Combination of Haar Wavelet and Karhunen Loeve Transforms for Medical Images Watermarking, and developed a novel watermarking method to embed the patient's data into the corresponding image or set of images used for the diagnosis [4]. Sun and Meinl stated a new wavelet-based denoising algorithm for high-frequency financial data mining [5]. Ghosh and Chaudhuri have been explained about the Fractal Investigation and Maximal Overlap Discrete Wavelet Transformation (MODWT) based Machine Learning Framework for Forecasting Exchange rates. Zitong Zhang et al. have analyzed different Wavelet Methods, Filters, and Lengths for Functional Brain Network Construction [6, 7].

3. Related work

3.1 Haar wavelet transform

In discrete form, Haar wavelets are related to a mathematical operation called the Haar transform. The Haar transform serves as a prototype for all other wavelet transforms. Haar wavelet is a sequence of rescaled square-shaped functions which together form a wavelet family or basis. The technical disadvantage of the Haar wavelet is that it is not continuous, and therefore not differentiable. The advantage of Haar transform advantage is it can be used for analyzation of signals with sudden transition and for localized feature of signals. The orthogonal property of the Haar function helps to analyze the frequency components of input signal. The Haar wavelet's mother wavelet function can be represented as,

$$\psi(t)=\left\{\begin{matrix} 1 & 0\leq t\leq 1/2 \\ -1 & 1/2\leq t\leq 1 \\ 0 & otherwise \end{matrix}\right\} \quad (1)$$

The 2 × 2 Haar matrix that is associated with the Haar wavelet is,

$$H_2=\begin{bmatrix} 1 & 1 \\ 1 & -1 \end{bmatrix}$$

It requires only additions and there are many elements with zero value in the Haar matrix, so the computation time is short. Input and output length are the same. However, the length should be a power of 2, i.e. N= $2^K, K \in N$. It can be used to analyze the localized feature of signals. Due to the orthogonal property of the Haar function, the frequency components of input signal can be analyzed. The equation of the Haar transform is $B_n = H_n A_n H_n^{\,T}$, where A_n is a $n \times n$ matrix and H_n is n-point Haar transform. Haar matrix consists of only real elements and it can be defined as non-symmetric matrix.

3.2 Maximal overlap discrete wavelet transform (MODWT)

The MODWT is a linear filtering operation that transforms into coefficients related to variations over a set of scales. It is used to inspect the scale-dependent signal behaviors. The MODWT is a time shift-invariant method, where a translation in the signal results in a translation of wavelet coefficients by the same amount. The MODWT is different and has several advantages when compared to DWT and it improves the alignment of the decomposed wavelet and scaling coefficients at each level with the original time series. This is the transform that aligns the wavelet coefficients at each time interval with the original signal. So, it is easy to analyze the localized signal variation with respect to scale and time. MODWT can be used to obtain scale based additive decomposition and a scale based energy decomposition.

The function f(x) is a linear combination of scaling function and wavelet function where j_o is the number of levels of the decomposition. The output is the combination of detailed and scaling coefficients. The detailed coefficients are produced by the transform at each level but the scaling coefficients are produced at the final level

$$f(x) = \sum_{K=0}^{N-1} C_k 2^{\frac{-j_o}{2}} \o\left(2^{-j_o} x - k\right) + \sum_{j=1}^{j_o} f_j(x) \quad (2)$$

$$f_j(x) = \sum_{k=0}^{N-1} d_{j,k} 2^{-\frac{j}{2}} \psi\left(2^{-j} x - k\right) \quad (3)$$

MODWT returns the N-many coefficients $\{c_k\}$ and $(j_o * N)$ many detailed coefficients $\{d_{j,k}\}$ of the expansion. The MODWT partitions the energy across the scaling coefficients and various scales.

$$\|x\|^2 = \sum_{j=1}^{j_o} ||w_j||\text{^}2 + ||v_{j_o}||\text{^}2 \quad (4)$$

Where x is the input data, w_j are the detail coefficients at scale j and v_{j_o} are the final level scaling coefficients.

4. Results and discussions

4.1 Haar wavelet transform

Figure 1 represents Haar approximation of EEG signal where the noise present in the signal has been removed by the Haar transformation effectively without changing the peak values of the original signal.

Haar transform has been filtered the detailed coefficients of the original signal where the detailed coefficients are shown in **Figure 2**.

Maximal overlap discrete overlap transform filters the input signal based on the number of levels where in each and every level the transform able to remove the noise coefficients present in the signal. **Figure 3** represents the output of Maximal overlap discrete wavelet transform. **Table 1** explains about the parameters of the signal like mean, standard deviation and variance and **Table 2** represents the parameters of the signal using daubechies external phase wavelet.

4.2 MODWT using daubechies extremal phase wavelet

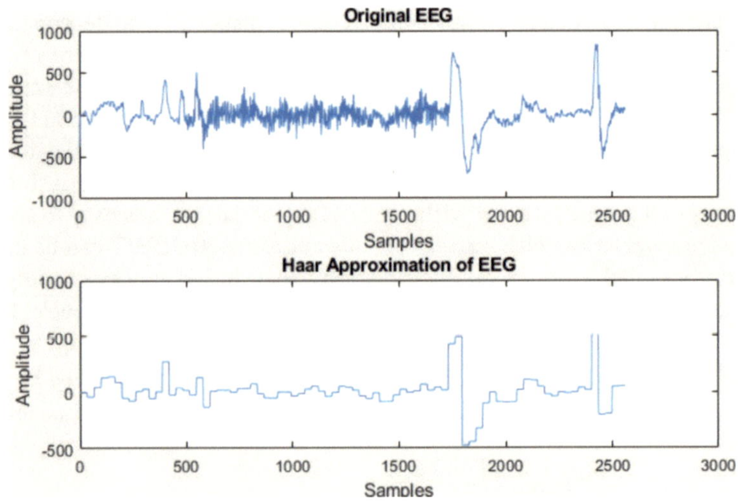

Figure 1.
Haar approximation of EEG signal.

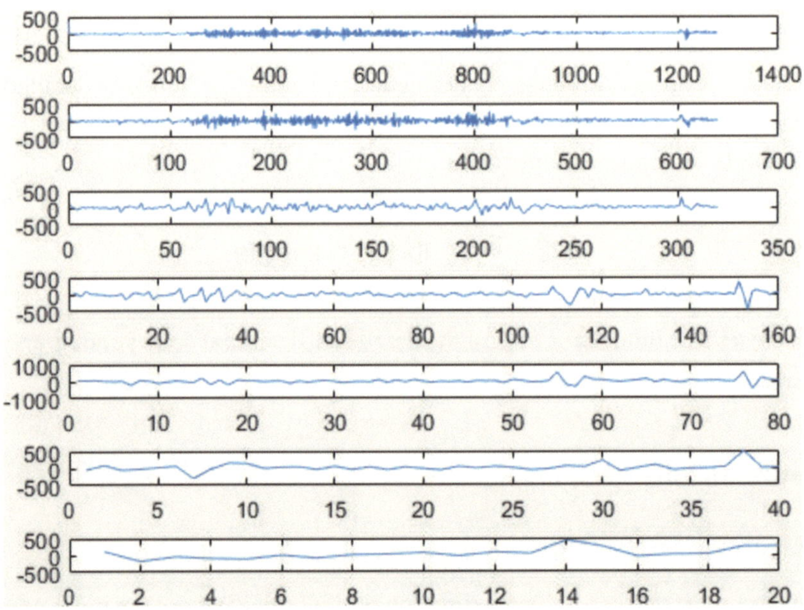

Figure 2.
Detailed coefficients of the EEG signal.

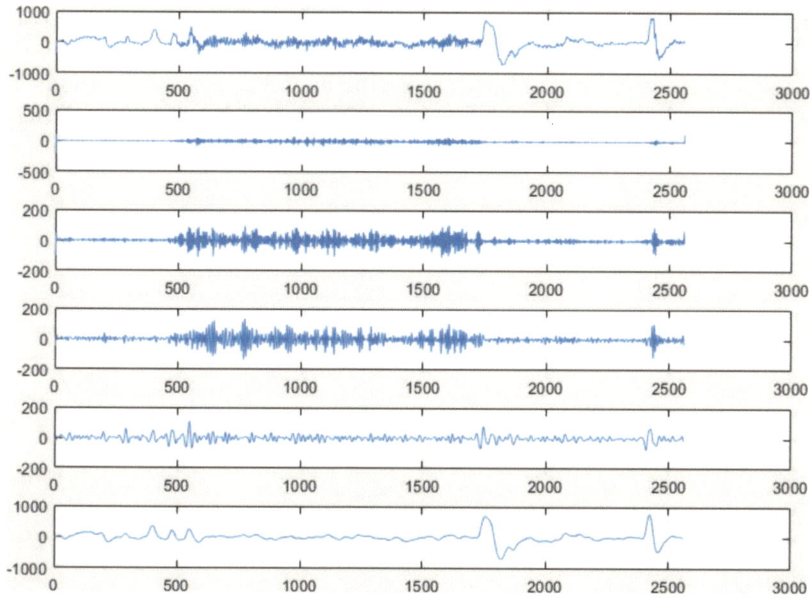

Figure 3.
Maximal overlap discrete wavelet transform.

Parameters	Original	Haar	MODWT
Mean	3.9176	3.9625	3.9176
Standard Deviation	172.0907	140.6722	156.6592
Varaiance	2.9615e+04	1.9789e+04	2.4542e+04

Table 1.
Parameters of the signal.

Parameters	db5	db10	db45
Mean	3.9176	3.9176	3.9176
Standard Deviation	159.2136	159.7792	160.1462
Variance	2.5349e+04	2.5529e+04	2.5647e+04

Table 2.
Parameters of MODWT using Daubechies Extremal phase wavelet.

5. Conclusion

In this paper, EEG signal has been analyzed with the help of transformation techniques like Haar Transform and with Maximal Overlap Discrete Wavelet Transform for the analysis of Epilepsy. It has been observed that the mean of the filtered signal and the input signal was approximately same after applying the transformations. These transforms are the processing algorithms to filter the noisy coefficients of the original signal. The structure of the signal should be same after the application of the algorithms especially in the case of biomedical applications where it has been achieved with the help of these Haar and Maximal Overlap Discrete Wavelet Transform (MODWT) for the identification of Epilepsy.

Acknowledgements

All the authors would like to thank Department of Science and Technology (DST), Cognitive Science Research Initiative (CSRI). Ref. No.: SR/CSRI/370/2016.

Author details

Sasikumar Gurumoorthy[1*], Naresh Babu Muppalaneni[2] and G. Sandhya Kumari[1]

1 Sree Vidyanikethan Engineering College (Autonomous), Tirupati, India

2 National Institute of Technology Silchar, Silchar, Assam, India

*Address all correspondence to: dr.gurumoorthy@ieee.org

References

[1] Ozaydin S, Alak IK. Speech enhancement using maximal overlap discrete wavelet transform. Gazi University Journal of Science, Part A. 2018;**5**(4):159-171

[2] Kumar A, Joshi LK. MODWT based time scale decomposition analysis of BSE and NSE indexes financial time series. International Journal of Mathematical Analysis. 2011;**5**(27):1343-1352

[3] Hostalkova E, Vysata O, Prochazka A. Multi-dimensional Biomedical Image De-Noising Using Haar Transform. In: 15th International Conference on digital signal processing. Cardiff, UK: IEEE Explorer, IEEE; July 2007. pp. 1-4. DOI: 10.1109/ICDSP.2007.4288547

[4] Hajjaji MA, Bourennane E-B, Abdelali AB, Mtibaa A. Combining Haar wavelet and Karhunen Loeve transforms for medical images watermarking. BioMed Research International. vol. 2014. Article ID: 313078, 15 pages. 2014. DOI: 10.1155/2014/313078

[5] Sun EW, Meinl T. A new wavelet-based denoising algorithm for high-frequency financial data mining. European Journal of Operational Research. 2012;**217**(3):589-599. DOI: 10.1016/j.ejor.2011.09.049

[6] Ghosh I, Chaudhuri TD. Fractal investigation and maximal overlap discrete wavelet transformation (MODWT)-based machine learning framework for forecasting exchange rates. Studies in Microeconomics. 2017;**5**(2):105-131. DOI: 10.1177/23210 22217724978

[7] Zhang Z, Telesford QK, Giusti C, Lim KO, Bassett DS. Choosing wavelet methods, filters, and lengths for functional brain network construction. PLoS ONE. United States. 2016;**11**(6):e0157243. DOI: 10.1371/ journal.pone.01572433

Chapter 9

Epileptic Seizure Prediction

Shaik Jakeer Hussain and Gurajapu Raja Sumant

Abstract

Epilepsy is a nervous disease which causes seizures. Electroencephalography (EEG) gives complex information about the brain dynamics but its visual inspection is difficult and requires skilled interpreters. Source localization means identifying the area of the brain where a seizure can occur. In general, source localization is necessary for patients with a special condition in epilepsy, i.e. when their disease is resistant to drugs. One-third of the people having epilepsy are drug resistant and the latest anti-epileptic drugs cannot stop the seizures completely. Unexpected occurrence of seizure disturbs the quality of life and causes physical damage and thus epilepsy should be predicted. This study will use various signal processing methods to extract features by studying the pre-ictal and inter-ictal periods, localize the source and then finally predict epilepsy with the help of Artificial Neural Networks. The knowledge thus derived can help in preparing a wearable brain - computer interface.

Keywords: electroencephalography (EEG), epileptic seizure, neural networks, epileptic source, localization, epileptic seizure prediction

1. Introduction

Epileptic seizure detection deals with the process of detecting a seizure when it occurs. The need of the day is to take forward this work to eventually predict a seizure much before it is detected as it the very nature of the seizure that it is random. This chapter discusses various methods to do the same.

The cause of disorder will remain unexplained unless a complete cure is possible and available. Two practical engineering approaches are used to research in epilepsy. The first approach involves monitoring the brain activity on multiple scales which gives us a base to understand the generation of seizures. The second approach is to model the natural properties of the brain network and manipulate these for the modulation of seizure generation.

This work mainly concentrates on amalgamation of the above approaches towards developing a closed loop device which has a feedback of brain signals to the device so that it can control interventions that stop seizures.

The main objective in this chapter is a search for a precursor for seizure prediction mainly in the preictal phase as shown in the **Figure 1**. This may have form of an identifiable, significant pattern, feature or a pattern to extract the feature.

Five techniques are used to achieve this objective. They are:

Using Lyapunov exponents.

Using Cross wavelets [1].

Fourier Bessel function [2].

Wavelets [3].

EMD [4].

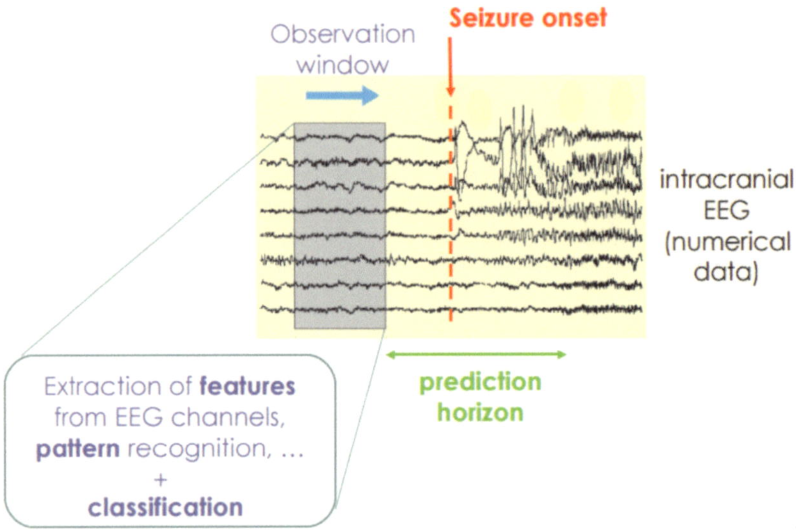

Figure 1.
Seizure prediction methodology.

2. Epileptic seizure prediction using cross wavelets, Lyapunov exponents and neural networks

A seizure prediction method to predict the transitions between Inter ictal and pre ictal states using cross wavelet and Lyapunov exponent features and neural network for binary classification had been proposed [1]. The CHB-MIT database was used.

2.1 Cross wavelet transform

The cross wavelet transform (XWT) of two time series xn and yn is defined as WXY = WXWY∗, where * denotes complex conjugation. We further define the cross wavelet power as $|W_{XY}|$. The complex argument $\arg(W_{XY})$ can be interpreted as the local relative phase between x_n and y_n in time frequency space [1].

2.2 Lyapunov exponent

A mathematical function which detects chaos is the Lyapunov exponents. Lyapunov exponents are the average exponential rates of divergence or convergence of nearby orbits in phase space.

$$\lambda_i = \lim_{t\to\infty} \log_2 \frac{p_i(t)}{p_i(0)} \tag{1}$$

Where λ_i are ordered from largest to smallest.

2.3 Application of cross wavelets, Lyapunov exponents and neural networks in prediction

The data is divided into Preictal and interictal as per the information of expert. Three types of preictal data is considered for experimentation. The methods adopted for prediction system are as shown in the block diagram below (**Figures 2** and **3**):

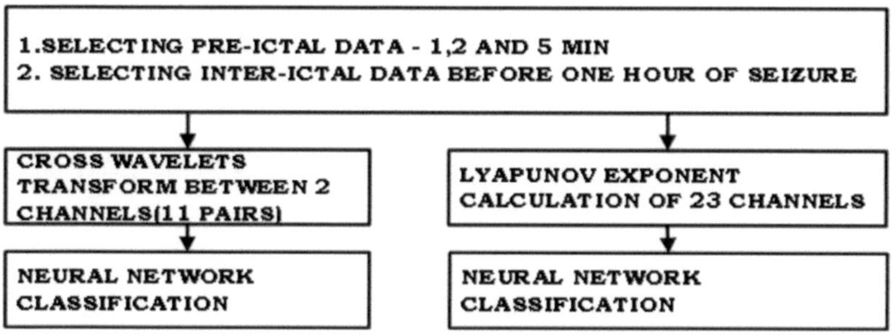

Figure 2.
Block diagram of epilepsy prediction system using cross wavelets, Lyapunov exponents and neural networks.

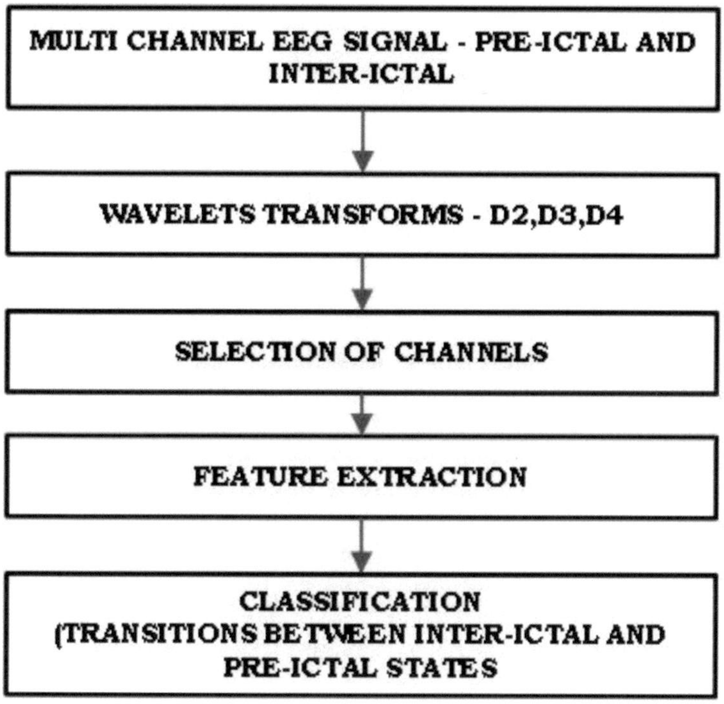

Figure 3.
Block diagram showing flow of seizure prediction using wavelet.

Pair Number	Left side Electrodes	Channel Number	Right Side electrodes	Channel Number
1	Fp1 -F7	1	Fp2-F8	13
2	Fp1-F3	5	Fp2-F4	9
3	T7-P7	3	T8-P8	15
4	C3-P3	7	C4-P4	11
5	P3-O1	8	P4-O2	12
6	P7-O1	4	T8-O2	16

where F:Frontal P:Posterior T:Temporal C:Central O:Occipital.

Table 1.
Division of channels into 11 pairs to calculate cross wavelet coefficients.

Data	True positive (TP)	False positive(FP)	Sensitivity (%)	Specificity (%)
Preictal (1 min)	152	28	8x.4	—
Preictal (2 min)	295	65	81.9	—
Preicta (5 min)	634	86	88.05	—
	TN	FN		
Inter Ictal	902	34		96.36
	Over all accuracy (%)		90.3	

Table 2.
Prediction performance of neural network with cross wavelet features.

Data	True positive (TP)	False positive(FP)	Sensitivity (%)	Specificity (%)
Preictal	180	0	100	—
Inter Ictal	297-TN	3-FN	—	99
	Overall accuracy (%)		99.37	

Table 3.
Prediction performance of neural network with lyapunov features.

The data is having 23 channels. The channels are selected as per standard bipolar montage, electrode placement and channel information is provided in **Table 1** in which channels are divided as 11 pairs to calculate cross wavelet coefficients.

Cross wavelet features are extracted from 11 channel pairs which are applied to Feed forward Back propagation neural network having two layers with 11 input neurons as input layer and one output neuron as one output layer. +1 is assigned as target for pre ictal features and − 1 for inter ictal features. The network trained and tested for various feature vectors and the results are tabulated in **Table 2**.

The above table can be interpreted as follows:

For the consideration of interictal period, it is the TN and FN values which are taken into consideration as we need to minimize false alerts. It can be seen that the TN and FN values were 902 and 34 respectively with 96.36% specificity. The preictal data on the other hand had 88.05 sensitivity for 5 minutes data.

The lyapunov exponent is calculated from 23 channels, the extracted features are given to Feed forward back propagation neural network. 23 input nodes and one output node. The network is trained with preictal and interictal features the training performance is evaluated and results are tabulated in **Table 3**.

From the above **Table 3**, we can notice that the number of TP values for preictal period is 180 whereas there were no FP and 100% sensitivity when prediction was done with lyapunov features. In comparison, the inter ictal period had shown 287 TN and 3 FN with 99% specificity. The overall accuracy was 99.37%.

3. Epileptic seizure prediction using wavelet transforms and neural networks

Feature extraction is done using DWT. EEG signals contain all the useful information below 30 Hz and for this reason 4 decomposition levels D1-D4 and one final approximation, A4 are chosen [3].

DECOMPOSED SIGNAL	FREQUENCY BANDS(HZ)	DECOMPOSITION LEVEL
D1	128—256	1(NOISES)
D2	64–128	2(HIGHGAMA)
D3	32——64	3(GAMA)
D4	16—32	4(BETA)
D5	8———16	5ALPHA)
D6	4 ———8	6(THEETA)
A6	0—4	6(DELTA)

Table 4.
Frequency bands and corresponding decomposition levels.

Based on EEG Ictal period marking of experts selected preictal and interictal periods. These data is decomposed using discrete wavelet transform [3]. Out of 7 sub bands selected three sub bands D2, D3, Dx. These decomposition details are mentioned in **Table 4**.

From these sub bands 4 features power, covariance, inter Quartile Range (IQR) and median absolute deviation (MAD) are extracted from 23 channels of pre ictal and interictal EEG data. Three channels are selected and the feature vector size is Equal to 36 = 3 (channels) x 3 (sub bands D2, D3, D4) x4 (features-power, covariance, IQR, and MAD) from each epochs of preictal and Interictal EEG data. These features are applied to feed forward back propagation neural network as shown in **Figure 4**. Two layers are used hidden layer 36 neurons and output layer having 36 neurons. It is binary classification target +1 is assigned for preictal (Epiliptic) data and − 1 is assigned to Inter Ictal (normal). Total 1588 epochs (1 second) are used for classification 800 for training and 788 used for testing. The performance is evaluated in terms of sensitivity, Specificity and Overall accuracy.

For comparison of performance, Elman Back propagation neural network is used. The performance of Elman Network is tabulated in **Table 5**. Sensitivity in Elman network is high, specificity and overall accuracy are low. By comparisons of

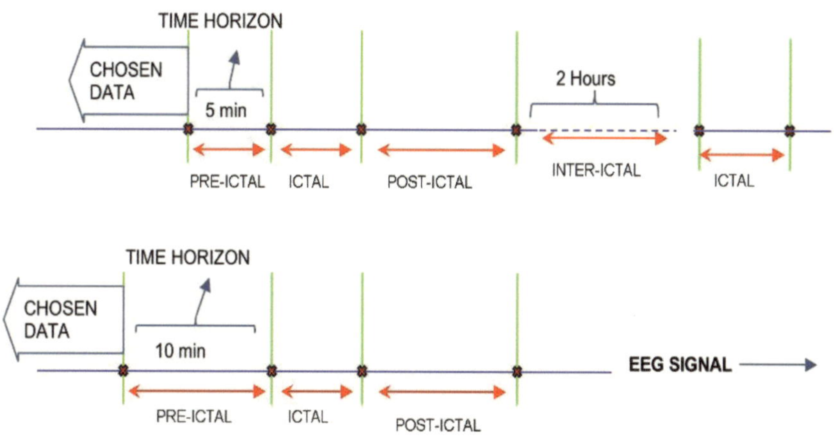

Figure 4.
Two types of data is chosen. First data has a time horizon of around 5 minutes for the pre-ictal period while the second has the time horizon for 10 minutes. The inter-ictal period is considered to be around 2 hours in order to nullify the post-ictal or seizure effects.

(TP)	(FP)	Sensitivity(%)	(TN)	(FN)	Specificity (%)	Overall accuracy (%)
296	4	98.6	381	107	78.1	85.9

Table 5.
Elman back propagation neural network performance.

(TP)	(FP)	Sensitivity (%)	(TN)	(FN)	Specificity (%)	Overall accuracy(%)
273	27	91	462	62	87	88.71

Table 6.
Feed forward neural network performance.

two types of neural networks feed forward network having better overall performance as the overall accuracy is about 88.71% compared to 85.9% of Elman back propagation (**Table 6**).

4. Epileptic seizure prediction based on Fourier-Bessel function

Any signal can be represented in terms of Fourier Bessel series due to its decaying nature. An EEG signal is expanded into a Fourier Bessel series [2]. In this way, an EEG signal can be segmented and periods interictal and ictal are classified to predict the occurrence of seizure.

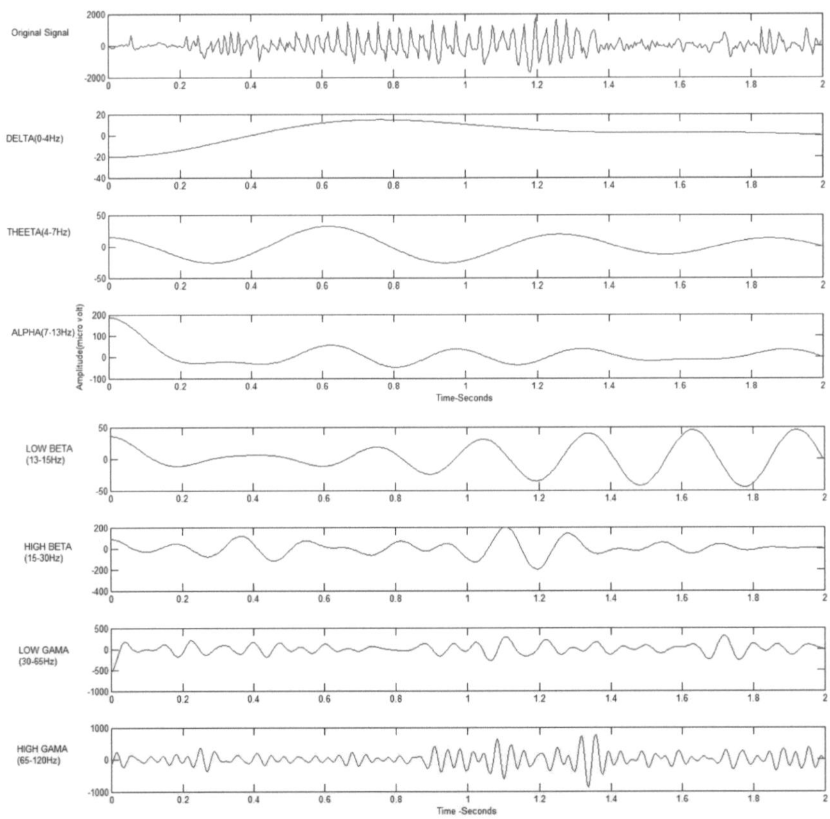

Figure 5.
First plot shows original signal followed by segmented EEG seizure signal of ictal period.

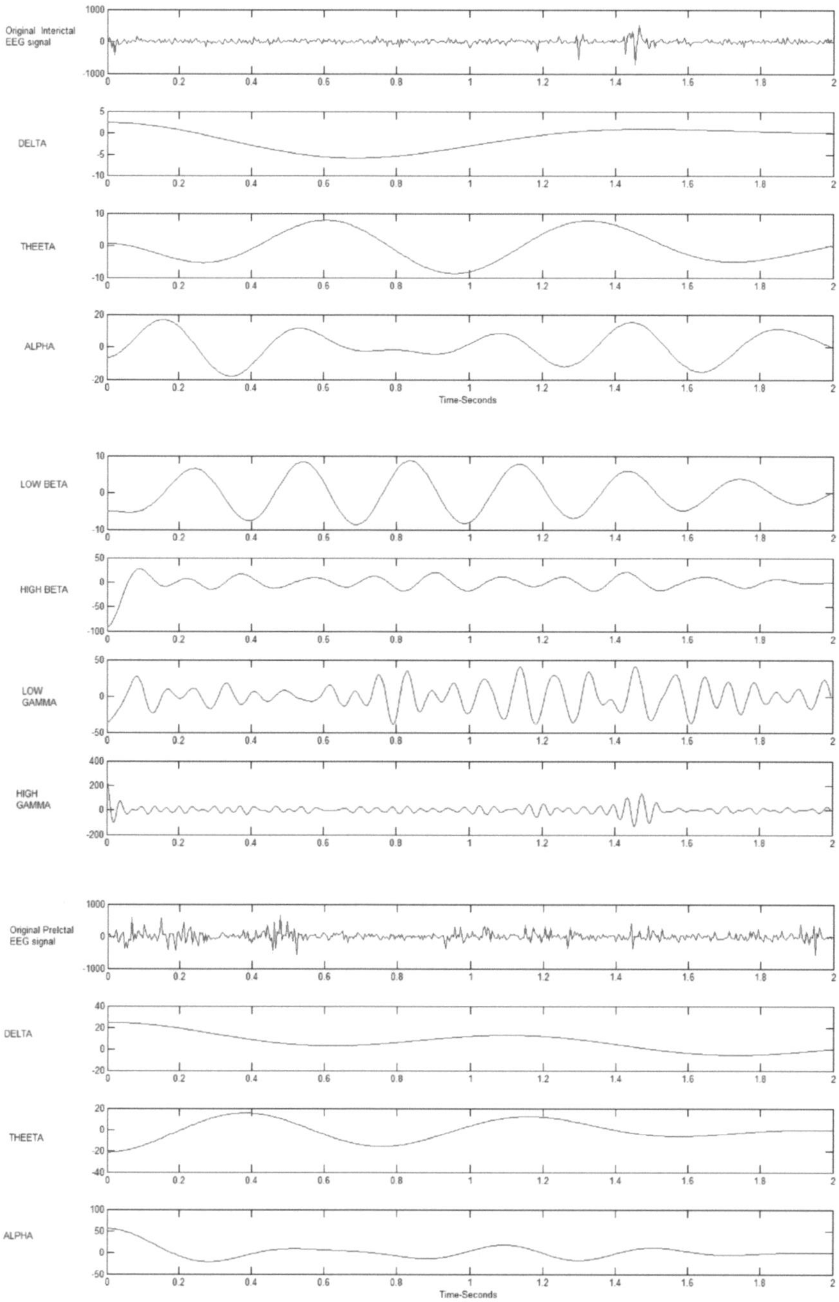

Figure 6.
First plot shows original signal followed by segmented EEG seizure signal of inter ictal period.

A 1–1 mapping exists between the frequencies and the coefficients. f_s = 256 and n = 128 (number of Fourier Bessel Coefficients).

All the **Figures 5–7** show the segmented bands of a seizure signal.

The five features energy in each sub band, fmean, IQR and MAD are extracted from each sub band.

The **Figure 8** shows the sum of all Bessel coefficients the preictal and interictal features are discriminating.

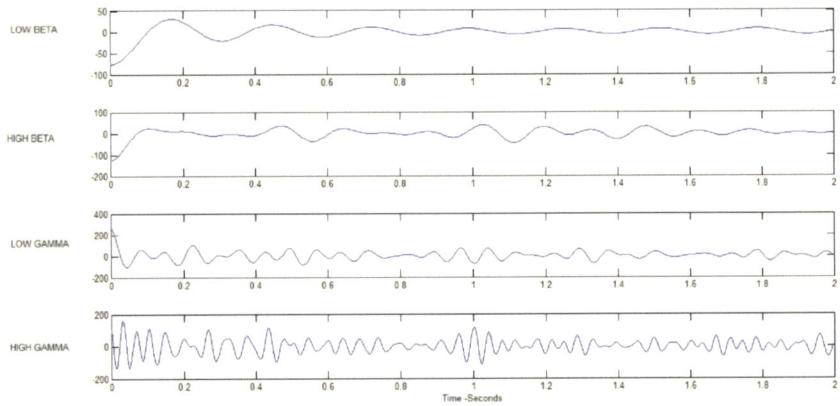

Figure 7.
First plot shows original signal followed by segmented EEG seizure signal of pre-ictal period.

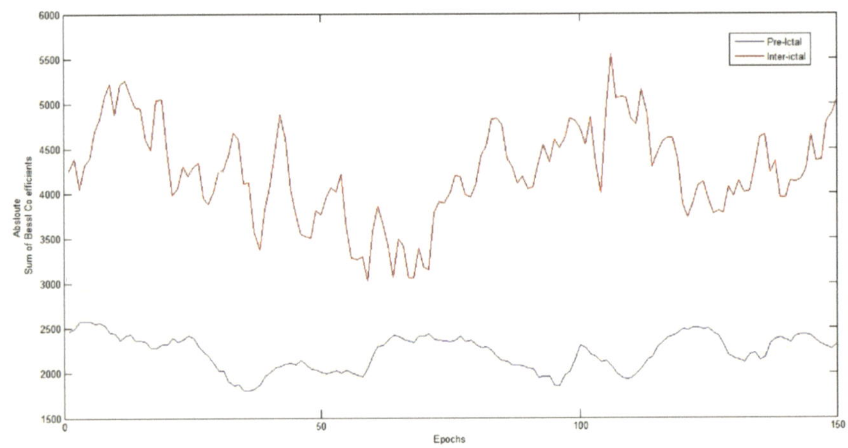

Figure 8.
Absolute sum of Bessel coefficients with red being Preictal and blue being Interictal EEG signals.

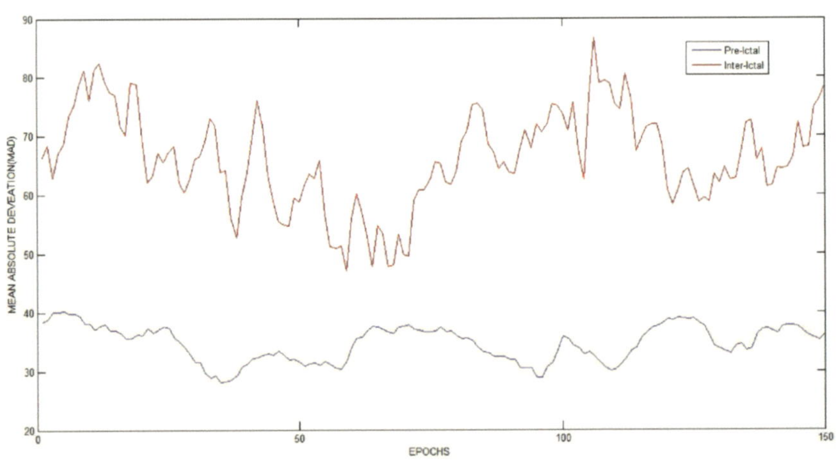

Figure 9.
MAD of coefficients with red being Preictal and blue being Interictal EEG signals.

From the **Figure 9** it can be observed that the feature, Median absolute deviation of Fourier Bessel coefficients for the Interictal and preictal are discriminating.

The inter ictal and pre ictal data is prepared as per the information in **Table 7**. The calculated Fourier-Bessel Coefficients from inter ictal and pre ictal data is given to Neural Network with 64 input neurons, one output neuron and one hidden layer. The Feed Forward Back propagation algorithm was used as shown in **Figure 10**. The network is trained −1 as target for inter -ictal and + 1 for pre-ictal.

The trained network is simulated with Inter-ictal and Pre-ictal data. There was one epoch as false negative and zero epochs as false positives. The simulation results had garnered 150 epochs of inter -ictal and 150 epochs of pre-ictal data. Inter ictal period is used to study sensitivity where as the pre ictal data is used for specificity.

The number of false negative values should be low so that it should have high sensitivity. The specificity must be high with lower false positive values. From **Table 8**, it is observed that sensitivity, specificity and accuracy of the

EEG Sub Band	Frequency Range (Hz)	Fourier-Bessel Coefficient(m)
DELTA	0–4	0–4
THEETA	4–7	4–7
ALPHA	7–13	7–13
LOW BETA	13–15	13–15
HIGH BETA	15–30	15–30
LOW GAMA	30–65	30–65
HIGH GAMA	65–120	65–120

Table 7.
Mapping of frequencies to the Fourier-Bessel coefficients.

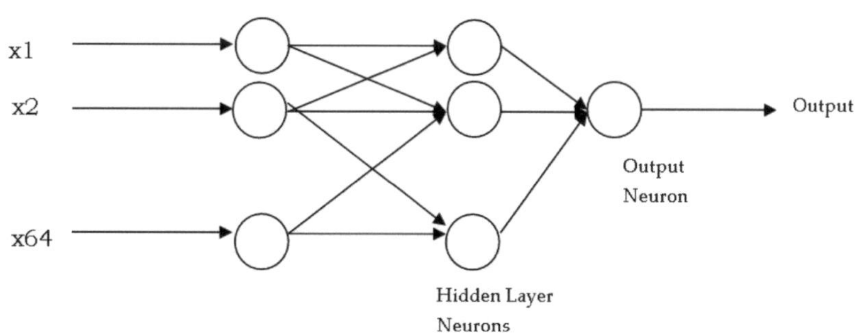

Figure 10.
The neural network architecture used above contains three layers: 64 neuron input layer, 1 neuron output layer and a hidden layer in the middle which also has 64 neurons.

File Name	File Start Time	File End Time	Number of Seizures	Seizure start seconds	Seizure End seconds
chb01_01	11:42:54	12:42:54	0	—	—
chb01_03	13:43:04	14:43:04	1	2996	3036
chb01_15	01:44:44	2:44:44	1	1732	1772

Table 8.
Seizure information of Subject-1 with timing in seconds.

TP	FN	Sensitivity	TN	FP	Specificity	TCA
149	01	99.33	150	0	100%	99.6%

Table 9.
Sensitivity, specificity and classification accuracy.

File Name	Number of Seizures	Seizure Start(seconds)	Seizure End(seconds)
chb24_13	1	3288	3304
chb24_14	1	1939	1966
chb24_15	1	3552	3569

Table 10.
Seizure information of Subject-2 with timing in seconds.

TP	FN	SE	TN	FP	SP	TCA
150	0	100%	150	0	100%	100%

Table 11.
Sensitivity, specificity and classification accuracy.

proposed method is superior and the seizure is predicted before 5 minutes for subject 1 (**Table 9**).

The inter-ictal and pre ictal data is prepared as per the information in **Table 10**. The trained network is simulated with inter-ictal and pre-ictal data. There were zero epochs as false negative and zero epochs as false positives.

The simulation results of 150 epochs of inter-ictal and 150 epochs of pre-ictal data have been tabulated as above in **Table 11**.

The number of false negative and false positive values was minimum due to the fact that the testing was done for shorter periods.

From **Table 11** it is observed that for shorter periods under consideration seizure is predicted before 5 minutes for subject 2 with 100% accuracy.

5. Epileptic seizure prediction based on localization

The selection of data was done a bit different from the previous works. Care has been taken to reduce the effects of post seizure by taking a minimum gap of 2 hours in the inter-ictal period.

Using the EEG data as compiled from above, IMF's are extracted using the EMD technique. Using these IMF's, features such as Kurtosis, Inter-quartile range and Median Absolute Deviation are extracted. The following **Figure 11** shows the steps involved in the study for prediction. The extracted features are used for training the Neural network and the results are tabulated.

For patient 8, source has been localized as discussed in the topic of source localization. It has been observed that 4 channels 6,8,20 and 21 have been the most significant channels. These channels are decomposed into 4 IMF's out of which 3 significant features are extracted thus a total of 4x4x3 = 48 features are extracted.

600 preictal and interictal epochs of 2 second duration are considered respectively, which means 1200 epochs (600 + 600 = 1200) with 48 features add up to a total input vector of 1200x48 to the neural network. This is tabulated as shown below in **Table 12**.

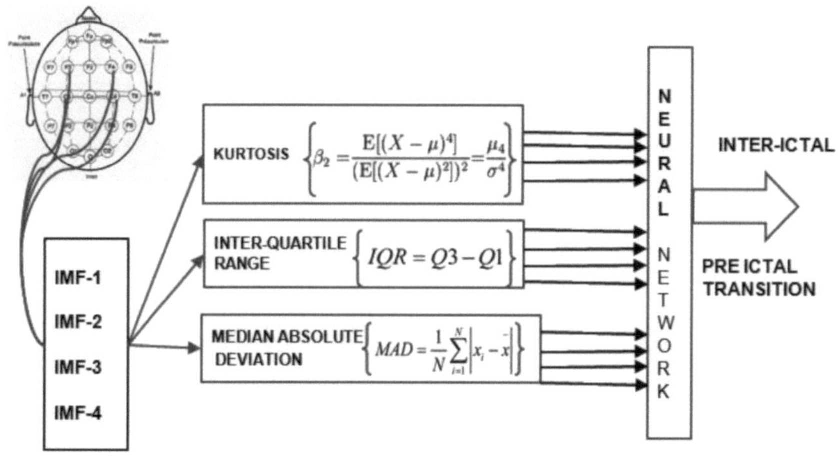

Figure 11.
Steps involved in epileptic seizure prediction using epileptic zone. It is divided into three parts. 1) the first part extracted the IMF's while in the second part 2) features are extracted from these IMF's. These features are given as 3) input to the neural network in the third part.

FEATURE	VECTOR LENGTH
CHANNELS	4 (6,8,20 and 21)
INTRINSIC MODE FUNCTIONS	4 levels
FEATURES	3 (MAD, IQR, Kurtosis)
TOTAL FEATURE VECTOR	4 X 4 X 3 = 48
PRE-ICTAL EPOCHS [2 SECOND]	600
INTER-ICTAL EPOCHS [2 SECOND]	600
TOTAL INPUT VECTOR TO NN	(1200) X 48

Table 12.
An overview of the input vector to neural network.

The following results were obtained in this method (**Table 13**):

The concept is extended to all the patients whose source has been localized as shown in below **Table 14**.

The prediction method is run on the entire channels localized from the source as derived from **Table 14**. The results are as shown in the **Table 13**. The above results are obtained for data of short intervals (**Table 15**). A testing has been run for continues data whose results are as shown in the figures below.

When a seizure free data is considered, there is a chance for false alarm. Consider the **Figure 12** where the result of testing of continuous seizure free data is shown.

	True Positive (TN)	False Negative (FP)	Sensitivity (%)	True Negative (TN)	False Positive (FP)	Specificity (%)	Over all accuracy
[5 Min]	289	11	96.33	290	10	96.67	96.5
[10 Min]	300	—	100	295	5	98.33	99.16

Table 13.
Sensitivity, specificity and classification accuracy using epileptic zone for prediction.

Patient	Channels
1	1, 5, 9, 13, 14, 15 and 21
2	1,12,15 and 9
3	1,4,6,8,14,20 and 21
5	2,3,9,15,19 and 23
8	6,8,20 and 21
24	5,6,20 and 21

Table 14.
Source localization results.

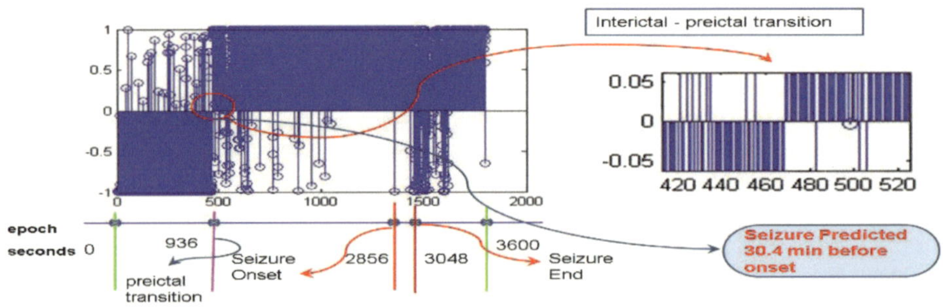

Figure 12.
The testing for continuous seizure data where seizure is predicted 30.4 min before onset.

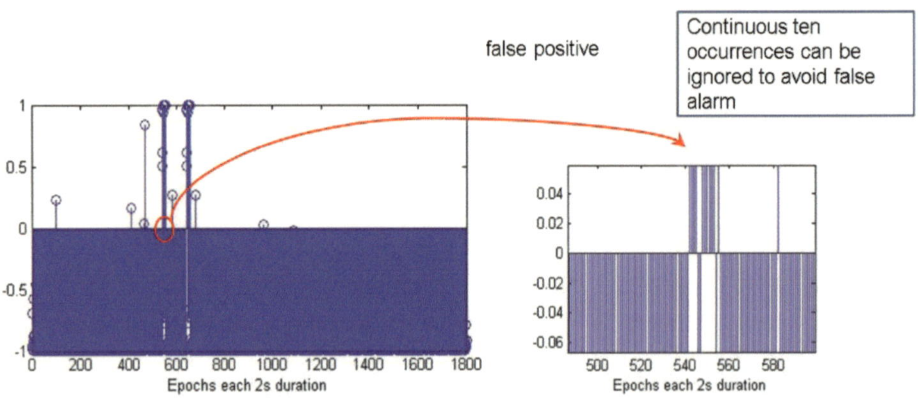

Figure 13.
A continuous seizure free data is used for testing. Since it is seizure free no transition should occur. There can be some spikes observed from the above zoomed in figure.

This false positive problem in seizure free data cannot be taken as a chance for seizure. Thus a false alarm avoidance methodology should be used (**Figures 13** and **14**).

A continuous occurrence of around 10 can be ignored so that no false alarm is triggered. In the above **Figures 9** and **10** continuous occurrences happen. Thus, it can be ignored.

6. Generalization of prediction

A new method is proposed for generalization of prediction. There are a few limitations using generalization of epileptic seizure prediction. One of the limitations is the variation issue. Focal seizures are particular to the part of the brain.

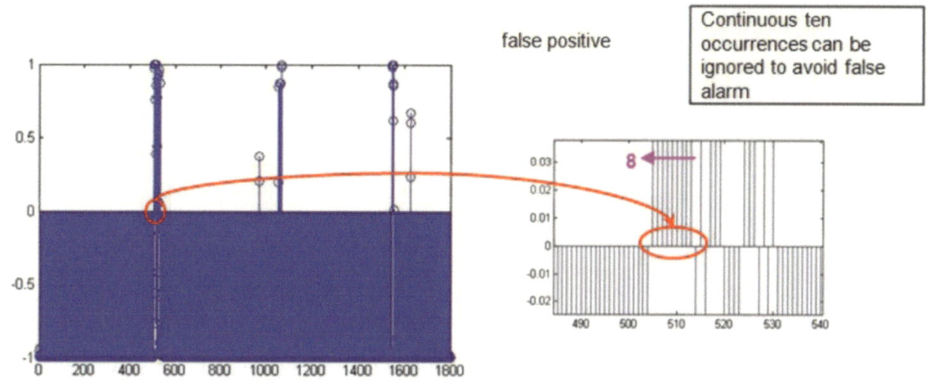

Figure 14.
Continuous seizure data with false positive values.

	True Positive (TP)	False Negative (FN)	Sensitivity (%)	True Negative (TN)	False Positive (FP)	Specificity (%)	Over all accuracy
[chb01]	290	10	96.66	277	33	89	92.8
Chb02	282	18	94	290	10	96.66	95.3
Chb03	284	16	9x.66	288	12	96	95.3
Chb05	270	30	90	264	36	88	89
Chb24	288	12	96	286	14	95.33	95.6

Table 15.
Sensitivity, specificity and classification accuracy using epileptic zone for prediction for all patients from source localization in ***Table 14****.*

Subjects	Sensitivity (%)	Specificity (%)	Over all accuracy (%)
Multiple(6)	81.7	76.2	79.75

Table 16.
Sensitivity, specificity and over all accuracy obtained for generalization of prediction.

Generalization of seizure prediction is possible with the help of epileptic source localized perfectly with clinical support using PET, FMRI, etc. For this work, the results of source localization are used. **Table 14** shows the results obtained from source localization. The data of these six patients are considered and a generalization is applied by averaging of the each level. The results obtained are as tabulated above in **Table 16**.

From the above table it can be noticed that the sensitivity obtained by generalization is 81.7%, while the specificity is 76.2%. The overall prediction accuracy stands at 79.75%.

7. Summary of the conclusions

EMD proves to be a good technique for seizure prediction. The main distinguishing attribute of this work is that it has been able to forecast the seizure about 30 minutes in advance. This might be a result obtained due to the preictal

S No	Author	year	Data Base	Algorithm	Prediction Time	Specificity	Sensitivity	Accuracy
1	Haddad, T [5]	2014	EEG	graph theory	30 min	—	—	72%
2	Nai-Fu Chang [6]	2012	CHB-MIT	wavelet coherence	—			70%
3	Christopher J. James [7]	2009	—	ICA, Phase Synchronization	35 min	65–80%	65–100%	—
4	Maryann D'Alessandro [8]	2003	EEG	intelligent genetic search process		90.47%	62.5%	
5	Leon D. Iasemidis [9]	2003	EEG	Lyapunov exponents	71.7 min			
6	Piotr Mirowski [10]	2009	EEG	cross correlation			71%	
7	Chisci [11]	2010	Freiburg ECOG	SVM classifier based on the Kalman filter,	—	100%	100%	—
8	Dorai, Arvind [12]	2010	EEG	Lyapunov exponents	65 seconds			8x.17%
9	Yang Zheng [13]	2014	EEG	bivariate empirical mode decomposition	—	—		
10	Peyvand Ghaderyan [14]	2014	Freiburg EEG	KNN-SVM	—	86.1%	91.11%	—
11	present work	2013	CHB-MIT	Lyapunov exponents	2 min	99%	100%	99.37%
12	present work	2013	CHB-MIT	Wavelets	5 min	100%	91%	88.71%
13	present work	2014	CHB-MIT	Fourier Bessel	5 min	100%	99.33%	99.6%
14	present work	2014	CHB-MIT	Localization-EMD-ANN	5 min	96.67%	96.33%	96.5%
15	present work	2014	CHB-MIT	Localization-EMD-ANN	10 min/30 min	98.33%	100%	99.16%

Table 17.
Comparison of prediction results.

period being much longer and the effects being nullified. The other existing prediction works were capable of only a few minutes. This gives the work much weight in the field of medicine as an alarm can be raised much well in advance and the life of a patient can be saved by alerting either the doctors or the patient himself to take necessary precautions. The concept of generalization can be improved with the help of other existing source localization techniques which make use of PET, FMRI, etc.

8. Comparisons of prediction results

The existing works for prediction using Lyapunov exponents as seen in S.no "5" had a prediction time of 71.7 minutes. The present work done using Lyapunov exponents was able to achieve a staggering result of 2 minutes prediction time with 99% specificity, 100% sensitivity and an overall classification accuracy of 99.97%.

S.no "2" had got a classification accuracy of 70% using wavelet coherence. The present work achieved a classification accuracy of 88.71% with 100% specificity and 91% sensitivity. The present works using Fourier Bessel as well as the EMD techniques have got good results

The above table is an indicator that progressive improvement has taken place in both the prediction time and prediction accuracy after the employment of localization and selecting only certain electrodes of interest (**Table 17**). Most of the previous literature is incomplete and this work aimed to bridge the gap. There has been significant success achieved in this segment.

Author details

Shaik Jakeer Hussain[1]* and Gurajapu Raja Sumant[2]

1 Vignan's Foundation for Science, Technology and Research (Deemed to be University), Guntur, India

2 Muffakham Jah College of Engineering and Technology (MJCET), Hyderabad, India

*Address all correspondence to: jk.shaik@gmail.com

References

[1] Shaik.Jakeer Hussain, "Epileptic Seizure Preidction using Cross Wavelets,Laypunove Exponents and Neural Networks", NCICN 2013

[2] Shaik.Jakeer Hussain and K.S.Rao, "A Neural Network Model for Predicting Epileptic Seizures based on Fourier-Bessel Functions", International Journal of Signal Processing, Image Processing and Pattern Recognition. Vol.7, No.5 (2014), pp.299–308.

[3] Shaik.Jakeer Hussain, "Epileptic Seizure Prediction Using Wavelet Transforms and Neural Networks", PGP-ACM, NCIC, 2013, pp 14–18.

[4] Shaik.Jakeer Hussain and K.S.Rao, "An Artificial Neural Network Model for Classification of Epileptic Using Huang-Hilbert Tranform", International Journal on Soft Computing (IJSC), ISSN: 2229–6735 (Online); 2229–7103

[5] Haddad, Tahar, Larbi Talbi, Ahmed Lakhssassi, Ben-Hamida Naim, and Sadok Aouini. "Epilepsy seizure prediction using graph theory." New Circuits and Systems Conference (NEWCAS), IEEE, 2014, pp. 293-296.

[6] Chiang, Cheng-Yi, Nai-Fu Chang, Tung-Chien Chen, Hong-Hui Chen, and Liang-Gee Chen. "Seizure prediction based on classification of EEG synchronization patterns with on-line retraining and post-processing scheme." Engineering in Medicine and Biology Society, EMBC, Annual International Conference of the IEEE, 2011, pp. 7564-7569.

[7] James, Christopher J., and Disha Gupta. "Seizure prediction for epilepsy using a multi-stage phase synchrony based system." Engineering in Medicine and Biology Society, EMBC, Annual International Conference, IEEE, 2009, pp. 25-28.

[8] D'Alessandro, Maryann, Rosana Esteller, George Vachtsevanos, Arthur Hinson, Javier Echauz, and Brian Litt. "Epileptic seizure prediction using hybrid feature selection over multiple intracranial EEG electrode contacts: a report of four patients." Biomedical Engineering, IEEE Transactions, 50(5), 2003, pp. 603-615.

[9] Iasemidis, Leon D. "Epileptic seizure prediction and control." Biomedical Engineering, IEEE Transactions, 50(5), 2003, pp. 549-558.

[10] Mirowski, Piotr, Deepak Madhavan, Yann LeCun, and Ruben Kuzniecky. "Classification of patterns of EEG synchronization for seizure prediction." Clinical neurophysiology, 120(11), 2009, pp. 1927-1940.

[11] Chisci, Luigi, Antonio Mavino, Guido Perferi, Marco Sciandrone, Carmelo Anile, Gabriella Colicchio and Filomena Fuggetta. "Real-time epileptic seizure prediction using AR models and support vector machines." Biomedical Engineering, IEEE Transactions, 57(5), 2010, pp. 1124-1132.

[12] Dorai, Arvind, and Kumaraswamy Ponnambalam. "Automated epileptic seizure onset detection." Autonomous and Intelligent Systems (AIS), International Conference, IEEE, 2010, pp. 1-4.

[13] Zheng, Yang, Gang Wang, Kuo Li, Gang Bao, and Jue Wang. "Epileptic seizure prediction using phase synchronization based on bivariate empirical mode decomposition." Clinical Neurophysiology, 125(6), 2014, pp. 1104-1111.

[14] Ghaderyan, Peyvand, Ataollah Abbasi, and Mohammad Hossein Sedaaghi. "An efficient seizure prediction method using KNN-based undersampling and linear frequency measures." Journal of neuroscience methods, 2014.

Chapter 10

The Dynamic of EEG Characteristics in Epileptic Children during the Treatment with Valproic Acid

Irma Khachidze

Abstract

Anticonvulsant drug (AED) treatment in epileptic children should be optimized through the anticipation of AED effectiveness at the beginning of the treatment. Researchers thought that the complex EEG analysis should identify the AED treatment's output in children with epilepsy. The research purpose is to study the different EEG pattern bases on AED treatment. A total of 43 patients with ages of 3–9 years were studied. Three EEGs' registration took place: before valproic acid-depakin (Dep) treatment, second (3 months), and third (6 months) after treatment. The background EEG pattern was investigated as a quantitative [absolute power spectra (APs)] and brain mapping. In addition, epileptiform EEG and the clinical characteristics of patients were evaluated. Valproic acid reduces Aps in high-amplitude slow waves and spontaneous epileptic patterns decrease and spike-wave complex (3/s) reduces; spikes-polyspikes, sharp waves, and generalized paroxysms during functional tests decreased. The rhythmic monomorphic theta waves (RMT) of tempo-parietal region were studied using brain mapping. The RMT correlated with the recurrence of seizures if Dep was withdrawn. The AED treatment effectiveness had been shown by decreases of slow waves and suppression of epileptiform EEG pattern and clinical improvement. The effective AED therapy should consider the analysis of the base EEG pattern, power spectra, and EEG mapping.

Keywords: EEG pattern, epileptic children, therapy

1. Introduction

Depakin is an anticonvulsant drug (AED) [1, 2] according to the International League Against Epilepsy (ILAE) recommendations [3, 4]. Depakin increases the GABA-ergic inhibition in the neuronal networks of the CNS [5]. VPA derivative depakine (Dep) [6] exerts a combined influence on the brain's neurons. It increases the GABA content through GABA transfers inhibition, reducing the reuptake of GABA in the brain tissue and activating the GABA receptors. [5].

The EEG study during Dep treatment depends on the form of epilepsy [7]. EEG investigation in pediatric population during Dep treatment should be considered as a better approach [8–10] as brain malination is not completed [11–13].

Moreover, nowadays no data base analysis is done to study the correlation between EEG and AED treatment [14]. Another problem is that there are more data on the EEG morphology compared to the quantitative EEG analysis [15–18].

A quantitative analysis of the EEG should reflect the effectiveness of the AED treatment since the EEG disorders are connected with clinical exacerbation [14, 19–21]. Thus, this work's purpose is to investigate the alteration of EEG in epileptic children during AED treatment.

2. Materials and methods

2.1 Epileptic children

Forty-three patients with ages of 3–9 years and with different forms of epilepsy were recruited. Three EEGs' registration took place: before treatment, second (3 months), and third (6 months) after treatment with valproic acid-depakin (Dep), 30–50 mg/kg treatment. They appealed at the Center of Experimental Biomedicene.

The diagnosis was done based on the International Classification of Epilepsy and Syndromes [4], clinical history, and neurological and MRI investigations. Classification of patients by seizure types and epileptic syndromes accurately identified the patients at risk for Dep-exacerbated epilepsy [22, 23]. Study involved both EEG and clinical analyses. Patients were characterized for the Dep dose, type and frequency of seizures, and EEG and Dep plasma levels [24, 25], both before and during the treatment. Out of 45 patients who received treatment, three of them developed undesirable effects. Although the physician adjusted the Dep dose, it did not improve the clinical outcome in two patients. Thus, these patients were excluded from the study. In summary, the present study included only 43 children of 3–9 years of age (**Table 1**).

The EEG investigation followed international performance standards [26] as part of the prescribed therapy plan. This plan was also approved by the parents and institutional ethics committee.

2.2 The EEG recording and methods of analysis

All patients underwent EEG recording three times: once—before administration of Dep (first visit) and twice—during Dep treatment, (i) 3–4 months later (the second visit) and (ii) 6–8 months later (the third visit).

The EEG registration was done with closed and open eyes. Functional test was performed with rhythmic photostimulation; hyperventilation and registration were ended with closed eyes. The duration of registration was 35–55 min.

The EEG signals were digitally recorded using a set of 19 scalp electrodes according to the International 10–20 system [26] and ENCEPHALAN 131–03, professional version "MEDICOM."

For an individual patient, a 10 s, artifact-free EEG pattern was analyzed.

A qualitative assessment of the EEG characteristics was performed in accordance of the age standards [27].

A quantitative EEG pattern of signal processing and the power spectrum was obtained for each lead. The spectral analysis was used to calculate the absolute value [28] of power (AVP, μV^2s) within six frequency bands: delta (0.5–4.0 Hz), theta-1 (4.0–6.0 Hz), theta-2 (6.0–8.0 Hz), alpha (8–13 Hz), beta-1 (13–24 Hz), and beta-2 (24–50.8 Hz) (**Figure 1**).

Number of patients	43 (26 male, 17 female)
Age (year)	
Mean ± SD	5.3 ± 1.23
Range	2.11–8.10
Onset of epilepsy	
Age (year)	4.3 ± 1.1
Range	2.00–5.37
Interval from the first to second seizures	
<1 week	3
1 week–1 month	14
1 month–1 year	21
>1 year	3
Unknown	2
Seizure types	
GS	
ABS	14
TN	5
CL	7
TN-CL	8
PS	
SPS	2
CPS	3
PSG	4
Etiology	
Post-traumatic	2
Perinatal	18
Neonatal	5
Febrile	8
Unknown	10
EEG findings	
Generalize	20
ABS	13
Focal (sharp waves, spikes, SW, etc.)	5
PSG	5

GS: generalize seizure; ABS: absence; SPS: simple partial seizure; CPS: complex partial Seizure; and PSG: partial, sometimes with secondarily generalization.

Table 1.
Characteristic of patients.

Alpha, beta, delta, and theta frequency bands were characterized by the wave amplitude, stability, and domination area.

Brain topography was conducted for the quantitative study.

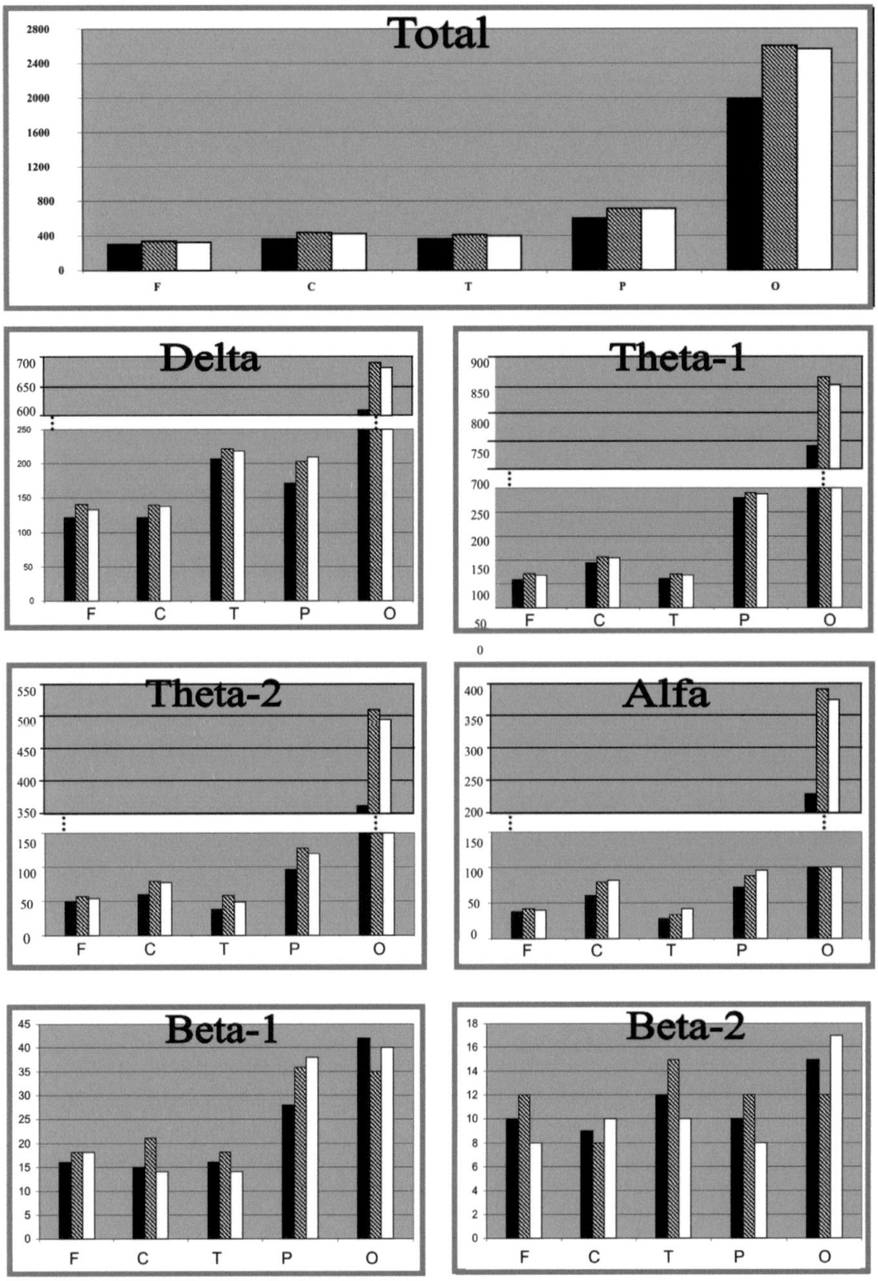

Figure 1.
Dynamics of absolute values of power spectra (AVP) at different stages of treatment. Summarizes results obtained from the quantitative analysis of the EEG dynamics, total of AVP (TAVP), and below the AVP of different frequency bands. X-line: F-frontal, C-central, T-temporal, O-occipital, and P-parietal regions of the brain cortex. Black columns—before treatment, shaded columns—3 months, and white columns—6 months after the initiation of Dep treatment. Y-line: power value—μV^2s.

2.3 Statistical analysis

Statistical significance for each endpoint measures was assessed using Mann–Whitney U-test (BIOSTAT). The data obtained before treatment served as a baseline for assessing the dynamics of EEG characteristics during treatment. Thus, each subject served as its own control in the evaluation of EEG during treatment.

The changes in the EEG characteristics were assessed using Wilcoxon signed-ranks test [29]. The significance was set at $p < 0.05$.

3. Results

EEG before administration of Dep can be described as the deceleration of the background EEG due to augmentation of the high-amplitude poly- and monomorphic waves within the low-frequency range. Quantitative spectral analysis (brain mapping) of interictal EEG revealed that, in the total EEG spectrum, the most dominant are the oscillations of 3–8 Hz with a prevalent amplitude of 60–120 μv.

Dep reduced the amplitude in the low-frequency range ($p < 0.05$).

3.1 Qualitative EEG study

The qualitative analysis revealed that the Dep therapy reduced the number of spontaneous paroxysmal discharge (by 76%) in the resting EEG and suppressed primarily the typical epileptiform complexes of spike-waves (SW) (3/s) (absence) [30, 31].

3.2 Quantitative EEG study

The quantitative analysis showed reduction of frequency ($p < 0.05$).

The Aps dynamics revealed the reduction of the incidence of low-frequency waves ($p < 0.05$), especially this effect was more prominent for the theta range.

Following the initial reduction of APs' alpha activity, especially in the occipital region ($p < 0.05$), this index did not show any further decline ($p < 0.05$).

Dep treatment produced a decreased brain activity within the range of beta ($p < 0.05$) [32].

The presence of a rhythmic monomorphic mid-/high-amplitude theta waves despite clinical improvements (seizure-free and no epileptiform EEG correlates) can provoke seizures after the Dep withdrawal. Seizures recurred due to not only Dep withdrawal but also due to dose reduction in patients. This aggravation of epilepsy was found in 64% of patients [33–35]. The rhythmic monomorphic mid-/high-amplitude theta waves can be observed using brain mapping and power spectra. Such a pattern is not visible in the visual EEG observation.

Dep therapy did not show a EEG clinical aggravation that was diagnosed with the criteria of Genton and McMenamin [33].

Dep treatment decreased the number of seizures. The clinical signs and EEG pattern are described in **Table 2**.

Clinical follow-up	EEG				
	Complete normalization EEG	Improve EEG	No EEG change	EEG worse	Total
Clinical improvement number (%)	33 (80%)	8 (18%)	1 (2%)		42
No clinical change number (%)			1 (2%)		1
Clinical aggravation number (%)					
Total number (%)	33 (80%)	8 (18%)	2 (3%)		43

Table 2.
Clinical outcome and EEG record in 46 patients.

4. Discussion

Antiepileptic therapy in children can be optimized via the anticipation of the efficacy of AED during the early stages of therapy. Since EEG provides rich information about the brain activity, we hypothesized that the comprehensive EEG evaluation during Dep therapy in the children with epilepsy can be a sensitive indicator of the efficacy of the treatment.

Dep therapy induced decreases of APs of low-frequency waves, which is an indicator of reducing of CNS excitation. Dep reduces beta bends in the posterior lobes, which is related with the CNS dysfunction [32].

Dep reduces spike-waves (3/s), which is related to the absence of epilepsy that is triggered from the thalamocortical pathway. Dep was considered as an effective drug in such cases [31, 36, 37].

Dep does not have an effect on irregular single spike-wave complexes, sharp waves, spikes-polyspikes, and paroxysmal bursts provoked by functional trials. These cases reflect certain specificity of epileptogenesis [7, 38]. Dep differently acts on the generation of epileptiform elements with various morphologies—particularly, it suppresses SW complexes (3/s) but does not have a good effect on irregular single spike-wave complexes, sharp waves, and spikes. Such a picture allows us to suggest the differences in the morphology of epileptiform elements that may reflect different neurophysiological and neurochemical mechanisms [3, 7, 39]. Revealing of selectivity represents certain theoretical and practical interests as it can serve as an indirect evi dence of assumptions in the genesis of various epileptiform EEG elements and accordingly different types of epileptic attacks [39, 40]. Other researchers like Truccolo et al. [41] apparently pay attention to the morphological pictures of background EEG [13].

VPA was shown different activity and is not effective of any type of epilepsy [38]. The possibility of Dep treatment of non-epileptic paroxysmal conditions in children and adolescents [42–45] and the investigation of children with partial epilepsy during carbamazepine (CBZ) treatment were described in our previous investigation [46].

Brain mapping revealed the essential prognostic value of morphology of the theta waves and its distribution upon the cortical surface. The EEG pattern was revealed before treatment initiation and was persistent during Dep therapy. The presence of rhythmic monomorphic mid-/high-amplitude theta waves on the EEG, especially of the temporoparietal regions, despite clinical improvements (seizure-free and no epileptiform EEG correlates) may suggest the possible recurrence of seizures after withdrawal of Dep. Not only withdrawal but even reduction of doses can lead to a recommencement of the attacks in this group of patients. Such a feature of VPA suggests that its antiepileptic effect is achieved via neurophysiological and molecular mechanisms, which partly differ from the action mechanisms of other AEDs [33, 34]. Analysis of basic characteristics of EEG during the treatment suggests that the rhythmic monomorphic mid-/high-amplitude theta waves are predicting signs of aggravation. Such an EEG pattern is revealed based on the evaluation of background EEG characteristics, spectral analysis, and EEG mapping using a quantitative EEG approach.

AED treatment should be done under a regular EEG control due to aggravation of the EEG pattern, which sometimes predicts the clinical signs of exacerbation [47, 48].

Reduction of slow wave concomitant with decreases of epileptiform pattern and clinical signs at 3 months after DEP treatment suggests that the treatment is effective in these cases [49].

5. Conclusions

The EEG study suggests that the presence of rhythmic monomorphic theta waves with the tempo-parietal region should anticipate the recurrence of epilepsy in children with epilepsy, if the Dep dose would be reduced or if the Dep therapy would be withdrawn. The efficacy of Dep treatment should be correlated with decreases of high amplitude, low frequency, and suppression of epileptiform EEG parallel to the clinical improvement. Thus, optimal therapy suggests of evaluation of baseline EEG, power spectra, and brain topography mapping using EEG methods.

Acknowledgements

The authors have no conflict of interest to declare.

Author details

Irma Khachidze[1,2]

1 Department of Behavior, Cognitive Functions and Human Psychophysiology, I. Beritashvili Center of Experimental Biomedicine, Tbilisi, Georgia

2 SEU University, Tbilisi, Georgia

*Address all correspondence to: irmakha@yahoo.com

References

[1] Goodridge PMG, Shorvon SD. Epileptic seizures in a population of 6000. II: Treatment and prognosis. British Medical Journal. 1983;**1**:645-647

[2] Hart YM, Sander JWAS, Johnson AL, Shorvon SD. National general practice study of epilepsy: Recurrence after a first seizure. Lancet. 1990;**1**:1271-1274

[3] Glauser T, Ben-Menachem E, Bourgeois B, Cnaan A, Chadwick D, Guerreiro C, et al. ILAE treatment guidelines: Evidence-based analysis of antiepileptic drug efficacy and effectiveness as initial monotherapy for epileptic seizures and syndromes. Epilepsia. 2006;**47**:1094-1120

[4] Comission on Classification and Terminology of the International League against Epilepsy. Proposal for revised classification of the epilepsies and epileptic syndromes. Epilepsia. 1989;**30**(3):389-399

[5] Dichter MA, Brodie MJ. Antiepileptic Drugs. The New England Journal of Medicine. 1996;**334**(24):1583-1590

[6] Zenkov LR. Anticonvulsive pharmacotherapy may aggravate epilepsy course. Zhurnal Nevrologii i Psikhiatrii Imeni S.S. Korsakova. 2005;**105**(10):52-54

[7] Stefan H, Fraunberger B. Valproate sustained release in the treatment of epilepsy. Fortschritte der Neurologie-Psychiatrie. 2005;**73**:681-686

[8] Besser R, Hornung K, Theisohn M, Rothacher G, Kramer G. EEG changes in patients during the introduction of carbamazepine. Electroencephalography and Clinical Neurophysiology. 1992;**83**:19-23

[9] Miyauchi T, Endo K, Yamaguchi T, Hagimoto H. Computerized analysis of EEG background activity in epileptic patients. Epilepsia. 1991;**32**:870-881

[10] Kalviainen R, Aikia M, Partanen J, Sivenius J, Mumford J, Saksa M, et al. Randomized controlled pilot study of vigabatrin versus carbamazepine monotherapy in newly diagnosed patients with epilepsy: An interim report. Journal of Child Neurology. 1991;**6**(Suppl 2): 60-69

[11] Fonseca LC, Tedrus GM, Chiodi MG, Cerqueira JN, Duran MH. Quantitative electroencephalography in children with benign childhood epilepsy with centrotemporal spikes: Analysis of band power. Arquivos de Neuro-Psiquiatria. 2004;**62**:455-458

[12] Camfield P, Gordon K, Camfield C, Tibbles J, Dooley J, Smith B. EEG results are rarely the same if repeated within six months in childhood epilepsy. The Canadian Journal of Neurological Sciences. 1995;**22**:297-300

[13] Konishi T, Naganuma Y, Hongou K, Murakami M, Yamatani M, Okada T. Effects of antiepileptic drugs on EEG background activity in children with epilepsy: Initial phase of therapy. Clinical Electroencephalography. 1995;**26**:113-119

[14] Perucca E, Gram L, Avanzini G, Dulac O. Antiepileptic drugs as a cause of worsening seizures. Epilepsia. 1998;**39**(1):5-17

[15] Clemens B, Menes A, Piros P, Bessenyei M, Altmann A, Jerney J, et al. Quantitative EEG effects of carbamazepine, oxcarbazepine, valproate, lamotrigine, and possible clinical relevance of the findings. Epilepsy Research. 2006;**70**:190-199

[16] Salinsky MC, Oken BS, Storzbach D, Dodrill CB. Assessment of CNS effects of antiepileptic drugs by using quantitative EEG measures. Epilepsia. 2003;**44**:1042-1050

[17] Neufeld MY, Kogan E, Chistik V, Korczyn AD. Comparison of the effects of vigabatrin, lamotrigine, and topiramate on quantitative EEGs in patients with epilepsy. Clinical Neuropharmacology. 1999;**22**:80-86

[18] Specchio LM, Beghi E. Should antiepileptic drugs be withdrawn in seizure-free patients? CNS Drugs. 2004;**18**(4):201-212

[19] Schmidt D, Löscher W. Uncontrolled epilepsy following discontinuation of antiepileptic drug in seizure free patients: A review of current clinical experience. Acta Neurologica Scandinavica. 2005;**111**:291-300

[20] Salinsky MC, Oken BS, Morehead L. Intraindividual analysis of antiepileptic drug effects on EEG background rhythms. Electroencephalography and Clinical Neurophysiology. 1994;**90**:186-193

[21] Herkes GK, Lagerlund TD, Sharbrough FW, Eadie MJ. Effects of antiepileptic drug treatment on the background frequency of EEGs in epileptic patients. Journal of Clinical Neurophysiology. 1993;**10**:210-216

[22] Trimble MR, Thompson PJ. Sodium valproate and cognitive function. Epilepsia. 1984;**25**:604

[23] Dreifuss FE, Langer DH, Moline KA, Maxwell JE. Valproic acid hepatic fatalities. III: US experience since 1984. Neurology. 1989;**39**:201-207

[24] Schneble H, König SA, Elger CE, Bergmann A. Recommendations for blood studies and clinical monitoring in early detection of valproate-associated liver failure. Klinik für Epileptologie, Universität Bonn Blutalkohol. 1993;**30**(1):1-20

[25] Marvin M. Goldenberg. Overview of drugs used for epilepsy and seizures. Etiology, Diagnosis, and Treatment Pharmacy and Therapeutics. 2010;**35**(7)

[26] American EEG Society. Guidelines in EEG. Journal of Clinical Neurophysiology. 1994;**11**:1-143

[27] Benninger C, Matthis P, Scheffner D. EEG development of healthy boys and girls. Results of a longitudinal study. Electroencephalography and Clinical Neurophysiology. 1984;**57**:1-12

[28] Harmony T, Hinojosa G, Marosi E, Becker J, Rodriguez M, Reyes A, et al. Correlation between EEG spectral parameters and educational evaluation. The International Journal of Neuroscience. 1990;**54**:147-155

[29] Wilcoxon F. Individual comparisons by ranking methods. Biometrics Bulletin. 1945;**1**:80-83

[30] Manning JP, Richards DA, Bowery NG. Pharmacology of absence epilepsy. Trends in Pharmacological Sciences. 2003;**24**:542-549

[31] Panayiotopoulos CP. Absence epilepsies. In: Engel JJ, Pedley TA, editors. Epilepsy: A Comprehensive Textbook. Philadelphia: Lippincott-Raven Publishers; 1997. pp. 2327-2346

[32] Niedermeyer E, da Silva FL. Electroencephalography: Basic Principles, Clinical Applications, and Related Fields. Philadelphia: Lippincott Williams & Wilkins; 2005. pp. 684-687

[33] Genton P, McMenamin J. Aggravation of seizure by antiepileptic drugs: What to do in clinical practice. Epilepsia. 1998;**39**:26-29

[34] Wu X, Xiao CH. Quantitative pharmaco-EEG of carbamazepine in volunteers and epileptics. Clinical Electroencephalography. 1996;**27**:40-45

[35] Salinsky MC, Binder LM, Oken BS, Storzbach D, Aron CR, Dodrill CB. Effects of gabapentin and carbamazepine on the EEG and cognition in healthy volunteers. Epilepsia. 2002;5(43):482-490

[36] Holmes MD, Brown M, Tucker DM. Are "generalized" seizures truly generalized? Evidence of localized mesial frontal and frontopolar discharges in absence. Epilepsia. 2004;**45**:1568-1579

[37] Sarkis RA, Loddenkemper T, Burgess RC, Wyllie E. Childhood absence epilepsy in patients with benign focal epileptiform discharges. Pediatric Neurology. 2009;**41**:428-434

[38] Stefan H, Lopes da Silva FH, Löscher W, Schmidt D, Perucca E, Brodie MJ, et al. Epileptogenesis and rational therapeutic strategies. Acta Neurologica Scandinavica. 2006;**113**:139

[39] Meeren HK, Pijn JP, Van Luijtelaar EL, Coenen AM, de Silva L. Cortical focus drives widespread cortithalamic networks during spontaneus absanse seizures in rats. The Journal of Neuroscience. 2002;**22**:1480-1495

[40] Pinault D. Cellular interactions in rat somatosensory thalamocortical system during normal and epileptic 5-9 Hz oscillation. The Journal of Physiology. 2003;**552**:881-905

[41] Truccolo W, Donoghue JA, Hochberg LR, Eskandar EN, Madsen JR, Anderson WS, et al. Single-neuron dynamics in human focal epilepsy. Nature Neuroscience. 2011;**14**:635-641

[42] Geladze N, Maloletnev V, Natriashvili G, Khachidze I, Kharatishvili I. Use of computer EEG for the assessment of the threshold of seizure readiness of the brain in epileptic children during interictal period: Collection of scientific works. Tbilisi State Medical University. 2003;**39**:469-471

[43] Clemens B, Piros P, Bessenyei M, Hollody K. Lamotrigine decreases EEG synchronization in a use-dependent manner in patients with idiopathic generalized epilepsy. Clinical Neurophysiology. 2007;**1**(118):910-917

[44] Geladze N, Maloletnev V, Khachidze I, Gugushvili M. The possibility of using of depakine in the management of non-epileptic paroxysmal conditions in children and adolescents. Proceedings of the Georgian Academy of Sciences. 2007;**N6**(33):341-347

[45] Khachidze I, Maloletnev V, Guguhvili M. Alteration of EEG characteristics in epileptic patients during the treatment with antiepileptic drugs. Journal of European College of Neuropsychopharmacology. 2008;**18**:557

[46] Khachidze I, Gugushvili M, Maloletnev V. Analysis of EEG dynamics in epileptic children during carbamazepine therapy. Asian Biomedicine. 2010;**4**(1):37-49

[47] Hedstrom A, Olsson I. Epidemiology of absence epilepsy: EEG findings and their predictive value. Pediatric Neurology. 1991;**7**:100-104

[48] Massa R, de Saint-Martin A, Carcangiu R, Rudolf G, Seegmuller C, Kleitz G, et al. EEG criteria predictive of complicated evolution in idiopathic rolandic epilepsy. Neurology. 2001;**57**:1071-1079

[49] Berg AT, Berkovic SF, Brodie MJ, Buchhalter J, Cross JH, van Emde Boas W. Revised terminology and concepts for organization of seizures and epilepsies: Report of the ILAE commission on classification and terminology, 2005-2009. Epilepsia. 2010;**51**:676-685

Section 4

Pharmacological, Surgical and Experimental Therapies for Epilepsy

Chapter 11

Cognitive and Psychological Side Effects of Antiepileptic Drugs

Katja Eva Brückner

Abstract

Among well-known side effects such as dizziness, nausea, headache and diplopia medical treatment of epilepsy may cause side effects on cognition, mood and behavior. In special constellations this can profoundly affect compliance with the medication as well as quality of life. Some patients are more vulnerable to side effects than others. Side effects can have profound impact on the development and future life of a patient. Some antiepileptic drugs (e.g. topiramate, zonisamide) show a more severe side effect profile than others (e.g. lamotrigine, levetiracetam). Thus, in the treatment of epilepsy, it is crucial to consider such possible side effects – especially in the beginning of or while changing the medical treatment. Specific neuropsychological examinations can monitor side effects on cognitive functions like concentration, memory or speech function. If this is not possible in an ambulant setting, specific screening instruments and repeated and precise interviews of patients and/or relatives can help to discover potential side effects. Because most side effects can be reversible, dosage modification or drug replacement is required as soon as incompatibilities are discovered.

Keywords: epilepsy, antiepileptic drugs, cognitive side effects, psychological side effects

1. Introduction

As one of the most common chronic neurological disorders, epilepsy affects many people across all population groups and ages. A prevalence rate of 0.5–1% of the population has been assumed [1]. More recent studies on large cohorts report even significantly higher rates: there is evidence of a prevalence rate of 1.2% of active epilepsy in the population [2]. Active epilepsy means that people diagnosed with "epilepsy" have had a seizure within the last 12 months, have seen a doctor because of their epilepsy, and/or have been treated with anticonvulsant medication. Before starting therapy, it must be clarified whether epilepsy is actually present. 20–30% of all patients with non-epileptic seizures are incorrectly diagnosed with epilepsy [3]. Therefore, differential diagnoses - such as psychogenic non-epileptic seizures, cardiovascular fainting, sleep behavior disorders, paroxysmal movement disorders or metabolic diseases have to be excluded. A differentiation from non-disease-relevant, paroxysmally occurring phenomena that do not require therapy (e.g. sleep myoclonus) is necessary before initiating therapy.

After a precise diagnosis, clarification of possible differential diagnoses and a positive therapy decision, drug treatment is usually the first choice in the treatment of epilepsy. Drug therapy is never curative, because the selected medication only

IntechOpen

prevents or reduces seizures in the sense of symptom prophylaxis. The underlying cause of epilepsy is not cured with drug treatment. Most patients with epilepsy can be easily being treated with medication and, depending on the epilepsy syndrome, become seizure-free with monotherapy or combination therapy [4]. Meanwhile, many agents with different mechanisms have been approved for the treatment of epilepsy. In addition to the desired effect - successful seizure control or a significant reduction of seizure frequency - as with all medications, there are also undesirable effects with anticonvulsants that are only tolerable to a certain extent and then only with a significant improvement in the seizure situation. The tolerable extent of these interference effects differs individually and depends on the individual situation. In addition to "classic" physical disturbances such as dizziness, nausea, headache and double vision, negative effects on cognitive performance and mental health are the least tolerated effects. Since drug therapy ideally leads to seizure freedom but does not cure epilepsy, in most cases drug treatment is a long-term therapy.

2. Medical treatment

There is a large number of anticonvulsants for drug therapy of epilepsy, although those of more recent and of latest generations are not inferior to those of the older generation in their anticonvulsant effects. Therefore, a choice must be made on the basis of possible interference and interaction profiles and taking into account the individual situation of each patient.

Special attention in the treatment decision requires certain patient groups such as women of childbearing age because certain anticonvulsants have increased teratogenicity. For example, Valproic acid should be avoided due to an increased risk of malformation and an unfavorable effect on the later intellectual development of the unborn child, especially in higher doses during pregnancy. However, other patient groups also need specific consideration: Patients with intellectual disabilities may experience an increase in their existing limitations due to paradoxical disturbances or drug-related negative effects on cognitive performance. Older patients are particularly susceptible to drug interferences due to various co–/multi-morbidities, various concomitant medications and the resulting interactions that may not always be foreseeable, as well as pharmacodynamics that change due to age.

3. Cognitive side effects of antiepileptic drugs

At the onset of epilepsy and prior to treatment cognitive impairment can be already observed in a large number of patients. Frequently detectable deficits can be found early in the course of the disease in attention, memory and executive functions [5].

Basically, all anticonvulsants can have a negative impact on cognitive performance. If any cognitive deficits before treatment existed, these deficits may be exacerbated. The most common negative effect of anticonvulsants is a decrease in information processing speed, reaction speed and concentration. Most treatment related cognitive disorders are reversible and fade after dose reduction or completely disappear after a change in substance. Only visual field defects with vigabatrine are irreversible, which is why this substance has been used only in individual cases and under strict ophthalmological control.

Among the anticonvulsants of the older generation valproic acid, carbamazepine and phenytoin have the most favorable cognitive side effect profile with comparatively little effects on concentration, memory, information processing speed or word fluency. The newer generation of anticonvulsants with a rather minor influence on cognitive performance are lamotrigine, levetiracetam, gabapentin, perampanel, lacosamide, oxcarbazepine, eslicarbazepine and pregabalin [6, 7]. For lamotrigine and lacosamide - in individual cases also for oxcarbazepine and perampanel - improvements in cognitive partial performance (e.g. information processing speed, concentration, vigilance) have been described [8–11]. In Contrast, topiramate and zonisamide are anticonvulsants with a relatively unfavorable cognitive disturbance profile. However, bromine, phenobarbital and primidone can also be associated with cognitive disturbances (e.g. cognitive slowing), whereby these substances are rarely used in everyday clinical practice. In combination therapies, a frequently condition in refractory epilepsy, undesirable interference effects can accumulate.

Topiramate relatively often and sometimes very impressively leads to deterioration in language skills such as verbal fluency and word finding, to a slowdown in the speed of reaction and to decline in working memory. In general, these interference effects occur even at relatively low doses and also if the dosage is very slow. In addition, there does not seem to be a habituation effect, so that the disturbance effects persist even with long-term therapy. Patients with intelligence impairment react to topiramate with the same cognitive disturbances as intellectually unaffected patients: Slow reactions, reduced language skills and reduced working memory can be found [12]. Even if these patients already have cognitive impairments, an additional drug-related deterioration should not be neglected, as this can have a fundamental impact on everyday competence and independence.

The following case study is intended to illustrate the possible scope of these cognitive effects caused by topiramate: A 20-year-old man introduced himself to the epilepsy centre. He developed epilepsy when he was 14 years old. At that time he attended the 8th grade of a secondary modern school (in German: Realschule). His former neuropediatric put him on topiramate, which he had tolerated subjectively well to this day (a current daily dose at admission 400 mg). He did not remember negative cognitive effects during school and did not complain about it when he was admitted. Soon after onset of epilepsy, the patient switched from secondary modern school to secondary school (in German: Hauptschule –a school with a lower level of graduation). In the end, he left school without graduating and subsequently found no apprenticeship training position, so at the time of admission to the epilepsy centre, he has been working in a supermarket as a temporary helper. While treatment optimization he was given an alternative anticonvulsant. Before changing his mediaction, he underwent neuropsycholgical examination (**Figure 1**).

With a dosage of 400 mg topiramate, the patient displayed significant performance deficits in speech fluency, working memory and reaction speed were striking. These cognitive functions are associated with a successful performance in school: Linguistic skills are required to express yourself concretely and correctly in class and exams, to understand learning content and tasks and to apply or implement them. Working memory functions include the short-term holding and simultaneous manipulation of information – fundamental achievements to understand spoken language. If these skills are impaired or even slowed down, a student will not be able to adequately follow the lessons, which can lead to an overall failure in school. Though epilepsy can be accompanied with cognitive impairments or even global impairments of intelligence regardless of the medication, it is likely that a slight intellectual disability has caused the failed educational/professional career of our patient. After several months he came back to the epilepsy centre for further medication changes. At this point topiramate was completely discontinued.

The patient did not report any cognitive changes. However, he has started to catch up on the secondary school graduation. He even planned the next higher school graduation as well, to start apprenticeship as a car mechanic. We examined our patient again (**Figure 2**).

In contrast to the first neuropsychological examination, cognitive performances that have previously been below range (verbal fluency, reaction speed and working memory), were now within normal range. So, there were significant improvements in cognitive performance after stopping topiramate, which suggests that the deficits

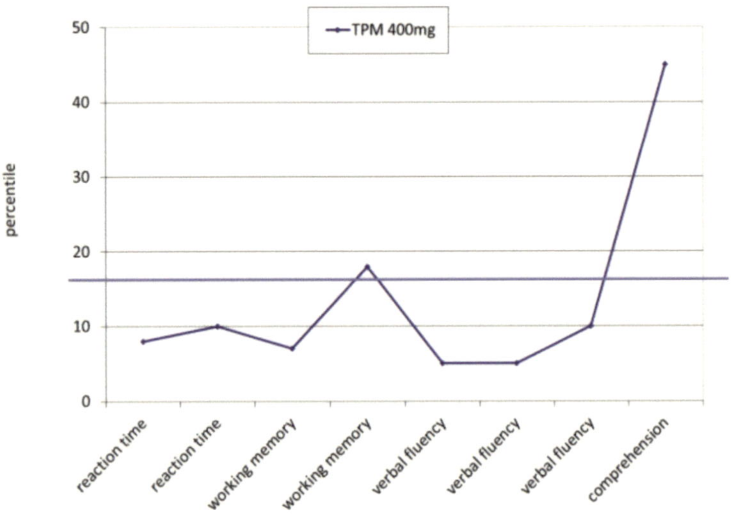

Figure 1.
Note: Percentile rank 16 = lower average limit compared to a healthy control group; reaction time = tasks on reaction speed, comprehension = task to understand language, TPM = topiramate; with 400 mg TPM, the patient's performance in almost all of the cognitive areas examined is below average compared to a healthy control group.

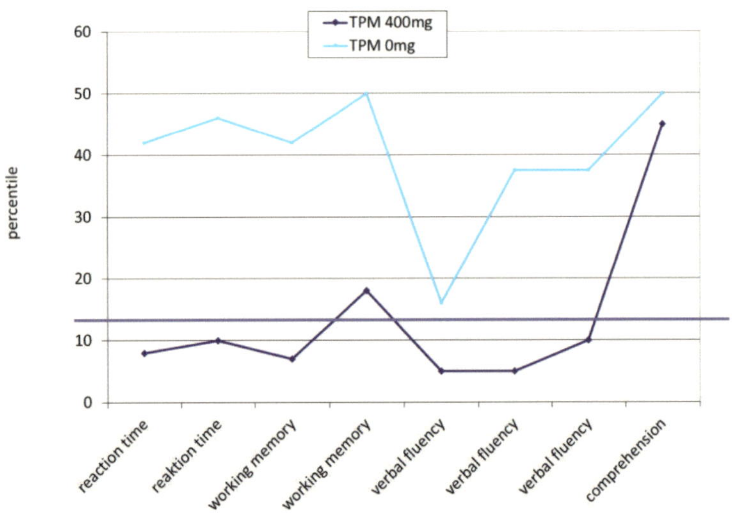

Figure 2.
Note: Percentile rank 16 = lower average limit compared to a healthy control group; reaction time = tasks on reaction speed, comprehension = task to understand language, TPM = topiramate; after discontinuing TPM (0 mg), all examined cognitive areas showed normal findings and thus shows a clear improvement compared to the previous examination (400 mg TPM).

found earlier (and thus probably also the failure in school) are related to the drug topiramate. Based on this case study, the possibly life-long social consequences due to the decision in favor of a certain drug at a certain point in patient patient's life, is very impressive.

Zonisamide - similar to topiramate - can lead to cognitive disturbances with memory disorders, cognitive slowdown and word finding disorders [13]. In contrast to topiramate, a dose effect can be observed here (the higher the dose, the more serious the impairment). It is supposed that the negative interference effects fade, but this is not reported in all studies [14], so that under certain circumstances a therapy attempt could be considered despite the initial interference effects (e.g. if other anticonvulsants have not led to the desired therapeutic success despite increasing them to the limit of interference).

Benzodiazepines (clobazam, clonazepam, diazepam, lorazepam) are a group of anticonvulsant drugs with well-known and sometimes clear cognitive side effects (sedation, fatigue, concentration disorders). Apart from this, additional problems such as development of tolerance and the risk of addiction rule out these drugs for long-term therapy in epilepsy treatment. Apart from individual cases, they are used only as a bridge drug in medication changes and as an emergency medicine with one-time dose.

4. Cognitive side effects in children

Most studies examining unwanted interference effects mainly focus on adults. For the treatment of children there are often no separate data available. Transferring the study results just to children and adolescents is not advisable. Naturally, a child's brain can, on the one hand, be restricted in its function by anticonvulsants, analogous to an adult brain. However, what is more is that unwanted interference effects can also adversely affect the further cognitive development. Disruptions in cognitive performances (e.g. working memory performance) can prevent or hinder the acquisition of new abilities and skills and may slow down the entire development. Especially child epilepsy syndromes can be associated with severe intellectual disabilities and developmental delays. Additional negative interference effects of the medication are detrimental, so that the child may not be able to exploit its entire and eventually already reduced development potential.

Not all available anticonvulsants are approved for the treatment of epilepsy in children Compared to adults, children are more sensitive to the undesirable effects of drugs. Lamotrigine, levetiracetam, rufinamide, and gabapentin appear to have a rather minor effect on cognitive performance - Lamotrigine is said to even improve concentration disorders in children [8, 15]. Topiramate and zonisamide, however, can also have a negative effect on cognitive performance in children. Both substances lead to the cognitive interference effects in children that have been observed in adults as well: word-finding disorders, cognitive slowdown, memory and working memory disorders [12]. In contrast to adults deteriorations in information processing speed, linguistic abilities, verbal learning and memory processes have also been described for valproic acid, oxcarbazepine and carbamazepine in children [16].

In contrast to adults, the drug-related cognitive deterioration is more serious in children, as further development and potential development in childhood and adolescence can be negatively influenced. Since school performance in particular plays an immense role in setting the course for later professional and social careers, the relevance of drug-related cognitive disruptive effects in childhood needs to be emphasized again, as the case study from the beginning illustrates very vividly.

As mentioned earlier, there is a connection between valproic acid during pregnancy and the intellectual abilities of the unborn child [17]. Compared to children who were exposed to carbamazepine during pregnancy, children after exposure to valproic acid (especially in higher doses) achieve an IQ value up to 10 points lower in the 6th year of life [18, 19]. Therefore this must be assessed as an irreversible, undesirable cognitive interference effect of valproic acid, even if this does not have a direct effect on the performance of the patient being treated, but rather on the unborn child who is been treated to. Since an association was also found between valproic acid during pregnancy and a later autism disorder in the child [20], therapy with valproic acid for women of childbearing age should be avoided.

5. Control of possible cognitive side effects

As the case study shows, the patient - and also the clinicians - are not always aware of the cognitive interference effects of anticonvulsants. In order to control possible influences on cognitive performance, it is therefore advisable - at least for certain substances (topiramate, zonisamide), to record the performance in a standardized manner before starting therapy, after reaching the target dose and if the patient reports any of new subjective cognitive complaints that occur during adjustment respectively. In specialized centres, this is carried out by experienced neuropsychologists as part of neuropsychological follow-up examinations with change-sensitive test procedures. In the outpatient neurological setting, however, a neuropsychological examination accompanying the drug setting is often not possible. Therefore, it is important to monitor potential changes by a detailed and repeated questioning of the patients or their caregivers about tolerability, including specific questions about possible changes/failures in school or work since the medication changeover, as well as test instruments specially designed for this question, such as EpiTrack and EpiTrack Junior (only available in German [21, 22]). Many different neuropsychological tests are available to control cognitive functions. The following cognitive performances should always be recorded: Attention (especially information processing speed), executive functions, language functions (especially verbal fluidity) and working memory. When selecting tests, care should be taken to ensure that the tests can be used repeatedly (e.g. parallel versions). In addition, possible mood changes should always be recorded.

In summary, because of their low negative impact on cognitive performance, certain anticonvulsants (e.g. lamotrigine, levetiracetam) are superior to others (topiramate, zonisamide, valproic acid). A monotherapy is always preferable to a combination therapy and a low dose to a high one, since most of the undesirable interfering effects described are both dose-dependent (lower dose - fewer or less interfering effects) and can tend to accumulate in combination therapies. In some cases, negative interfering effects can be counteracted by slowly increasing the medication (start low – go slow). However, this does not apply to all substances (see topiramate). In the case of drugs known to have undesirable cognitive interferences, the start of therapy should, if possible, be accompanied by neuropsychological follow-up examinations.

The best possible seizure control or seizure reduction is necessary for both the quality of life and the general performance of a patient. Therefore, substances with cognitive interference effects may sometimes be preferable to others (e.g. when other substances are not effective). In these cases, an individual assessment of the cost–benefit profile is necessary.

6. Psychological side effects of anticonvulsant medication

Like people with other chronic diseases, patients with epilepsy suffer significantly more often from psychological comorbidities such as depression or anxiety than healthy people. Treatment-refractory epilepsy and epilepsy with a seizure origin in temporal structures are affected with particular frequency [23]. Psychological complaints represent a significant impairment of the quality of life for those affected and require both precise diagnostics and consistent therapy. Treatment with mood-stabilizing, antidepressant drugs and accompanying psychological psychotherapy should therefore be considered for these patients. Concerns about possible proconvulsive effects of antidepressants are usually unfounded (with a single exception: amitriptyline) and should not prevent therapy.

However, before starting antidepressant therapy, it must be clarified whether the psychological complaints of the patient are possibly an undesirable interference of the anticonvulsant medication: Substances like topiramate, zonisamide, levetiracetam, and perampanel can have a negative impact on mood [13, 24]. Depressive and psychotic symptoms as well as increased aggressiveness were observed with topiramate. With levetiracetam, depressive symptoms can occur in individual cases as an undesirable drug interference effect as well. Much more common with this substance, however, are increased irritability and aggressiveness, which can unsettle both patients and relatives and in some cases lead to serious problems in the social environment. A dose reduction or a switch to another medication is advisable in both cases. For example, brivaracetam, which has been available since the beginning of 2016, promises to have a lower impact on psychological well-being with a similar mechanism of treatment [25–27].

With regard to psychological comorbidities, lamotrigine should be emphasized as an anticonvulsant with a probably additional antidepressant effect. Lamotrigine is therefore particularly recommended for patients with depression. However, lamotrigine can lead to unwanted sleep disorders, especially in the initial phase. This can be countered either by reducing the dose and then increasing it more slowly or by redistributing the individual doses during the day (higher dose in the morning, lower dose in the evening). In addition to lamotrigine, pregabalin also has a beneficial effect on psychological comorbidities, especially anxiety and sleep disorders. Topiramate, which is used in lower doses also for migraine prophylaxis and addiction therapy [28], can be used in patients with additional migraines - taking into account the above-mentioned factors relating to cognitive performance.

7. Psychological side effects in children

There is evidence that both topiramate and levetiracetam can lead to undesirable mood changes, particularly depression, irritability, personality changes, and hyperactivity in some children. Phenobarbital and primidone can lead to behavioral problems in children as well. Lamotrigine, on the other hand, has a mood-enhancing effect in children like in adults [29], and in children also has a positive effect on aggressiveness and impulsiveness [15]. Rufinamide appears to be unproblematic with regard to undesirable psychological disturbances [30].

In children and adolescents with intellectual disabilities, an increase in behavioral problems has occasionally been described with lamotrigine. Here, however, this might be due to the "lack of" sedation under lamotrigine compared to other anticonvulsants and the possible associated improved vigilance. If the medication switch to lamotrigine leads to behavioral problems, this might not be related to the medication but to the possibly underlying disease and then of course it requires another handling than that of a re-sedation.

In summary, it is advisable to check a possible relationship between a newly dosed anticonvulsant and the psychological complaints of a patient and then to counteract this by switching to an alternative medication. Since correlations between emotional side effects of anticonvulsants, a rapid dose escalation, an already existing mental illness and a family predisposition for mental illness were found, it is advisable to consider these aspects in drug selection [31].

8. Control of possible psychological side effects

To control possible psychological side effects, questionnaires can be used in addition to exploration and behavioral observation. The Beck Depression Inventory (BDI-II), Beck Anxiety Inventory (BAI) and the Hospital Anxiety and Depression Scale (HADS) are well-known and well established methods [32–34]. The Neurological Disorders Depression Inventory for Epilepsy (NDDI-E) was developed specifically for people with epilepsy to detect depressive symptoms [35]. For children, the Child Behavior Checklist (CBCL-4-18) is recommended [36].

9. Alternatives to drug therapy

Due to the diverse side effects of anticonvulsants, alternative treatment methods (e.g. epilepsy surgery) should be considered early if therapy refractivity is determined. Therapy-refractory epilepsy is present if two suitable anticonvulsants dosed up to the interference limit in monotherapy and a combination therapy has not led to seizure freedom. For a clearly defined group of patients, epilepsy surgery is a safe, well-established and very promising treatment option: For example, in the case of unifocal temporal lobe epilepsy due to proven hippocampal sclerosis, the chance of postoperative freedom from seizures is up to 80%. In comparison, the chances of success of a further drug change for these patients are significantly lower.

10. Conclusion for practice

Since drug-based epilepsy therapy is mostly a long-term – sometimes a lifelong – therapy, it is of particular importance to take undesirable interfering effects into account. In addition to the frequency of seizures, cognitive and psychological side effects are particularly serious for the quality of life of patients. Therefore, when treating epilepsy with drugs, the focus should not only be on the desired effects on the frequency and severity of seizures, but also on possible undesirable effects on cognitive performance and mental health. Both the individual living conditions of the individual patient (e.g. possible later desire for children, upcoming training/studies) as well as possible comorbidities (e.g. previous psychological comorbidity, intellectual impairment, cognitive partial performance disorders) must be taken into account when selecting drug therapy. Especially in children, patients with intellectual disabilities and elderly patients (due to the increased vulnerability to undesirable disturbances), it is recommended to start with a low dose and slowly increase the dose ("start low, go slow"). For certain substances, the monitoring of cognitive functions and mood before and during the change/adjustment is necessary, e.g. based on neuropsychological follow-up examinations, special screening procedures and a detailed and specific questioning of the patient and the caregivers (**Table 1**).

Abbreviations/anticonvulsants		**Possible cognitive side effects**	**Possible emotional side effects**
BR	Bromine	—	o
BRV	Brivaracetam	o	o
CBZ	Carbamazepine	(– In children)	+
CLB	Clobazam	—	Drug addiction problem
CLZ	Clonazepam	—	Drug addiction problem
DZP	Diazepam	—	Drug addiction problem
ESL	Eslicarbazepine	o	o
GBP	Gabapentine	o	(– In children)
LCM	Lacosamide	+	o
LEV	Levetiracetam	o	—
LTG	Lamotrigine	+	+
LZP	Lorazepam	—	Drug addiction problem
OXC	Oxcarbazepine	(+),(– In children)	o
PER	Perampanel	(+)	—
PB	Phenobarbital	—	(– In children)
PHT	Phenytoine	—	o
PGB	Pregabalin	—	+
PRM	Primidon	—	(– In children)
RFM	Rufinamide	o	o
TPM	Topiramate	—	—
VGB	Vigabatrin	Irreversible visual field defects	
VPA	Valproic acid	(– In children, – in the unborn child)	+
ZNS	Zonisamide	—	(–)

Legend: – negative interfering effect, + positive effect, o no known interfering effect.

Table 1.
Overview of possible cognitive and psychological side effects of anticonvulsants.

Author details

Katja Eva Brückner
Epilepsiezentrum Hamburg, Ev. Krankenhaus Alsterdorf, Hamburg, Germany

*Address all correspondence to: k.brueckner@eka.alsterdorf.de

References

[1] Hamer H, Lang J, Richter S, et al. Gesundheitsökonomie und Lebensqualität bei Epilepsie. Zeitschrift für Epileptologie. 2015;**28**:153

[2] Zack MM, Kobau R. National and state estimates of the numbers of adults and children with active epilepsy — United States, 2015. MMWR. Morbidity and Mortality Weekly Report 2017; 66:821-825. DOI: http://dx.doi.org/10.15585/mmwr.mm6631a1.

[3] Gates JR. Nonepileptic seizures: Classification, coexistence with epilepsy, diagnosis, therapeutic approaches, and consensus. Epilepsy & Behavior. 2002;**3**:28-33

[4] Shorvon SD, Goodridge DMG. Longitudinal cohort studies of the prognosis of epilepsy: Contribution of the National General Practice Study of epilepsy and other studies. Brain. 2013;**136**(11):3497-3510 https://doi.org/10.1093/brain/awt223

[5] Witt JA, Helmstaedter C. Should cognition be screened in new-onset epilepsies? A study in 247 untreated patients. Journal of Neurology. 2012;**259**:1727-1731

[6] Meador KJ, GEvins A, Loring DW, McEvoy LK, Ray PG, Smith ME, et al. Neuropsychologicalandneurophysiologic effects fo carbamazepine and levetiracetam. Neurology. 2007;**69**:2076-2084

[7] Meador KJ, Yang H, Pina-Garza JE, Laurenza A, Kumar D, Wesnes KA. Cognitive effects of adjunctive perampanel for partial-onset seizures: A randomized trial. Epilepsia. 2016;**57**(2):243-251. DOI: 10.1111/epi.13279

[8] Pressler RM, Binnie CD, Coleshill SG, Chorley GA, Robinson RO. Effekt of lamotrigine on cognition in children with epilepsy. Neurology. 2006;**8**(1):1495-1499

[9] Helmstaedter C, Witt JA. The longer-term cognitive effects of adjunctive antiepileptic treatment with lacosamide in comparison with lamotrigine and topiramate in a naturalistic outpatient setting. Epilepsy & Behavior. 2013;**26**:182-187

[10] IJff DM, van Veenendaal TM, Majoie HJM, de Louw AJA, Jansen JFA, Aldenkamp AP. Cognitive effects of lacosamide as adjunctive therapy in refractory epilepsy. Acta Neurologica Scandinavica. 2015;**131**:347-354

[11] Dirani M, Nasreddine W, Abdulla F, Beydoun A. Seizure control and improvement of neurological dysfunction in Lafora disease with perampanel. Epilepsy Behav Case Rep. 2014;**2**:164-166

[12] Brandt C, Lahr D, May TW. Cognitive adverse events of topiramate in patients with epilepsy and intellectual disability. Epilepsy & Behavior. 2015;**45**:261-264

[13] White JR, Walczak TS, Marino SE, Beniak TE, Leppik IE, Birnbaum AK. Zonisamide discontinuation due to psychiatric and cognitive adverse events: Acase-control study. Neurology. 2010;**75**(6):513-518

[14] Park SP, Kim SY, Hwang YH, Lee HW, Suh CK, Kwon SH. Long-term efficacy and safety of zonisamide monotherapy in epilepsy patients. Journal of Clinical Neurology. 2007;**3**:175-180

[15] Moavero R, Santarone ME, Galasso C, Curatolo P. Cognitive and behavioral effects of new antiepileptic drugs in pediatric epilepsy. Brain & Development. 2017 Jun;**39**(6):464-469.

DOI: 10.1016/j.braindev.2017.01.006 Epub 2017 Feb 13

[16] Fastenau PS, Johnson CS, Perkins SM, Byars AW, deGrauw TJ, Austin JK, et al. Neuropsychological status at seizure onset in children: Risk factors for early cognitive deficits. Neurology. 2009;**73**:526-534

[17] Meador KJ, Baker GA, Browning N, Clayton-Smith J, Combs-Cantrell DT, Cohen M, et al. Cognitive function at 3 years of age after fetal exposure to antiepileptic drugs. New England Journal of Medicine. 2009;**360**(16):1597-1605

[18] Loring DW, Marino S, Meador KJ. Neuropsychological and behavioral effects of antiepileptic drugs. Neuropsychological Review. 2007;**17**(4):413-425

[19] Meador KJ, Baker GA, Browning N, et al. Fetal antiepileptic drug exposure and cognitive outcomes at age 6 years (NEAD study): A prospective observational study. The Lancet Neurology. 2013:244-252. DOI: 10.1016/S1474-4422(12)70323-X

[20] Christensen J, Grønborg TK, Sørensen MJ, et al. Prenatal Valproinsäuree exposure and risk of autism spectrum disorders and childhood autism. JAMA. 2013:1696-1703. DOI: 10.1001/jama.2013.2270

[21] Lutz MT, Helmstaedter C. EpiTrack: Tracking cognitive side effects of medication on attention and executive functions in patients with epilepsy. Epilepsy & Behavior. 2005:708-714. DOI: 10.1016/j.yebeh.2005.08.015

[22] Helmstaedter C, Schoof K, Rossmann T, Reuner G, Karlmeier A, Kurlemann G. Introduction and first validation of EpiTrack junior, a screening tool for the assessment of cognitive side effects of antiepileptic medication on attention and executive functions in children and adolescents with epilepsy. Epilepsy Behav. 2010 Sep;**19**(1):55-64. DOI: 10.1016/j.yebeh.2010.06.042 Epub 2010 Aug 17

[23] Helmstaedter C, Aldenkamp AP, Baker GA, Mazarati A, Ryvlinf P, Sankar R. Disentangling the relationship between epilepsy and its behavioral comorbidities— The need for prospective studies in new-onset epilepsies. Epilepsy & Behavior. 2014;**31**:43-47

[24] Fritz N, Glogau S, Hoffmann J, Rademacher M, Elger CE, Helmstaedter C. Efficacy and cognitive side effects of tiagabine and topiramate in patients with epilepsy. Epilepsy & Behavior. 2005;**6**(3):373-381

[25] Asadi-Pooya AA, Sperling MR, Chung S, et al. Efficacy and tolerability of adjunctive brivaracetam in patients with prior antiepileptic drug exposure: A post-hoc study. Epilepsy Research. 2017;**131**:70-75

[26] Zhang L, Li S, Li H Zou X. Levetiracetam vs. brivaracetam for adults with refractory focal seizures: A meta-analysis and indirect comparison. Seizure 2016 (39): 28-33. https://doi.org/10.1016/j.seizure.2016.05.004

[27] Yates SL, Fakhoury T, Liang W, Eckhardt K, Borghs S, D'Souza J. An open-label, prospective, exploratory study of patients with epilepsy switching from levetiracetam to brivaracetam. 2015 Epilepsy & Behavior; 52: 165-168. https://doi.org/10.1016/j.yebeh.2015.09.005

[28] Johnson AB, Ait-Daoud N, Bowden CL, DiClemente CC, Roache JD, Lawson K, et al. Oral topiramate for treatment of alcohol dependence: A randomised controlled trial. Lancet. 2003;**361**:1677-1685

[29] Lee GP. Medical Treatmant of epilepsy. In: Neuropsychology of

Epilepsy and Epilepsy Surgery. Oxford Workshop Series. Oxford: Oxford University Press; 2010. pp. 73-93

[30] Resnick T, Arzimanoglou A, Brown LW, Flamini R, Kerr M, Kluger G, et al. Rufinamide from clinical trials to clinical practice in the United States and Europe. Epileptic Disorders. 2011;**13**(Suppl.1):S27-S43

[31] Mula M, Trimble MR, Lhatoo SD, Sander JWAS. Topiramate and psychiatric adverse events in patients with epilepsy. Epilepsia. 2003;**44**(5):659-663

[32] Beck AT, Ward CH, Mendelson M, Mock J, Erbaugh J. An inventory for measuring depression. Archives of general psychiatry 1961; 4: 561--571

[33] Beck AT, Epstein N, Brown G, Steer RA. An inventory for measuring clinical anxiety: Psychometric properties. J Consul Clin Psychol. 1988;**56**:893-897. DOI: 10.1037/0022-006X.56.6.893

[34] Zigmond AS, Snaith RP. The hospital anxiety and depression scale. Acta Psychiatrica Scandinavica. 1983;**67**(6):361-370. DOI: 10.1111/j.1600-447.1983.tb09716.x

[35] Gilliam FG, Barry JJ, Hermann BP, Meador KJ, Vahle V, Kanner AM. Rapid detection of major depression in epilepsy: A multicentre study. Lancet Neurology. 2006;**5**:399-405

[36] Achenbach TM. Manual for the Child Behavior Checklist/4-18 and 1991 Profile. Burlington: Department of Psychiatry, University of Vermont; 1991

Chapter 12

Challenges Related to Epilepsy Management in Sudan, an Example of Low-Middle Income Country

Ismat Babiker, Awab Saad, Basil Ibrahim and Mohamed Abdelsadig

Abstract

Epilepsy is one of the most common neurological diseases that require long-term healthcare, although it has no racial, gender, or geographical boundaries, certain populations and demographics face different challenges regarding management of epilepsy. These challenges include patients' and communities' misconceptions of epilepsy nature, treatment and outcome, various use of traditional and spiritual therapy in management of epilepsy, stigma of epilepsy, shortage of neurology facilities and specialists and their aggregation in the capital, and collapse of the healthcare system in Sudan. This chapter aims to highlight some of the difficulties facing people with epilepsy in Sudan, an example of a low middle-income country.

Keywords: difficulties, seizures, developing countries, Africa, treatment

1. Introduction

Epilepsy is a global health challenge, one that is responsible for a social and economic burden worldwide, it is estimated to be twice as common in low-income countries than that in the high-income countries, especially in a poor country like Sudan, resulting in unfair treatment, prejudice and stigma [1], and overwhelming decrease in quality of life [2]. People with epilepsy (PWE) in Sudan suffer from a collapsing and deficient health care system, and a community falling behind and lacking enough understanding towards their affliction, with a cultural heritage and misconceptions, and an educational system contributing to make it only that much more difficult for (PWE) to live a normal life, sometimes weighing them down and preventing them from seeking professional medical help altogether. The resultant treatment gab causes a mortality rate dwarfing that of first world countries [3]. On top of that, Sudan is lacking sufficient research and infrastructure to develop satisfying estimates about the situation on the ground, and recent data are scarce [3].

1.1 Sudan: background and population

Sudan is the third largest country in Africa that occupies almost 728,000 square miles of northeast Africa. It sits along the sub-Saharan crossroads and along the cost of the red sea that runs through its east-northern borders. In addition to Egypt, Sudan shares borders with six other countries, which are Ethiopia, chad, Libya, Eritrea, Central African Republic, and lastly South Sudan that had its secession from Sudan by July 2011. Sudan is mainly formed of flat plains interspersed by mountain ranges, and due to its immense area, Sudan has different climates and several rivers coursing through the country, mainly the blue and white Niles that join together to form the river Nile in Khartoum the capital city of Sudan.

Although it's an enormously sized country, it is sparsely populated compared to some of the African countries as it has an estimated census of 43 million people, the majority of which are rural in comparison to the urban population that is mainly centered in the capital.

Sudan is vastly enriched with different races, cultures and a blend of Arabic tribes that form the majority of the population and various African tribes and ethnicities, this enrichment may be contributing to its ever astounding cultural diversities and perhaps the fuel to political differences and the rather devastating civil wars that have crushed the country for ages, viciously affecting Sudan in every aspect possible. Sudanese people are still facing major challenges in everyday aspect of life duet to this overwhelming political instability through its history.

1.2 Healthcare system in Sudan

As a low middle-income country, Sudan is confronted with many brutal challenges, especially in health sector. Some of the challenges encountered are the poor assessment and execution of policies, lack of firm health informatics system, inadequate financial spending, centralized medical services and facilities in Khartoum and urban cities, and insufficient training for postgraduate doctors. To add more to the burden on medical care is the deficiency of preventive medicine application, poor referral system, problematic diaspora of physicians, lack of communities' awareness leading to the fixed stigma and spiritual misconceptions of diseases that are causative of delayed medical seeking behaviors and use of folk medicine. These difficulties robustly affect the quality of health care and specifically the management of chronic diseases as epilepsy.

2. Neurology in Sudan

Neurology practice in Sudan is affected by the weakened health care system, Adult and child neurology is confronted by extreme challenges affecting people with neurological diseases. Up to the year 2005 there were only three practicing neurologists that were delivering medical care for an unconceivable ratio of one neurologist to 12 million people [4]. In addition to the enlarging population, this ratio could be attributed to lack of neurology training programs for postgraduate doctors which has begun in the past 10 years, in addition the shortage of neurology clinics in Sudan as today there are 3 tertiary neurology centers that provide adult neurology services, all of which are located in the capital which only aggravates the problem of the ability to seek neurology consultations and follow-ups especially for patients living outside Khartoum. Other major setbacks are the shortage of neuro-physiologists, neuro-imaging facilities and neuroradiologists and the desperate need for neurology nursing and rehabilitation centers.

3. Epilepsy misconceptions in Sudan

There is a lot of stigma and misconceptions that befall (PWE) in Sudan, where epilepsy is perceived as demonic possession, Satanic rituals, spells and witchcraft [3], some cultures have superstitions similar to that of Saudi tribes where they consider (PWE) as a presentiment of evil, a manifestation of envy and "Evil Eye" [5], while in some cultures (PWE) are considered a grace and bringers of god-bliss to their families [6]. However, others believe PWE are infectious, mentally ill, impotent and should neither get married nor have a job. Some people consider epilepsy an incurable disease, while others think the condition will pass on its' own so they completely dismiss the therapeutic process as a futile endeavor. Some religious followers would resort to special forms of prayer involving rigorous movements to help alleviate the condition. Such beliefs direct people toward seeking traditional methods and healers, who antagonize demons, introduce herbs, ointments, cautery and prayers as stand-alone treatment for epilepsy.

A cross sectional study done in Sudan to evaluate the impact of spiritual and traditional believes of care givers on the management of children with epilepsy, it established that 80% of them were educated, one third of study population attributed epilepsy to supernatural causes. More than two thirds acknowledged use of both traditional and spiritual medicine, more than half used different religious methods to treat epilepsy. Almost half of participants believed that religious and or traditional treatment were truly effective in the management of epilepsy, and one third used herbs in the treatment of epilepsy [7].

4. Scarce personnel and trained physicians

In Sudan the number of centers where appropriate investigation tools has increased in the recent years, more cities are constructing new centers for neurology (like Madani neurology center, Aljazeera State), but it's in no way comparable to the increase in patients and the services that need to be provided [8].

Despite the increase in number of medical faculties and doctors, the number of physicians with specialty training in neurology remains lacking. The overall condition of freedom and civil rights in the country along with the increased costs of living, which are all factors contributing to the mass immigration of doctors and other healthcare professionals to seek a respected income that enables them to live a decent life. It is worth mentioning that some doctors in Sudan live off salaries ranging anything from the equivalent of 15 to 300 dollars per month.

5. Anti-epileptic drugs (AEDs) in Sudan

Currently, there are more than 25 licensed AEDs in clinical practice in the developed world, compared to few registered AEDS in Sudan, most of which are old generation AEDs, although older generation medications are still effective even in comparison to newer generation AEDs, the newer generation have less side effects and are more tolerable [9]. Tolerability and adverse effects are a major influence on compliance, and discontinuation of therapy, therefore increasing morbidity and mortality in people with epilepsy.

The use of AEDs is influenced by the pre-existing belief system that pushes people towards traditional herbals and local healers [3], with some believing the medication is useless while others consider s it to be undermining of the more trusted traditional methods. However, among those who would have access to proper medical help, and those who appreciate the need for medication, other factors further affect the treatment gap and challenge adherence to medication. Patients who are seizure free for a long duration or those taking more than one medication may fail to adhere to therapy or omit doses.

Descriptive analysis of cost-benefit for some patients indicates that their concern about the high price of the medication greatly outweighs the need for the drug, and would as a result seek free samples provided by charity organizations, while some patients fail to obtain the drug [10]. Antiepileptic drugs represent a tremendous economic burden on families of patients with epilepsy. The yearly cost of AEDs alone falls not less than 276 US dollars per patient per year, while visitations and consultations along with investigation could reach 51 dollars. Other indirect costs can include travel, for those who live far from the capital, reaching up to 90 dollars. Insurance rarely helps and patients find themselves forced to sell valuable assets like one's cow or shop to cover the expenses, and many find themselves in debt. All of these factors need to be accounted for by the patient and caregivers and affect adherence negatively [11].

6. The collapse of the health care system

Access to AEDs like other medications in Sudan was subject to variations related to inflation and other complex geopolitical factors, resulting in fluctuating prices in the period from 2009 to 2013 (6 times change in pricing). And while the general market dynamics in the country were somewhat fluctuant, the general indicators of regional macroeconomics have been declining steadily (e.g. GDP in dollars) following factors like change in market policies, conflicts in the south leading to loss of big fractions of the country's' resources, up to the more recent financial crisis in the country in the period 2018-2020, where cash was virtually inaccessible to the public, making all medications into a luxury, and culminating in an event of pharmaceutical scarcity of drugs, despite the government's best efforts to mitigate the impact of the economic situation [12]. Some policies had a relatively positive effect, like price liberalization privatization of the sector. And while reports and studies are yet to fully estimate the on-going catastrophe, the global status of lock-down and quarantine due to the COVID-19 pandemic certainly made it more challenging to get access to medical care or self-management for (PWE) in such a collapsing healthcare system [13].

7. Stigma

Stigma is the social outspoken or perceived labeling of an individual or a group of people according to true or presumed different characteristics attributed to specific health related and non-health related conditions, rendering these individuals incapable of leading equal lives to their peers in society [14, 15].

Components of stigma include behavioral, emotional and cognitive elements that are portrayed in patients responses or attitudes and their interaction with society [16]. The burden of stigma unfolds in both active and passive manners, those who discriminate and those facing discrimination can inflict stigma after being subjected to it. This gives rise to the different entities of stigma and its effects on different life attributes of stigmatized individuals in society [15].

The manifestations and impact of stigma in the attitude form further branches it into perceived, anticipated, and internalized stigmas, while the social form of stigma includes the enacted or experienced stigma. Perceived stigma describes one's thoughts or self-image perceived through the eyes of those surrounding one's life regarding an acknowledged distinguishing characteristic [16]. Anticipated stigma refers to a presumed inappropriate response in the form of an act of discrimination or labeling in a social setting to one's condition by others. Internalized stigma denotes self-inflicted discrediting and undermining due to awareness and acknowledgment of one's difference. Experienced or felt stigma refers to consequences of an act of labeling or discrimination that was made intentionally to point out a stigmatizing characteristic [14, 16, 17].

7.1 Health related stigma

Stigma is a major social determinant of health, attributing to disease morbidity, mortality and to the successfulness of healthcare services [18].

Elements that articulate the complex process of health conditions related stigma include illness nature, it's course, and characteristics that represent origins of stigma; population related elements; treatment modalities and healthcare providers sought for consultation; reactions as well as coping mechanisms of stigmatized individuals to social acts of discrimination that may take a toll on their identity, social life, and economic thriving [17, 19, 20].

What is not so clearly defined however, is the relationship between stigma and healthcare outcomes, attributing to stigma being an entity that while having similar grounds in most health related conditions, its effects can be as illness specific as exclusive features of that illness, often referred to as the hidden burden of an illness, and this is an area that is deficient in research data [21, 22].

7.2 Manifestation of stigma in high income vs. low-income countries

Health related stigma, can be visualized more clearly in communities where compensation of one's health condition related disability is lacking. These compensations aim towards minimizing the gap between individuals with disabling health conditions and their peers in community. Communities where efforts to minimize this gap are lacking are mostly those of low-income economical index [20].

Stigma adversely affects individual health outcomes as well as related life chances, including educational opportunities, employment, housing, and social relationships. It has also been shown to negatively affect help- and treatment-seeking behaviors, compromising the ability to treat and prevent stigmatized health conditions. Masking of research on illness specific stigma under the generalization of its nature has limited the ability to understand the overall impact of stigma on individual wellbeing and the overall disease burden, restricting the ability to develop interventions addressing stigma, and this masking is amplified especially in low-income countries, because of the lacking resources available to healthcare research and services in general [20, 23].

Stigma affects caregivers of individuals being stigmatized, be it their families, relatives or close companions. Caregivers of patients in low-income countries suffer a heavier burden due to lacking national health agencies support, which widens the gap between illness-limited individuals and their peers in society, further enforcing stigma as well as worsening the financial burden. All these elements associated with stigma in low income countries develop a synergistic effect, in which each element contributes to the vicious cycle of further reducing the quality of life of stigmatized individuals [23].

7.3 Stigma of epilepsy in low-income countries

The weight and burden associated with epilepsy in terms of stigma manifests with variable intensities and forms across different age groups and communities [6, 24].

Developmental aspects of one's life including physical, mental and social development, and their bases of parenting by one's family, education and an uninterrupted social learning experience, are affected differently with various onset age groups of epilepsy. For example, having a child with epilepsy puts tremendous pressure on the family and caregivers, especially in a low-income country where taking care of an illness free child can be troublesome. This leads to stressful parenting, creating many obstacles for a child who has epilepsy to develop at a normal rate. A child with epilepsy has a higher chance of academic underachievement, which would setback building of self-esteem and eventually in conjunction with other epilepsy related elements leads to enforcement of stigma and further disability and unsuccessful treatment, in contrast to adolescence onset of epilepsy which would have a different impact on their quality of life and would manifest in different aspects like social withdrawal despite being in a functional social and economic status. Adulthood onset of epilepsy and the manifestation of stigma associated with it could be less severe than childhood and adolescence onset and would affect one's ability to be involved in certain elements of society, but could also be devastating in certain low-income regions with plummeting education and awareness levels, for example not being able to have a spouse in a low-income community where having epilepsy is thought to be of demonic possession [1, 6, 24].

7.4 Stigma and mismanagement of epilepsy in Sudan

Epilepsy in Sudan accounts for 1.6 annual mortality rates and 238.7 disability adjusted life years per 100,000. It is associated with notable stigma and social burdens. Patients with epilepsy suffer a tremendous burden of social discrimination adversely affecting their quality of life [6]. These patients are subject to being denied equal chances to a dignified life following neglect, isolation and lack of national healthcare support.

As studies in Sudan regarding epilepsy are primarily focused on clinical presentation of epilepsy, no in depth illustration or correlation between stigma of epilepsy and the outcome of epilepsy healthcare have been conducted.

However, some of the magnitude of epilepsy stigma in the Sudanese population has been captured across the different age groups of patients with epilepsy in urban and rural areas.

A study conducted by Taha et al. to identify epilepsy related stigma in the Sudanese community and to find correlation between penetrance of the type of stigma on patients through stigma degree scoring, have detected that approximately 16% of both men and women with epilepsy suffer from highly precipitated felt stigma. 12.5% of remaining patients of epilepsy who did not suffer from felt stigma have noted the common belief in their communities of the contagious nature of epilepsy while 56.2% declared their communities believed epilepsy was of demonic possession, 13% mentioned people were afraid from them when they were having seizures in public and hence they do not help them. The Sudanese community surrounding patients with epilepsy also showed poor respect to patients' privacy evident with 77.4% of patients stating that despite not disclosing their condition, it was publicly known. Where expected least, Sudanese communities showed an alarming response to children with epilepsy from their teachers and mentors, as 22% of patients at primary school age mentioned that their teachers treated them badly. Two out of three patients with epilepsy were found to have either courtesy or coaching stigma, which represent enacted stigma of parents and guardians of patients with epilepsy, and this translates into a boosting effect for all forms of stigma being enforced in epileptic patients having their caregivers constantly reminding them of their condition. Patients who stated that their disease hindered their progress in life and those who expressed frustration and stress were found to be more than those who could cope with their condition, and this was significantly associated with a high seizure frequency. This shows that poor control of seizures inevitably diminishes the ability of patients to conceal their condition, leading to more discrimination and exacerbation of stigma [1].

An important implication of living in a resource-limited country is deficiencies that could be noted across all social services especially healthcare services. Muwada Bashir et al. portrayed a brilliant scope in their study of detecting the quality of life of Sudanese patients with epilepsy under the burden of inequalities of healthcare services, which showed that stigmatization, social discrimination and inadequate health services are major problems that Sudanese patients with epilepsy and their families confront in their daily life. The study concluded that stigma among other factors associated with epilepsy is worsening the burden on both patients and caregivers by crippling their healthcare services accessibility and by increasing efforts of coping with the disease in a society with a culture that is shaped by a low economic status [6].

8. Children with epilepsy

Children constitute the main domain of people with epilepsy; this subpopulation faces many challenges. These challenges begin with the different etiologies of epilepsy in Sudan and Africa, of these etiologies central nervous system infectious agents (malaria, onchocerciasis), and perinatal insults constitute the main causes of epilepsy. Such causes could explain why the majority of people with epilepsy are in Africa. In addition, these causes along with other factors contribute to the poor outcome of epilepsy in the developing world.

Children with epilepsy have comorbidities including autism, intellectual disability that could be caused by perinatal insults and cerebral palsy; they are also more vulnerable to physical and sexual abuse. Studies from Sudan demonstrated that 10% of children with epilepsy have associated attention deficit hyperactivity disorder (ADHD) [25], one third had learning disabilities, and 10% had motor disabilities [26], theses comorbidities represent the difficulty in the management of these children, as a multidisciplinary approach is required in management, which is usually unavailable in Sudan and the developing world.

Since the 1950s, children with neurological disorders were seen in adult neurology clinics, as pediatric neurology training program in Sudan has recently been initiated, with a few pediatric neurologists available.

Currently there is one pediatric neurology tertiary center and four specialized child neurology clinics in Sudan, 3 of them are located in the capital, these 4 clinics serve the whole of Sudan, as well as referred patients from neighboring countries including: Chad, Eretria, and South Sudan where facilities for neurological investigations are limited. The shortage of pediatric neurologists and pediatric neurology centers and their location mainly in the capital, along with the high cost of transportation to the center, long waiting lists till evaluation by a specialist, further complicate the management of children with epilepsy [8].

8.1 Epilepsy in schools

It is important to review epilepsy status in school settings where children spend most of their time. Schools in Sudan rarely have dedicated clinics to accommodate children's health needs, and while school teachers should act as caregivers, most of them are usually ill-informed or lacking appropriate knowledge about epilepsy, and none of them have had any sort of training to help in case of a seizure, so a considerable proportion does not know what to do when a child develops a seizure [27, 28].

Many teachers fall as victims of the communities' misconceptions and could even play a passive role in the stigma, contributing to the child's anxiety. Many had no idea about possible causes of epilepsy and guessed that parents would not sign up their children with epilepsy to school due to suspected mental sub-normality, stigma, or fear of unattended falls or attacks. On the other hand, figures demonstrated a significant amount of children ditch school altogether because of the illness. Other students do not mind having a classmate with epilepsy at school but they share their teachers' beliefs and misconceptions, and would sometimes, as a result, engage in bullying and discriminatory behaviors against them. The condition is barely touched in school curriculums and students do not undergo any sort of training to help them act properly around their peers who have epilepsy.

9. Women with epilepsy

Globally, 50% of women and girls with epilepsy are in the reproductive age range [29]. Epilepsy in the developing countries has a slight male predominance; this is likely due to underreporting of epilepsy in women due to negative attitudes and stigma facing them, that include difficulties in getting married, increased divorce rates, having children or even being abandoned by their families because of their illness, and harder chances of being employed. This underreporting of epilepsy in women leads to deficits in health care seeking behavior, hence contributing to the epilepsy treatment gap in women.

Apart from the aforementioned social difficulties, women with epilepsy are challenged with many issues that include the effect of epilepsy and AEDs on their sexual function, contraception, pregnancy, fetal abnormalities, childbirth, and breastfeeding [30–33].

Due to the shortage of neurologists in Sudan, the majority of women with epilepsy are managed and counseled by non-specialized doctors. A study conducted in Sudan to assess doctors' knowledge of women issues and epilepsy using standardized knowledge of women issues and epilepsy (KOWIE II) questionnaire concluded that the majority of Sudanese doctors' knowledge was unsatisfactory. They were unaware of sexual dysfunction among women with epilepsy, that women with epilepsy should continue taking their AEDs when they are pregnant, and that women can safely breastfeed while taking AEDs [34].

10. Conclusion

Sudan has been a victim of war, poverty, substandard infrastructure, and a failing healthcare system. These factors along with epilepsy stigma, misconceptions and false believes represent major challenges in epilepsy management in Sudan.

11. Recommendations

All these challenges must be approached systematically to ensure the best management for patients with epilepsy. Such approaches include the need for a mass movement against epilepsy headed by individuals experienced in the field, and fundamental governmental partnership and aid to provide organizational efforts and funding for instituting and decentralizing neurology facilities outside Khartoum, and ensuring the availability and affordability of investigations and medications especially the new generation AEDs. Epidemiologic studies are needed to outline the treatment gap of epilepsy and guide nationwide strategies and efforts to increase the awareness of communities about epilepsy are needed especially in the rural areas to fight disease stigma, Special groups need further attention such as making efforts for prevention of infections leading to epilepsy in children, the involvement of other healthcare providers such as social workers, speech and language therapists, nutritionists, and special teachers in the management of children with epilepsy can never be overemphasized. Lastly, telemedicine should be implemented in the management of epilepsy in Sudan.

Authors' contribution

Ismat Babiker wrote the following sections: children with epilepsy, women with epilepsy, co-wrote AEDs in Sudan, and contributed in chapter editing.

Awab Saad wrote Sudan: background and population, healthcare system in Sudan, Neurology in Sudan, co-wrote epilepsy misconceptions in Sudan, and contributed in chapter editing.

Basil Ibrahim wrote stigma, health related stigma, manifestation of stigma in high vs. low-income countries, stigma in low-income countries and in Sudan, and contributed in chapter editing.

Mohamed Abdelsadig wrote the collapse of the healthcare system in Sudan, epilepsy in schools, scarce personnel and trained physicians, co-wrote AEDs in Sudan, epilepsy misconceptions in Sudan, and contributed in chapter editing.

Conflict of interest

The authors declare no conflict of interest.

Author details

Ismat Babiker*, Awab Saad, Basil Ibrahim and Mohamed Abdelsadig
University of Medical Sciences and Technology, Khartoum, Sudan

*Address all correspondence to: ismatbabiker94@gmail.com

References

[1] Hamid O, Taha MAO, Balla SA, Hussien A. Stigma of epilepsy among patients and their relatives attending charity clinic, Omdurman — Sudan. J Neurol Sci. 2013;333:e61-2.

[2] Sokrab M, Sokrab A, Elzubeir M. Quality of life in people with epilepsy in Sudan: An example of underserved communities in developing countries. Qatar Med J. 2012;2012(2):59-63.

[3] Newton CR, Garcia HH. Epilepsy in poor regions of the world. Lancet. 2012;380(9848):1193-201.

[4] Seidi O, Hussein A. Sudan. Practical Neurology 2005;5:311-314.

[5] Chowdhury S, Chakraborty P pratim. Universal health coverage - There is more to it than meets the eye. J Fam Med Prim Care. 2017;6(2):169-70.

[6] Bashir MBA, Cumber SN. The quality of life and inequalities in health services for epilepsy treatment among patience in the urban cities of Sudan. Pan Afr Med J. 2019;33:10.

[7] Mohammed IN, Babikir HE. Traditional and spiritual medicine among Sudanese children with epilepsy. Sudan J Paediatr. 2013;13(1):31-7

[8] Elseed MA, Mohammed IN, Hamed AA. Paediatric neurology service in Sudan: Current situation and future challenges. Sudan J Pediatric. 2015;15(1):114.

[9] Osman M, Babiker E, Oe Babiker M. Highlight and Opinion Managing childhood epilepsy in a resource-limited setting: A pragmatic approach. Vol. 15, S. Sudan Association of Paediatricians; 2015.

[10] Elsayed M, El-Sayed N, Badi S, Ahmed M. Factors affecting adherence to antiepileptic medications among Sudanese individuals with epilepsy: A cross-sectional survey. J Fam Med Prim Care. 2019 8(7):2312.

[11] Abdelrahim MA, Alfaki MM, Alsherif RA, Dafaalla MD, Alfaki MI, Ahmed MS, et al. Estimation of the direct cost of epilepsy among Sudanese patients attending charity clinic in Omdurman 2014. J Neurol Sci. 2015 Oct 15;357:e30.

[12] Omer AM. The health system in Sudan is characterized by heavy reliance on charging users at the point of access. J Med Res Heal Sci. 2019;2(2):515-39.

[13] Miller WR, Von Gaudecker J, Tanner A, Buelow JM. Epilepsy self-management during a pandemic: Experiences of people with epilepsy. Epilepsy Behav. 2020;111:107238.

[14] Link BG, Phelan JC. Conceptualizing stigma. Annu Rev Soc. 2001;27(1):363-85.

[15] The evolving understanding of stigma - Harvard Health. Available from: https://www.health.harvard.edu/newsletter_article/the-evolving-understanding-of-stigma.

[16] Penn DL, Judge A, Jamieson P, Garczynski J, Hennessy M, Romer *D. Stigma*. In: Evans DL, Foa EB, Gur RE, Hendin H, O'Brien CP, Seligman MEP, et al., editors. Treating and preventing adolescent mental health disorders. Oxford University Press; 2005.

[17] Ablon J. The nature of stigma and medical conditions. Epilepsy Behav. 2002 Dec;3(6):2-9.

[18] Sartorius N. Stigmatized illnesses and health care. Croat Med J. 2007 Jun;48(3):396-7.

[19] Nyblade L, Stockton MA, Giger K, Bond V, Ekstrand ML, Lean RM, et al. Stigma in health facilities: Why it matters and how we can change it. BMC Med. 2019 Feb 15;17(1):25.

[20] Kane JC, Elafros MA, Murray SM, Mitchell EMH, Augustinavicius JL, Causevic S, et al. A scoping review of health-related stigma outcomes for high-burden diseases in low- and middle-income countries. Vol. 17, BMC Medicine. Bio Med Central Ltd.; 2019. p. 17.

[21] Stangl AL, Earnshaw VA, Logie CH, Van Brakel W, Simbayi LC, Barré I, et al. The Health Stigma and Discrimination Framework: A global, crosscutting framework to inform research, intervention development, and policy on health-related stigmas. BMC Med. 2019 Feb 15;17(1):31.

[22] Van Brakel WH. Measuring health-related stigma--a literature review. Vol. 11, Psychology, health & medicine. Routledge ; 2006. p. 307-34.

[23] Scambler G, Hopkins A. Being epileptic: coming to terms with stigma. Sociol Health Illn. 1986 Mar 1;8(1):26-43.

[24] de Boer HM, Mula M, Sander JW. The global burden and stigma of epilepsy. Vol. 12, Epilepsy and Behavior. Academic Press; 2008. p. 540-6.

[25] Ahmed EE, Mohamed IN, Mohammed N. Spectrum of attention deficit hyperactivity disorders (ADHD) among Sudanese children with epilepsy. Vol. 15, S. Sudan Association of Paediatricians; 2015.

[26] Ohaeri JU, Awadalla AW, Farah AA. Quality of life in people with epilepsy and their family caregivers. An Arab experience using the short version of the World Health Organization quality of life instrument. Saudi Medical Journal. 2009; 30(10): 1328.

[27] Elhassan MA, Alemairy AA, Amara ZM, Hamadelneel AA, Mohamed AH, Elaimeri AA. Epilepsy: Knowledge, Attitude, and Practice Among Secondary School Teachers in Khartoum State. Neurol Ther. 2017 Dec 1;6(2):225-35.

[28] Babikar H, Abbas I. Knowledge, practice and attitude toward epilepsy among primary and secondary school teachers in South Gezira locality, Gezira State, Sudan. J Fam Community Med. 2011;18(1):17.

[29] Gooneratne IK, Wimalaratna M, Ranaweera AKP, Wimalaratna S. Contraception advice for women with epilepsy. BMJ 2017;357:j2010.

[30] Zahn CA, Morrell MJ, Collins SD, Labiner DM, Yerby MS. Management issues for women with epilepsy: a review of the literature. Neurology 1998;51(4):949-56.

[31] Morrell MJ, Sarto GE, Shafer PO, Borda EA, Herzog A, Callanan M. Health issues for women with epilepsy: a descriptive survey to assess knowledge and awareness among healthcare providers. JWomens Health Gend Based Med 2000;9(9):959-65.

[32] Mawer G, Briggs M, Baker GA, Bromley R, Coyle H, Eatock J, et al. Pregnancy with epilepsy: obstetric and neonatal outcome of a controlled study. Seizure 2010;19(2):112-9.

[33] Kaufman KR, Wong S, Sivaraaman K, Anim C, Delatte D. Epilepsy and AED-induced decreased libido — the unasked psychosocial comorbidity. Epilepsy Behav 2015;52:236-8.

[34] Elnaeim AK, Elnaeim MK, Babiker IBA. Knowledge of women issues and epilepsy among doctors in Sudan. Epilepsy Behav. 2018 Jul 1;84:79-82.

Chapter 13

Presurgical Evaluation of Epilepsy Surgery

Tak Lap Poon

Abstract

Drug-resistant epilepsy (DRE) is defined as failure of two adequate trials of appropriately chosen and administered antiepileptic drugs. Approximately about 30% of epilepsy patients are drug resistant. Accountable reasons to treatment failure including failure to recognize epilepsy syndrome, poor drug compliance, lifestyle factors, etc. In modern era of medicine, DRE patient should be encouraged to have early referral to tertiary epilepsy centre for presurgical evaluation. Comprehensive neurophysiology, structural neuroimaging, and neuropsychological and psychiatric assessment are regarded as essential elements. Invasive electroencephalography (EEG) monitoring in terms of subdural electrodes, depth electrodes, foramen ovale electrodes, and more advanced technique using stereoelectroencephalography (SEEG) are strong armamentarium for epilepsy surgeon. Epilepsy surgery in terms of resection, disconnection, or neuro-modulation should be recommended after a multi-disciplinary agreement.

Keywords: epilepsy surgery, drug resistant epilepsy, presurgical evaluation, anatomo-electro-clinical hypothesis

1. Introduction

Drug-resistant epilepsy (DRE) is defined as failure of two adequate trials of appropriately chosen and administered antiepileptic drugs. Approximately about 30% of epilepsy patients are drug resistant. Accountable reasons to treatment failure including failure to recognize epilepsy syndrome, poor drug compliance, lifestyle factors etc. In modern era of medicine, DRE patient should be encouraged to have early referral to tertiary epilepsy centre for presurgical evaluation. Comprehensive neurophysiology, structural neuroimaging, neuropsychological and psychiatric assessment are regarded as essential elements. Invasive electroencephalography (EEG) monitoring in terms of subdural electrodes, depth electrodes, foramen ovale electrodes, and more advanced technique using stereo-electroencephalography (SEEG) are strong armamentarium for epilepsy surgeon. Epilepsy surgery in terms of resection, disconnection or neuro-modulation should be recommended after a multi-disciplinary agreement.

2. Background and definition of drug-resistant epilepsy (DRE)

Patients with epilepsy whose seizures do not respond successfully to anti-epileptic drug (AED) therapy are considered to have drug-resistant epilepsy (DRE).

IntechOpen

The prior equivalent term included medically intractable epilepsy or pharma-resistant epilepsy. This group of patient have the greatest burden of epilepsy related disabilities, and also added the significantly the healthcare resources expenses.

In 2010, a consensus proposal from task force of the International League Against Epilepsy (ILAE) commission on therapeutic strategies. A framework comprises two "hierarchical" levels is proposed for definition of drug-resistant epilepsy (DRE). Level 1 is categorization of outcome to a therapeutic intervention and level 2 is core definition of DRE based on how many "informative" trials of antiepileptic drugs (AEDs) resulted in a "treatment failure" outcome. The definition of DRE usually requires failure of two adequate trials of appropriately chosen and administered antiepileptic drugs (be it sequential monotherapy or combined polytherapy) [1]. It is also important to include the impact of seizure factors (frequency, severity, associated behavioural problem) on individual psychosocial wellbeing. Such impact will lead to the physicians' decision on drug options and the urgency of considering non-medical therapies.

Other important areas in the clinical assessment of DRE include the following.

2.1 The epidemiology

The prevalence of epilepsy patients aged 15 years or over in Chinese communities has been estimated at about 3–5.7 per 1000 [2], and about 40,000 Hong Kong people could be expected to have active epilepsy. The cumulative probability of a second attack at 1, 2, and 3 years was 30, 37 and 42% respectively. DRE comprised about one third of all epilepsy patients. A more recent study in 2008 showed the crude prevalence of active epilepsy and seizure disorder were estimated to be 3.94/1000. So the cases that should have under tertiary care for consideration of intensive work up will be around 1000 cases annually. There existed a treatment or referral gap of 20 years in the United States for this group of patient [3, 4]. It is foreseen that the local condition will be similar and an unmet need should call for more escalated awareness.

2.2 The pathogenesis

Prospective studies with chronic epilepsy patients suggested that 70–80% of patients retain their status as intractable versus in remission [5]. In other words, a minority, around 20% of initial intractable seizure cases will archive seizure freedom in long run and vice versa. Postulated mechanism leading to intractability includes glial proliferation and dendritic sprouting with synaptic recognition [6] in mesial temporal sclerosis. The concept of paroxysmal depolarization shift (PDS) is cellular events in which rapidly repetitive action potentials are not followed by the usual refractory period, thereby generating a prolonged membrane depolarization. Repetitive neuronal firing probably underlies the interictal and ictal unit and local field recording of high frequency oscillations (HFO).

Another compelling theory is the build-up of epileptic "neuronal network" (NN), via alternation in neuronal circuitry [7, 8]. A well-defined NN example is the limbic network with sequential propagation path via hippocampus, amygdala, lateral temporal neocortex and entorhinal cortex, medial thalamus and frontal inferior lobes. The interest on neuronal network analysis in epilepsy had gained strength with the use of high resolution recording techniques. Seizures start in a well-defined brain area and spread at great speed to connected brain area recruiting specific neuronal networks into typical oscillatory behaviour. Therefore, epilepsies should be considered as resulting from disturbed network interactions that implies "multi-targeted treatments" [9–13].

2.3 Clinical course or trajectories and complications

In a recent study using incident cohort of drug resistant epilepsy, which adopt ILAE DRE criteria, there are different patterns of disease progression or trajectories observed [14]. The 30% proportion of patient eventually suffered from DRE was again observed. A long delay from disease onset to failure of second AED was also found. This finding might give insights to the pathogenesis as mentioned earlier.

The mortality and morbidity of DRE, is in general, believed to be higher than that of seizure free patients or patient with good seizure control [15–17]. Even in those that suffered from infrequent seizure, their daily life and subjective well-being are also jeopardized in various extents [18].

2.4 The classification

It is a common practice, among epileptologist, to subdivide the refractory epilepsy cases into temporal lobe epilepsy (TLE) and non-temporal lobe epilepsy (NTLE). The former also constitute two distinct groups, namely, mesial temporal lobe epilepsy (mTLE) and neocortical temporal lobe epilepsy (NeTLE), according to the clinical and radiological manifestations. Both mTLE and NTLE shared similar pathological substrates (**Table 1**) apart from the mesial temporal sclerosis only found in the former. The TLE patients usually present with complex partial seizures, with or without generalized seizure, depending on the neuronal network involved. Though a minority of these TLE will became seizure free after repeated drug trials [15], most of the patients will run a clinical course of refractory seizure attack, and indeed, they form the most well-known surgically remediable epilepsy syndrome [19].

For the non TLE cases, the clinical and radiological features are diverse and also depend on the underlying etiologies or pathological substrates. In general, the seizure semiology is less well defined and the MRI abnormalities are variable and they are challenging in the perspective of seizure focus localization. Usually concerted effort and multi modalities investigations (in phase 1 of presurgical evaluation) are required [20].

Pathological substrate	Mesial TLE	Neocortical TLE
Mesial temporal sclerosis	Most common	Not present
The others: present in both		
Neoplastic	High grade or low grade glioma	
Developmental	Focal cortical dysplasia	
Infective	Viral encephalitis	
Vascular	Cavernous angioma	
Migrational disorder	DNET, ganglioglioma	
Trauma	Encephalomalacia	

Table 1.
Temporal lobe epilepsy (TLE) pathology.

3. Approach to drug treatment failure

Before considering referral to tertiary centre for work up of DRE for surgical intervention, there are certain reasons of treatment failure that should be considered:

1. Failure to recognize a generalized epilepsy syndromes e.g. West's syndrome, Rasmussen's syndrome, autosomal dominant nocturnal frontal lobe epilepsy (ADNLE), early myoclonic encephalopathy (EME) etc.

2. Inappropriate choice of first line anti-epileptic drug (e.g. carbamazepine) that will aggravate seizures.

3. Poor drug compliance and lifestyle factors contributing to seizure recurrence.

These factors are often quoted as "pseudo-resistance" [21–23].

3.1 Guideline

There has been a number of regional and international consensus and guidelines related to comprehensive management of epilepsy surgery. In Hong Kong, the first guideline, *The Hong Kong Epilepsy Guideline 2009*, was published by the Hong Kong Epilepsy Society with the aim as a general guideline for the medical practitioner [24]. The Guideline included the following aspects:

1. Diagnosis, review, and referral

2. Patient education

3. Following a first seizure

4. Investigations

5. Classification

6. Principles of management

7. Pharmacological or AED management

8. Management of drug-resistant epilepsy

9. Side-effects of AEDs

10. Presurgical evaluation of drug-resistant epilepsy

11. Other forms of treatment

12. Prolonged seizures in the community

13. Treatment of status epilepticus

14. Perioperative management of seizure

15. Older people with epilepsy

16. Children and young people with epilepsy

The guidelines had the updated version in 2017–2018 and the whole guideline was divided into four sections addressing the following aspects including use of antiepileptic drugs, guideline on status epilepticus, drug resistant epilepsy, and woman and epilepsy [25].

3.2 Selection of eligible candidate

There is observation that the longer the delay between the onset of DRE and the surgery, the lower the chance of postoperative seizure freedom and improved psychosocial outcome [26]. So a timely referral is mandatory for quality care of such group of patients.

Anyhow, before recruiting the patient, the first step is to identify the appropriate candidate. Conceptually, the eligibility criteria will include the following:

1. Patient and patient's family understand and accept the surgical treatment and the potential risk

2. The seizure is disabling despite adequate and appropriate drug trial

3. The available imaging and neurophysiological data should be consistent with the possibility of a surgical remediable epileptic syndrome.

3.3 Presurgical evaluation

The first objective is to identify the epileptogenic zone, EZ by various invasive and non-invasive modalities of investigations. The more sophisticated or invasive approach will also depend on the clarity of structural identifiable pathologies in neuroimaging and the link with the clinical semiology.

The second objective, after screening of the potential epileptogenic zone, is to develop strategies to safeguard the lesion can be safely resected with no significant physical or cognitive sequelae.

The ultimate goal in presurgical evaluation is to identify the concept of "Six cortical zones" (**Figure 1**).

From pragmatic point of view, detailed interview of patient and patient's family and friends who can give detailed witness history and past background is mandatory. The interview should aim for recapitulating all relevant past history and probably risk factor or etiological factors. The latter will also give insights to prognosis of the epileptic disorder with respect to surgical treatment. A good example will be a case of post encephalitic epilepsy will render surgical intervention less successful [27].

There should be a multi-disciplinary team and the respective investigations should include neuroimaging, psychiatric, neuropsychological and electrophysiological assessment. A tertiary level or above epilepsy centre should have the available epilepsy surgery presurgical investigations of in two different levels:

- Level 1 investigations are compulsory to all epilepsy patients for better localization of epileptogenic zone by means of: (1) improvement of detection of structural lesion on MRI, (2) mapping the source of interictal epileptiform discharges, (3) detection of focal interictal brain dysfunction, and (4) detection of ictal focal brain hyperperfusion, and for assessment of risk of postoperative deficits by means of: (1) determination of hemisphere dominant for language, (2) prediction of risk of postoperative memory decline, (3) reduction of risk of visual field deficit, and (4) reduction of risk of motor deficit.

- Level 2 investigations are indicated for possible epilepsy surgery candidates with no formal conclusion about the localization or extension of epileptogenic zone. They are generally referring to those invasive monitoring tools.

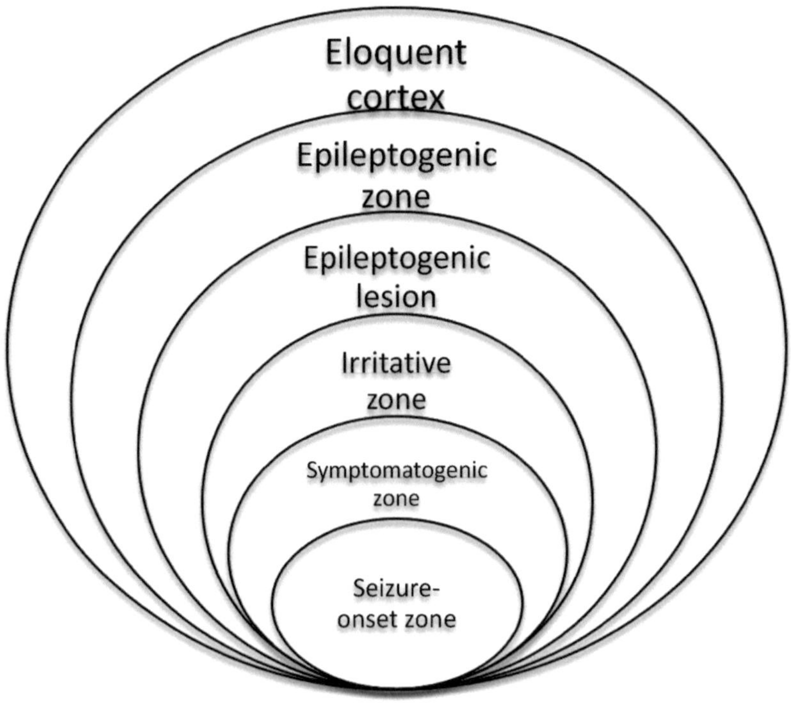

Figure 1.
Six cortical zones.

3.4 Neurophysiology

The neurophysiological evaluation includes interictal and ictal EEG sampling, which can be attained by non-invasive or invasive means in a long term recording manner.

The inter-ictal EEG will provide important hint to lateralization or localization of EZ. This is particularly true in cases of TLE solely unilateral anterior temporal spike is a strong predictor of post-operative seizure freedom [28]. Anyhow, it is not uncommon to have unilateral MTS with bitemporal interictal epileptiform discharges found [29]. Another interictal EEG pattern with good localizing value is short bursts of low-voltage, high frequency oscillations associated with focal cortical dysplasia [30].

Conceptually, the video EEG recording will capture the habitual seizures and the ictal EEG discharge and the lateralization and localization of the ictal onset zone can be deduced from analysis of adequate number of captured events.

After combined analysis of ictal and interictal EEG data, the irritative and ictal onset zones can be estimated [31].

Invasive recording is indicated when there is a hypothesis of epileptogenic zone that is not fully supported by the non- invasive diagnostic modalities results. These difficult scenarios are especially found in the non-lesional cases [32, 33].

3.5 Structural neuroimaging

Magnetic resonance imaging (MRI) of brain constitutes the basic, yet the most important investigation of choice in presurgical evaluation. It is particularly true in some epileptic disorder like temporal lobe epilepsy, of which mesial temporal sclerosis is the pathological substrate, got its unique radiological-anatomical correlates:

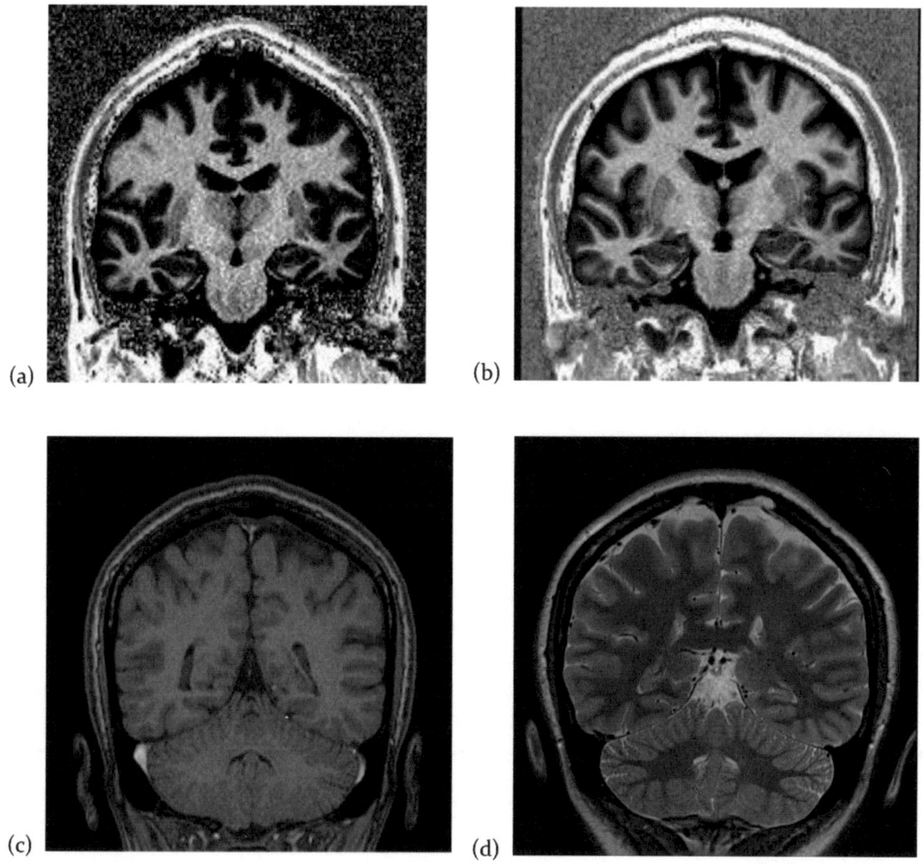

Figure 2.
Patient was regarded to be non-lesional epilepsy initially in 1.5 T MRI (a) and found to have cortical dysplasia in left temporal stem in 3 T MRI (b). Another epilepsy patient had very subtle lesion in right subependymal region in 1.5 T MRI (c) and confirmed to be subependymal heterotopia by 3 T MRI (d).

The MRI features of hippocampal sclerosis include (1) hippocampal atrophy on T1, (2) increased signal on T2-weighted images or fluid-attenuated inversion recovery (FLAIR) sequences, and (3) decreased signal on inversion recovery sequences [34, 35].

The detection of these abnormalities should be carried out with optimized imaging techniques, which include angulated coronal sections obtained perpendicular to the long axis of the hippocampal structures.

For the extratemporal substrates, MRI can also define hemimegalencephaly, schizencephaly, and focal subcortical heterotopia. Focal cortical dysplasia is the most common developmental pathology in children with extratemporal lobe seizures, and there is an international classification to define the underlying histopathology and foretell the outlook of surgical success [36].

3 T MRI system has better signal-to-noise ratio, spatial and tissue contrast resolution than a 1.5 T system. Studies have shown that for initially nonlesional cases scanned by 1.5 T system with standard MRI brain protocol, more than half had new findings after rescanned by 3 T MRI system with multichannel phased-array coils (**Figure 2**).

The recommended MRI epilepsy protocol includes:

1. Volume acquisition T1W sequence acquired in oblique coronal orientation, orthogonal to long axis of hippocampus, covers whole brain in 0.9–1 mm partition

2. Oblique coronal T2WTSE an T2W FLAIR sequences, orientated perpendicular to long axis of hippocampus, 2–3 mm slice thickness

3. Axial T2W or T2W FLAIR sequence of 3 mm slice thickness of whole brain

Diffusion tensor imaging (DTI) and tractography can be used for fiber tracking and noninvasive structural network mapping and is an optional imaging sequence to aid preoperative planning for surgical trajectory. Recent study reported identification of significant diffusion abnormalities of tract sections in ipsilateral dorsal fornix and contralateral parahippocampal white matter bundle in patients with poor postoperative seizure control. Though more studies are warranted to make conclusion, these results may help in understanding the mechanism of postoperative persistent seizure and may act as imaging prognosticator for operation outcome.

However, there are pathological substrates that go beyond the detection of MRI analysis. As a result, multi-modality imaging of the brain will come into play [37–39].

There are some functional neuroimaging modalities, namely PET, SPECT, fMRI and magnetoencephalography (MEG). Some of these scans can be co-registered with MRI to give more detailed structural-functional correlated imaging analysis. They will aid the localization of epileptogenic zone, and the sensitivity will largely depend on the epileptic syndrome. MEG helps to localize the epileptogenic zone and delineate the relationship between the suspected abnormality and the relevant regions in the brain. The placement of invasive electrodes can be guided by the MEG findings. A MEG-guided review of MRI may reveal subtle abnormalities and permit a precise surgical excision of the irritative zone. MEG is also indicated in patients with multiple intracerebral lesions, such as multiple cavernomas, in whom a sole epileptogenic lesion may be identified for lesionectomy [40–43].

With such information, the indication of further invasive studies will also be justified (**Figure 3**).

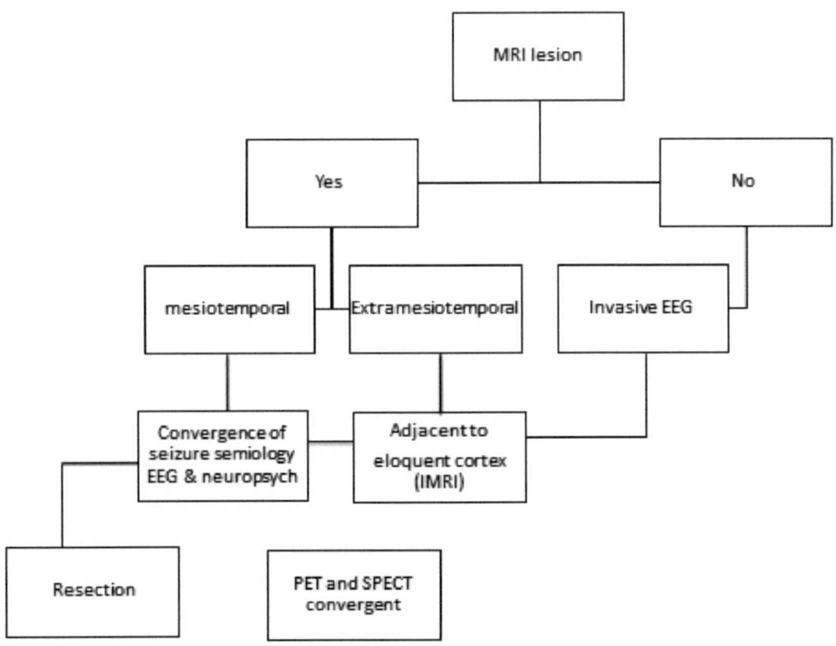

Figure 3.
Algorithm of workup of refractory epilepsy.

3.6 Neuropsychological assessment

Conceptually, the principle of neuropsychological batteries of test lies on the functional neuroanatomy(**Table 2**). It is controversial to state the prediction of postoperative cognitive outcome should be based on the side that was to be resected or the side that would remain following surgery.

There is always a long debate between the usage of WADA test and fMRI in determination of language dominance. In majority of cases, fMRI can clearly lateralize the language localization. However, in cases having agitation or mental compromise, or there is bilateral activations in fMRI, WADA test should be considered as a definitive test (**Figure 4**). Anyhow, the lower the mental reserve and the higher the functional adequacy of the resected tissue will preclude the surgical feasibility [44, 45].

3.7 Psychiatric assessment

It is recommended that the presurgical evaluation should include a thorough psychiatric assessment [32]. There are several reasons:

1. The prevalence of psychiatric disorder is prevalent in epilepsy patients, and psychopathology is common in patients with TLE.

2. Appropriate assessment might help to anticipate acute anxiety, delusions, and the latter symptoms might be aggravated in some temporal epilepsy cases, in perioperative period

3. The life time history of psychiatric disorder was associated with worst post-surgical seizure outcome, though the existence of stable psychiatric disorder does not preclude epilepsy surgery.

The areas of assessment should include four domains, namely, behavioural, psychiatric, self-esteem profile and quality of life.

3.8 Invasive EEG studies

In general, the indications to consider invasive EEG monitoring are as the followings:

1. To define precisely the epileptogenic zone when non-invasive data are not concordant

2. To conclude the divergence of non-invasive data in different regions

3. To map eloquent cortical and subcortical function for resective surgery planning

	Cognitive function	Remark
Temporal lobe	Memory and language	Left side represents verbal memory Right side represents visual memory
Frontal lobe	Executive and behavior	
Posterior part	Perception and higher sensory	

Table 2.
Functional neuroanatomy.

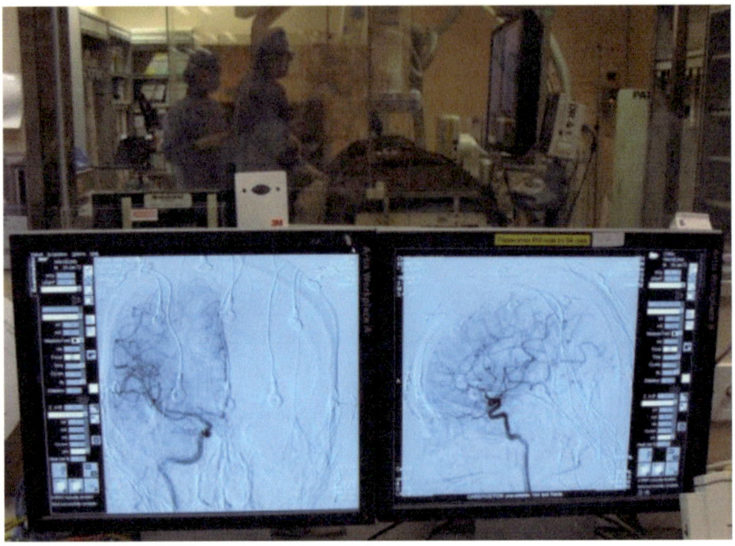

Figure 4.
Clinical photo showing the setup for WADA test.

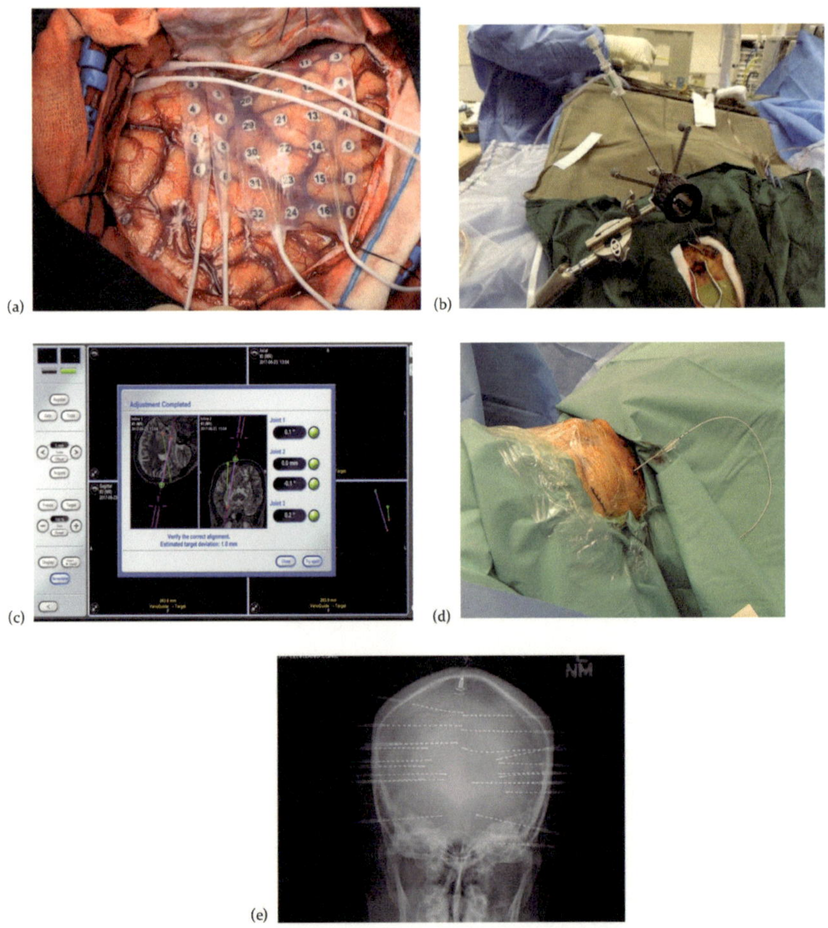

Figure 5.
Types of invasive EEG studies: (a) subdural strips and grids, (b) intracerebral depth electrodes, (c) insular depth electrodes insertion with neuro-navigation guidance, (d) foramen ovale electrodes, and (e) stereoelectroencephalography (SEEG).

4. To further validate the epileptogenic zone or provide information of prognostic value

5. To perform therapeutic treatment for active regions using thermocoagulation

Traditionally, modalities of invasive EEG monitoring include subdural electrodes, intracerebral depth electrodes, epidural peg electrodes and foramen ovale electrodes. A comprehensive review on risks and benefits in using subdural and depth electrodes showed that the related complications include epidural or subdural haemorrhage, intracerebral haemorrhage or contusion, meningitis, oedema around electrode, cerebral oedema, increased intracranial pressure etc. The overall complication rate ranges from 0.4% to 6.6%.

Stereoelectroencephalography (SEEG) is getting its popularity to enable precise recordings from deep cortical areas in bilateral and multiple lobes without subjecting the patients to have bilateral large craniotomies. The key and most important concept in considering SEEG is to test individualized *anatomo-electro-clinical hypothesis*. Based on clinical history, semiology, preoperative imaging and vEEG data, the findings of SEEG help the clinicians to understand the spatial and temporal dynamics of seizure i.e. where it starts, when and when it spreads. Study from Italian group showed that SEEG is a useful and relatively safe tool to localize the epileptogenic zone with procedure-related morbidity 5.6%. Other centres incorporate the neuro-robotic system in performing SEEG and showed comparable results. In general, SEEG had equivalent efficiency in determination of epileptogenic zone with lower operative morbidities and complications including CSF leak and intracranial haemorrhage, and better tolerance to patients. Current application of EEG recordings is not only limited to scalp EEG and intracranial EEG with subdural electrodes and depth electrodes (**Figure 5**) [46–49].

4. Epilepsy surgery for drug resistance epilepsy

The decision of surgical intervention is usually made in a consensus agreement among the discipline which carry out the investigation in a multi-disciplinary patient management conference in each epilepsy surgery centre. Basically it is a rational estimation of the precision of the epileptogenic zone (thus the success rate of seizure cure) and the risk benefit analysis of the potential post-operative risk.

In general, the outcome will be more favorable for lesional epileptic syndrome with concordance of investigation results and neuropsychological proof of "absence" of important cognitive function within the resected areas. On the contrary, the lack of concordance, the presence of important function in the pathological substrate will preclude the surgical feasibility. Besides the disease factor, there are also patient factors like seizure frequency, duration of illness, comorbidity that will govern the prognostication [50].

Conventionally, the operative outcome will be categorized in four classes according to Engel's classification [51] (**Table 3**).

Class I	Free of disabling seizures
Class II	Rare disabling seizures ("almost seizure-free")
Class III	Worthwhile improvement
Class IV	No worthwhile improvement

Table 3.
Engel's classification.

The rationale is to have complete resection of the epileptogenic zone. Broadly there are three types of epilepsy surgery

1. Curative, respective surgery in terms of resection surgery involves temporal lobe surgery and extratemporal lobe surgery. Among the different epileptic syndrome, the mesial temporal sclerosis usually has the most favorable seizure outcome: 70% of the patients have Engel's Class I [52, 53].

2. Palliative surgery in terms of disconnection surgery includes corpus callosotomy, hemispherectomy (anatomical/functional), hemispherotomy, multiple subpial transections. All these procedure are often performed in pediatric group of patients and they had been shown to have seizure reduction ranged from 40 to 50% [54].

3. Modulatory, in terms of deep brain stimulation (DBS), vague nerve stimulation (VNS), responsive neurostimulation (RNS) and gamma knife radiosurgery [55]

5. Long-term outcome after epilepsy surgery

Epilepsy surgery for temporal lobe epilepsy is usually recommended because of promising result. One study including 80 patients with temporal lobe epilepsy showed that the cumulative proportion of patients who were free of seizures impairing awareness was 58% in the surgical group and 8% in the medical group [56]. The Early Randomized Surgical Epilepsy Trial (ERSET) included 38 patients with mesial temporal lobe epilepsy and showed that zero of 23 participants in the medical group and 11 of 15 in the surgical group were seizure free during year 2 of follow-up [57]. Another study including more than 3000 patients from Germany concluded that the number of non-lesional patients and the need for intracranial recordings increased, and more than 50% of evaluated patients did not undergo surgery [58].

6. Treatment consideration for non-lesional epilepsy

There is always difficulty in identification of the epileptogenic zone in non-lesional neocortical epilepsy. Seizure free outcomes are about 55% for non-lesional temporal lobe epilepsy and 43% for non-lesional extratemporal lobe epilepsy patients. Concordance with two or more presurgical evaluations including interictal EEG, ictal EEG, FDG-PET, and ictal SPECT was significantly related to a seizure-free outcome. Another study showed that 38% of non-lesional epilepsy patients had an excellent outcome after resective epilepsy surgery after long-term intracranial EEG. In temporal lobe epilepsy with MRI negative and PET positive findings, surgery could achieve Class I surgical outcomes at postoperative 2 years in about 82% [59, 60].

7. Factors related to failure in epilepsy surgery

Failure of epilepsy surgery may be caused by wrong localization of the epileptogenic zone, very widespread epileptogenic zones and very limited resection of the suspected epileptogenic zone.

In patient after mesial temporal resection, seizure may arise from neocortical regions instead of from residual hippocampal structure. This may imply the existence of regional epileptogenicity. Hippocampus represents the area of cortex with the lowest threshold for seizure generation and the surrounding neocortical tissue also exhibiting epileptogenicity then becomes the site of ictal onset. About 25% of patients with seizure relapse after mesial temporal sclerosis may have seizure onset in the contralateral temporal region.

Extensive reevaluation of these patients is suggested for consideration of reoperation if epileptogenic focus can be localized.

8. Recent advance in epilepsy surgery

Minimally invasive intracranial endovascular EEG monitoring by means of nanowire and catheter and stent-electrode recordings is evolving [61]. High frequency Oscillations (HFOs) are believed as a potential marker for detection of epileptogenicity and predictive factor for epilepsy surgery outcome. However, a meta-analysis was able to show the significant but small relation between removal of HFO-generating brain region and outcome [62–64].

9. Conclusion

The prerequisite of seizure origin in a well circumscribed area of brain and the precision of localization of such epileptogenic zone by epilepsy work up make modern epilepsy surgery a promising treatment modality for refractory epilepsy.

The pre-operative assessment, which include multiple disciplines, however, should be focused on two important conceptual facets

1. Data concordance: the individual seizure pattern is ascribed to the hypothetical brain lesions, as suggested by neurophysiological and radiological data.

2. Functional reserve: the brain pathological region, if being resected, will not leave patient with significant morbidities

The advent of wide range of diagnostic tests and available surgical techniques has widened the applicability of surgical treatment. The success rate of these surgical interventions range from 10 to 20% of seizure reduction to more than 70% seizure freedom, depend on the different scenario.

In conclusion, epilepsy surgery for drug resistance epilepsy involves close collaboration and teamwork by multi-disciplinary specialties. Epilepsy surgery could be performed in different epilepsy centres. Patients should be referred early in their refractory disease course to a higher level epilepsy center for evaluation of the complex surgical options. Public education and promotion on management of refractory epilepsy by surgical treatments should be encouraged and lead by our local professional bodies and health organizations.

Author details

Tak Lap Poon
Department of Neurosurgery, Queen Elizabeth Hospital, Kowloon, Hong Kong

*Address all correspondence to: poontaklap@yahoo.com.hk

References

[1] Kwan P, Arzimanoglou A, Berg AT, et al. Definition of drug resistant epilepsy: Consensus proposal by the ad hoc task force of the ILAE commission on therapeutic strategies. Epilepsia. 2010;**51**:1069-1077

[2] Kwan P, Brodie MJ. Definition of refractory epilepsy: Defining the indefinable? Lancet Neurology. 2010;**9**:27-29

[3] Hui ACF, Kwan P. Epilepsy in Hong Kong: A literature review. Hong Kong Medical Journal. 2004;**10**:185-189

[4] Fong GCY, Kwan P, Hui ACF, Lui CHT, Fong Jason KY, Wong V. An epidemiological study of epilepsy in Hong Kong SAR China. Seizure. 2008;**17**:457-464

[5] Yoon HH, Kwon HL, Mattson RH, Spensor DD, Spensor SS. Long term seizure outcome in patients initially seizure free after resective epilepsy surgery. Neurology. 2003;**61**:445-450

[6] Jansky J, Janzky I, Schulz R, et al. Temporal lobe epilepsy with hippocampal sclerosis: Predictors for long term surgical outcome. Brain. 2005;**128**:395-404

[7] Brodie MJ, Kwan P. Staged approach to epilepsy management. Neurology. 2002;**58**:S2-S8

[8] Pitkanen A, Sutula TP. Is epilepsy a progressive disorder? Prospects for new therapeutic approaches in temporal-lobe epilepsy. Lancet Neurology. 2002;**1**: 173-181

[9] Holmes GL, Ben-Ari Y. Seizing hold of seizures. Nature Medicine. 2003;**9**:994-996

[10] Bragin A, Engel J Jr, Wilson CL, et al. Hippocampal and entorhinal cortex high-frequency oscillations (100-500 Hz) in human epileptic brain and in kainic acid-treated rats with chronic seizures. Epilepsia. 1990;**40**:127-137

[11] Garbelli R, Frassoni C, Condorelli DF, et al. Expression of connexin 43 in the human epileptic and drug-resistant cerebral cortex. Neurology. 2011;**76**: 895-902

[12] Spencer SS. Neural networks in human epilepsy: Evidence of and implications for treatment. Epilepsia. 2002;**43**:219-227

[13] Sefan H, Da Silva FHL. Epileptic neuronal networks: Methods of identification and clinical relevance. Frontiers in Neurology. 2013;**4**(8):1-15

[14] Choi H, Hayat MJ, Zhang R, et al. Drug-resistant epilepsy in adults: Outcome trajectories after failure of two medications. Epilepsia. 2016;**57**:1152-1160

[15] Tomson T. Mortality in epilepsy. Journal of Neurology. 2000;**247**:15-21

[16] Sperling MR, Feldman H, Kinman J, Liporace JD, O'Connor MJ. Seizure control and mortality in epilepsy. Annals of Neurology. 1999;**46**:45-50

[17] Shackleton DP, Westendorp RG, Kasteleijn-Noist Trenite DG, de Craen AJ, Vandenbroucke JP. Survival of patients with epilepsy: An estimate of the mortality risk. Epilepsia. 2002;**43**:445-450

[18] Luoni C, Bisuli F, Canevini MP, et al. Determinants of health-related quality of life in pharmacoresistant epilepsy: Results from a large multicenter study of consecutively enrolled patients using validated quantitative assessment. Epilepsia. 2011;**52**:2181-2191

[19] Spencer SS. When should temporal lobe epilepsy be treated surgically? Lancet Neurology. 2002;**1**:375-382

[20] Casino GD. From the American Epilepsy Society 2009 annual course non substrate-directed epilepsy and surgery: PRO and CON. Epilepsy & Behavior. 2011;**20**:190-193

[21] Smith D, Defalla BA, Chadwick DW. The misdiagnosis of epilepsy and the management of refractory epilepsy in a specialist clinic. QJM. 1999;**92**:15-23

[22] Perucca E, Gram L, Avanzini G, Dulac O. Antiepileptic drugs as a cause of worsening seizures. Epilepsia. 1998;**39**:5-17

[23] Cramer JA, Glassman M, Rienzi V. The relationship between poor medication compliance and seizures. Epilepsy & Behavior. 2002;**3**:338-342

[24] Fong KY, Kwan KLP, Chak WK, Fong CY, Fong D, Fung CW, et al. The Hong Kong epilepsy guideline 2009. Hong Kong Medical Journal. 2009;**15**(Supplement 5):6-28

[25] Poon TL, Lui CHT, Chan I, Siu DYW. Updated review: Drug-resistant epilepsy and presurgical evaluation of epilepsy surgery. Hong Kong Medical Journal. 2018;**24**:610-616

[26] Yoon HH, Kwon HL, Mattson RH, Spencer DD, Spencer SS. Long term seizure outcome in patient initially seizure free after respective surgery. Neurology. 2003;**61**:445-450

[27] Trinka E, Dubeau F, Andermann F, et al. Successful epilepsy surgery in catastrophic postencephalitic epilepsy. Neurology. 2000;**54**:2170-2173

[28] Tonini C, Beghi E, Berg AT, et al. Predictors of epilepsy surgery outcome: A meta-analysis. Epilepsy Research. 2004;**62**:75-87

[29] Ergene E, Shih JJ, Blum DE, So NK. Frequency of bilateral independent interictal epileptiform discharges in temporal lobe epilepsy. Epilepsia. 2000;**41**:213-218

[30] Gambardella A, Palmini A, Andermann F, et al. Usefulness of focal rhythmic discharges on scalp EEG of patients with focal cortical dysplasia and intractable epilepsy. Electroencephalography and Clinical Neurophysiology. 1996;**98**:243-249

[31] Rosenow F, Luders H. Presurgical evaluation of epilepsy: Invited review. Brain. 2001;**124**:1683-1700

[32] Sophia M, Sherman EMS, Forde S, et al. Psychiatric outcomes of epilepsy surgery: A systemic review. Epilepsia. 2011;**52**:880-890

[33] Jayakar P. Invasive EEG monitoring in children; when, where and what? Journal of Clinical Neurophysiology. 1999;**16**:408-418

[34] Cascino GD, Jack CR Jr, Parisi JE, et al. Magnetic resonance imaging-based volume studies in temporal lobe epilepsy: Pathological correlations. Annals of Neurology. 1991;**30**:31-36

[35] Cendes F, Andermann F, Glorr P, et al. MRI volumetric measurement of amygdala and hippocampus in temporal lobe epilepsy. Neurology. 1993;**43**:719-725

[36] Bae YS, Kang HC, Kim HD, Kim SH. New classification of focal cortical dysplasia: Application to practical diagnosis. Journal of Epilepsy Research. 2012;**2**:38-42

[37] Knake S, Triantafyllou C, Wald LL, et al. 3T phased array MRI improves the presurgical evaluation in focal epilepsies: A prospective study. Neurology. 2005;**65**:1026-1031

[38] Hiratsuka Y, Miki H, Kikuchi K, et al. Sensitivity of an eight-element phased array coil in 3 tesla MR imaging:

A basic analysis. Magnetic Resonance in Medical Sciences. 2007;**6**:177-181

[39] Keller SS, Glenn GR, Weber B, et al. Preoperative automated fibre quantification predicts postoperative seizure outcome in temporal lobe epilepsy. Brain. 2017;**140**(1):68-82

[40] Mamelak AN, Nancy Lopez REEGT, Akhtari M, Sutherling WW. Magnetoencephalography-directed surgery in patients with neocortical epilepsy. Journal of Neurosurgery. 2002;**97**:865-873

[41] Papanicolaou AC, Simos PG, Castillo EM, Breier JI, Sarkari S, Pataraia E, et al. Magnetocephalgraphy: A noninvasive alternative to the Wada procedure. Journal of Neurosurgery. 2004;**100**:867-876

[42] Makela JP, Forss N, Jaaskelainen J, Kirveskari E, Korvenoja A, Paetau R. Magnetoencephalography in neurosurgery. Neurosurgery. 2006;**59**: 493-511

[43] Poon TL, Cheung FC, Lui HTC. Magnetoencephalography and its role in evaluation for epilepsy surgery. Hong Kong Medical Journal. 2010;**16**:44-47

[44] Hans O. Luders. Textbook of Epilepsy Surgery. UK: Informa

[45] Schwartz TH, Jeha LE, Tanner A, Bingaman WE, Sperling M. Late seizures in patients initially seizure free after epilepsy surgery. Epilepsia. 2006;**47**:567-573

[46] Gonzalez-Martinez J, Bulacio J, Thompson S, Gale J, Smithason S, Najm I, et al. Technique, results, and complications related to robot-assisted stereoelectroencephalography. Neurosurgery. 2016;**78**:169-180

[47] Cardinale R, Rizzi M, d'Orio P, Casaceli G, Arnulfo G, Narizzano M, et al. A new tool for touch-free patient registration for robot-assisted intracranial surgery: Application accuracy from a phantom study and a retrospective surgical series. Neurosurgical Focus. 2017;**42**(5):1-7

[48] Wellmer J, Von Der Groeben F, Klarmann U, Weber C, Elger CE, Urbach H, et al. Risks and benefits of invasive epilepsy surgery workup with implanted subdural and depth electrodes. Epilepsia. 2012;**53**(8):1322-1332

[49] Kahane P, Landre E, Minotti L, Francione S, Ryvlin P. The Bancaud and Talairach view on the epileptogenic zone: A working hypothesis. Epileptic Disorders. 2006;**8**(Suppl 2):S16-S26

[50] Tellez-Zenteno JF, Dhar R, Wiebe S. Long-term seizure outcomes following epilepsy surgery: A systematic review and meta-analysis. Brain. 2005;**128**:1188-1198

[51] Engel J. Surgical Treatment of the Epilepsies. Lippincott Williams & Wilkins; 1993

[52] Wiebe S, Blume WT, Girvin JP, et al. A randomized, controlled trial of surgery for temporal lobe epilepsy. The New England Journal of Medicine. 2001;**345**:311-318

[53] Engel J Jr. The timing of surgical intervention for mesial temporal lobe epilepsy: A plan for a randomized clinical trial. Archives of Neurology. 1999;**56**:1338-1341

[54] Consensus Guidelines on the Management of Epilepsy 2010. Epilepsy Council, Malaysian Society of Neurosciences. Available from: http://www.neuro.org.my/

[55] Fisher R, Salanova V, Witt T, Worth R, Henry T, Gross R, et al. Electrical stimulation of the anterior nucleus of thalamus for treatment

of refractory epilepsy. Epilepsia. 2010;**51**(5):899-908

[56] Capraz IY, Kurt G, Akdemir O, Hirfanoglu T, Oner Y, Sengezer T, et al. Surgical outcome in patients with MRI-negative, PET-positive temporal lobe epilepsy. Seizure. 2015;**29**:63-68

[57] Engel J Jr, McDermott MP, Wiebe S, Langfitt JT, Stern JM, Dewar S, et al. Early surgical therapy for drug-resistant temporal lobe epilepsy. JAMA. 2012; **307**(9):922-930

[58] Noe K, Sulc V, Wong-Kisiel L, Wirrell E, Van Gompel JJ, Wetjen N, et al. Long-term outcomes after nonlesional extratemporal lobe epilepsy surgery. JAMA Neurology. 2013;**70**(8):1003-1008

[59] Cloppenborg T, May TW, Blumcke I, Grewe P, Hopf LJ, Kalbhenn T, et al. Trends in epilepsy surgery: Stable surgical numbers despite increasing presurgical volumes. Journal of Neurology, Neurosurgery, and Psychiatry. 2016;**87**(12):1322-1329

[60] Lee SK. Surgical approach in nonlesional neocortical epilepsy. Journal of Epilepsy Research. 2011;**1**:47-51

[61] Sefcik RK, Opie NL, John SE, Kellner CP, Mocco J, Oxley TJ. The evolution of endovascular electroencephalography historical perspective and future applications. Neurosurgical Focus. 2016;**40**(5):1-8

[62] Cossu M, Cardinale F, Castana L, Citterio A, Francione S, Tassi L, et al. Stereoelectroencephalography in the presurgical evaluation of focal epilepsy: A retrospective analysis of 215 procedures. Neurosurgery. 2005;**57**: 706718

[63] Gloss D, Nevitt SJ, Staba R. The role of high-frequency oscillations in epilepsy surgery planning. Cochrane Database of Systematic Reviews. 2017

[64] Holler Y, Kutil R, Klaffenbock L, Thomschewski A, Holler PM, Bathke AC, et al. High-frequency oscillations in epilepsy and surgical outcome. A meta-analysis. Frontiers in Human Neuroscience. 2015;**9**(574):1-14

Chapter 14

Pyramid Exploration Intervention, Environmental Enrichment, Aerobic Swimming Exercise and Brain Neuroplasticity in the Kainate Rat Model of Temporal Lobe Epilepsy

Vasavi R. Gorantla, Sabyasachi Maity and Richard M. Millis

Abstract

Previous studies have shown that environmental enrichment increases neurogenesis and reverses learning and memory deficits in rats with kainate-induced seizures. We tested the hypothesis that exploring a wooden pyramid for 3h/d augments neurogenesis and attenuates the learning and memory deficits following chemical lesioning of the hippocampus and motor cortex with kainic acid (KA). A pyramid exploration intervention (PEI) was created by subjecting rats to residing in a pyramidal wooden structure of 3 h/d for 30 d. We also compared the effects on neurogenesis for PEI to those for aerobic (swimming) exercise (EX) and environmental enrichment via exploration of a rectangular-shaped wooden cage. Following KA seizures, the PEI increased brain neurogenesis. Differences in measures of neurogenesis were not significantly different than those for EX and EE. Aerobic (swimming) exercise and novel environment exposures appear to increase neural plasticity and may be considered a complementary treatment for epilepsy.

Keywords: neurogenesis, neural plasticity, environment, learning, memory, behavior, amygdala, hippocampus, motor cortex, complementary and alternative medicine

1. Introduction

Previous studies from our laboratory have shown that regimens of short periods of daily swimming exercise and environmental enrichment increases brain neurogenesis, learning and memory in the kainate rat model of temporal lobe epilepsy [1–3]. Temporal lobe epilepsy (TLE) is associated with oxidative stress, a putative mechanism for neuronal apoptosis [1] and decrements in neural plasticity that impairs the brain's cognitive functions [2]. Oxidative stress is known to reduce neuronal antioxidant and anti-apoptotic activity which damages the brain's learning and memory networks [3]. Epilepsy is often resistant

IntechOpen

to treatment with antiepileptic drugs that are also known to produce oxidative stress and to promote neuronal apoptosis [4]. Manipulation of an animal's environment appears to have the potential for producing physiological, therapeutic effects and are purported to function as environmental enrichment schemes for improving responsiveness to drug treatments. We have reported increases in neurogenesis and improvements in performance of rats on learning and memory tasks associated with environmental enrichment by allowing rats to explore a novel cage with different objects in different configurations for 3 h/d, for 30 d. Another such environmental enrichment intervention involves subjecting rats to stress restraint in a pyramidal wooden structure. This environmental intervention is shown to reduce the physiological and oxidative stresses associated with immobilization and restraint [5].

Nikola Tesla was a mathematician-physicist and the inventor of many of today's most advanced electromagnetic technologies [6]. Among Tesla's hypotheses more, than a hundred years ago, is the prediction that the architectural design of the great pyramid of Egypt produces electromagnetic effects within its chambers [7]. Pyramids are reported to augment local electric fields via a lightning-rod effect [8] and function as electromagnetic conductors [7]; although, the mechanisms remain unclear. It may, therefore, not be an accident of nature that pyramidal-shaped neurons evolved to generate and focus electromagnetic energy in the brain. Pyramidal-shaped neurons comprise 12 billion of the 16 billion neurons in the human cerebral cortex [9]. A psychiatrist-inventor, Hans Berger, in the 1920s, was the first person to demonstrate electroencephalographically-measured brain waves (EEG) [10]. It is now known that each brain wave represents the synchronized action potentials of millions of pyramidal cells in the cerebral cortex [11]. In view of these interesting aspects of pyramids and pyramidal cells in the brain, the present study is designed to test the hypothesis that a pyramid exploration intervention (PEI) augments brain neurogenesis and improves the brain's learning and memory functions in an animal model of TLE.

2. Methods

These studies were approved by the institutional animal care and use review board of Manipal University, Bangalore India, in partnership with the American University of Antigua College of Medicine.

2.1 Animals

The animal subjects were 4-month-old male Wistar rats maintained under conditions of 12-hour light-dark diurnal cycles in Manipal University's Animal Research Facility. The animals were fed *ad libitum* with a normal balanced rat chow diet.

2.2 Experimental design

Figure 1 depicts the study design intended to determine the effects of a pyramid exploration intervention (PEI) on neurogenesis, learning and memory functions in rats. The animals were grouped as follows: 1. Normal control rats (NC); 2. Normal control rats with exposure to the PEI (NC + PEI); 3. Sham control rats with exposure to the PEI (SC + PEI); 4. Kainic acid-lesioned rats; and 5. Kainic acid lesioned rats with exposure to the PEI (KA + PEI). NC animals were undisturbed in their home cages. NC + PEI animals were subjected to the PEI for 3 h/d. SC + PEI

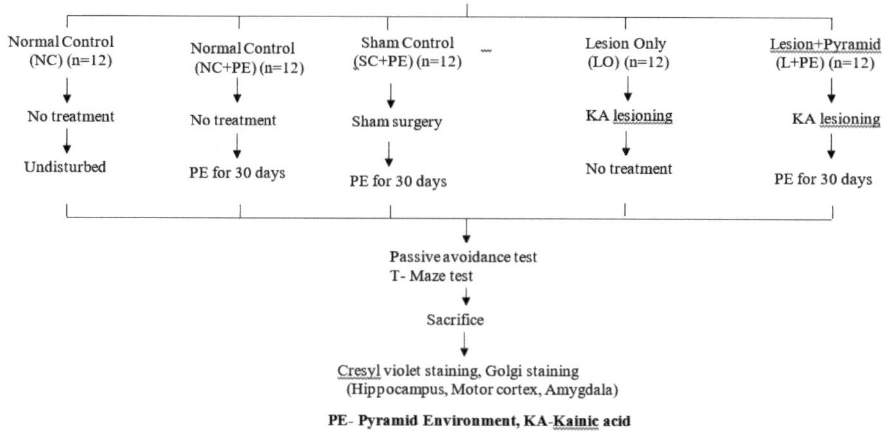

Figure 1.
Experimental design. Summary of the experimental design for demonstrating the effects of an environmental intervention involving exploration of the pyramid structure (PE) shown in ***Figure 1*** *in groups of 4-month-old male Wistar rats.*

animals were subjected to sham surgery followed by exposure to the PEI. The sham surgery involved fixing the rats in a stereotaxic apparatus under general anesthesia after which burr holes were drilled in the skull using stereotaxic coordinates for the lateral ventricles taken from a standard rat brain atlas. A Hamilton syringe was inserted into the lateral ventricles bilaterally and removed without administration of any fluids or drugs. Following suturing of the scalp wounds, the rats were placed back in their home cages and were subjected to the PEI 3 h/d for 30 d. KA animals were administered kainic acid (KA) bilaterally into the lateral ventricles using a Hamilton syringe. Animals in the KA lesioned + PEI group were administered KA and then underwent PEI for 3 h/d for 30 d. The PEI was initiated 1-d after grouping in the NC animals, 1-d after surgery SC + PEI animals and starting on the first postictal day in the KA + PEI group.

2.3 Surgical and related experimental procedures

SC and KA animals were anesthetized with a mixture of ketamine (50 mg/mL), xylazine (4.5 mg/mL) and acepromazine (0.4 mg/mL) at a dose of 0.70 mL/kg body weight and were fixed in the stereotaxic apparatus with the incisor bar situated 3.7 mm below the inter-aural line. The skull was exposed and a burr hole was drilled guided by the stereotaxic coordinates as follows: 3.7 mm from bregma, 4.1 mm lateral from the midline [12]. KA lesioning was accomplished using a Hamilton syringe needle filled with 0.5 μg/μL KA, 1.0 μl of which was administered slowly over 20 min. The KA-filled syringe was lowered from the stereotaxic syringe holder 4.5 mm to reach the lateral ventricles. After the needle was withdrawn, the skin was sutured and the animals were returned to their home cages.

2.4 Pyramid exploration intervention (PEI)

Exposure of animals to PEI was accomplished in a wooden cage of larger dimension than the steel home cage (**Figure 2**). Rats were allowed to explore the PEI environment for 3 h every d for 30 d, beginning immediately following either grouping (normal control group), sham operation (sham-operated control group) or KA + lesioning (kainate experimental group) for 3 h/d for 30 d beginning 1-d the grouping (normal controls), sham operation (sham controls) or KA lesioning.

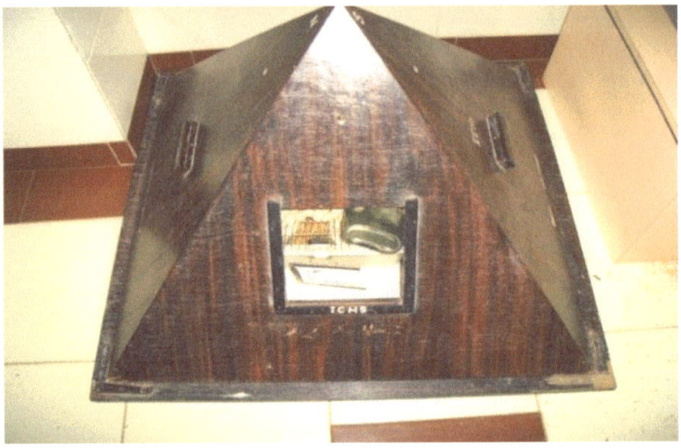

Figure 2.
Pyramid exploration environmental intervention. Rats were allowed to explore this pyramid-shaped wooden structure for 3 h every d for 30 d, beginning immediately following either grouping (normal control group), sham operation (sham-operated control group) or kainate lesioning (kainate experimental group).

2.5 Morphological procedures

Identification of surviving neurons. Surviving neurons were identified by cresyl violet staining of neuronal Nissl substance. Rats were deeply anesthetized with ether and fixation was performed by transcardial perfusion of the left ventricle with 15 ml of 0.9% heparinized saline at 1 mL/min, followed by perfusion with approximately 250 mL of 10% formalin at 1 mL/min. Brains were excised following decapitation. Coronal sections (5-6 mm thickness) were cut and were post-fixed for 24 h using 10% formalin. Tissues were then dehydrated in 70% alcohol for 2 h, 90% alcohol for 2 h, 3 changes in 100% alcohol for 2 h, clearing with xylene for 2 h and embedded in paraffin. A rotatory microtome was used to cut 5 μm thick sections from the mid-dorsal hippocampus and motor cortex. Sections were then mounted serially on gelatinized slides and stained with 0.1% cresyl violet at pH 3.5-3.8. Cresyl violet staining was followed by sequential treatment with 90% and 100% alcohol for 1-2 minutes each, xylene for 2 minutes, followed by mounting in DPX.

Cell counting. Surviving neurons were counted using light microscopy. Total number of surviving neurons were counted in 10 randomly-selected fields, at 40× magnification (Magnus, Olympus Pvt. Ltd. New Delhi, India) and were averaged. Cells with pyknotic nuclei were excluded from the count. The researcher doing the counting was blinded to the animal grouping and experimental treatment.

Identification of dendritic branch points and intersections. Dendritic branch points and intersection were identified by the Golgi-Cox staining procedure with some modifications [13]. Using the same procedure as described above for anesthetization, the brains were quickly removed and incubated in Golgi-Cox fixative, without perfusion or post-fixation. Tissue collected from individual animals were fixed in individual bottles as follows: Brains were maintained as fresh as possible, placed in clean bottles on glass wool or gauze, covered with Golgi-Cox solution and left at room temperature in a room without light to limit oxidation. After 2 days, the Golgi-Cox solution was changed. The brains were exposed to the fixative for 2 weeks followed by impregnation in Golgi-Cox solution and dehydration in the following order: 50% ethanol and 70% ethanol for 1 hour each, 90% ethanol for 2 hours, 100% ethanol for 1 hour. The tissue blocks were then blotted to remove the alcohol from their surface, after which they were carefully mounted on a tissue holder by applying 2 drops of Fevikwik adhesive on the wooden block and the tissue was fixed. Sections were then cut using a base sledge microtome to a thickness of 120 μm. Using a soft brush, sections were collected in 70% ethanol, washed in distilled water for 5 minutes, 5% sodium carbonate for 20 minutes, distilled water for 5 minutes, 70% ethanol–10 minutes consisting of 2 washes for 5 minutes each, 90% ethanol for 10 minutes consisting of 2 washes for 5 minutes each, 100% ethanol for 10 minutes consisting of 2 washes for 5 minutes each, Cedar wood oil for 1 hour, xylene for 10 minutes consisting of 2 washes for 5 minutes each. Sections were mounted on a glass slide using DPX.

Counting of dendritic branch points and intersections. The dendritic branch points and intersections of darkly-stained neurons throughout their arborizations were counted using camera lucida tracing equipment (Dutta Scientific, Bangalore). Neurons exhibiting truncated dendritic branches within a 100 μm radius of the soma were excluded. Interference from adjacent neurons was eliminated as described for neuronal counts. Counting of dendritic branch points and intersections was accomplished by Sholl's concentric circle method [14]. Concentric circles were drawn on a transparent sheet with 20 μm as the radial distance between two adjacent circles. The concentric circles template was placed on the camera lucida-traced neuron so that the center of the neuron's soma coincided with the center of a circle. Then, the number of branch points between the two adjacent circles were counted. Intersections were defined as points of dendrite touching or intersecting with a circle. Branch points and intersections were counted up to a radial distance of 100 μm from the neuronal cell body.

2.6 Behavioral testing

Behavioral tests were administered on the 42nd day following grouping for the NC group and on the 42nd day following surgery or KA-induced seizures for the other groups. All testing was done at approximately 7:00 PM to control for the diurnal variation of night-time activity in rodents.

The T–maze task. Rats were subjected to left-right discrimination, a spatial memory task testing the animal's ability to discriminate the left or right arm of a T-maze for a food reward. The animals were food-deprived for 2 days prior to testing to enhance motivation. The rats were subjected to an orientation period by being placed in the start box for 60 s. The animals were then permitted to explore the T–maze for 30 minutes and to ingest 15 pellets (10 mg/pellet) in each goal area. The animals were then returned to the start box. The orientation was done for 2 consecutive days followed by 6 trials/day for 4 consecutive days.

Spontaneous alternation test. Each animal, after being placed in the start box, was allowed to move into the maze structure where they selected one of the branches of the maze, and once they ingested a food pellet in the goal area they were placed back in the start box for the next trial. The interval between trials was one minute and the maze branch selected by the rat was recorded. At the end of the 4-day experimental period, the total number of branch alternations was used to compute percent bias as follows: (Number of selections of most frequently selected branch ÷ Number of trials) x 100.

Rewarded alternation test. One day after completing the spontaneous alternation test described above, six trials of the rewarded alternation test were performed daily. Each trial included two runs consisting of a forced and a selection run. For the forced run, the animals were forced into one of the branches of the maze by blocking the other branch and they were permitted to ingest the food pellets within the goal area. After eating the food in the goal area, they were placed back in the start box to perform the selection run. For the selection run, the goal area of the forced branch of the maze was kept empty and food pellets were placed in the goal area of the alternate branch. Both maze branches were accessible to the animals;

a one-minute pause separated each forced and selection run and there was another one-minute pause between each trial. Maze branch selection was predetermined and was the same for all animals on a given day; on the next day, the forced branch was changed. For the selection run, a correct response was recorded whenever the branch opposite to the forced branch was selected and *vice versa* for recording of an incorrect response. Percentage of correct responses was computed as follows: (Number of correct responses ÷ Number of trials) x 100.

Passive-avoidance learning and memory test. This test has the following 3 parts: i) an exploration test, ii) an aversive stimulation and learning phase (passive-avoidance acquisition), and iii) a retention test.

Exploration test. Each animal performed three exploration tests per day. The interval between trials was five minutes and each trial was three minutes in duration. Each animal was placed in the center of a large compartment facing away from the entrance to a dark small one. The door between the large and small compartments was open and the animal was permitted to explore both the large and small compartments for three minutes. Time within the large compartment, time within the small compartment and number of crossings from large to small compartments were recorded as a measure of exploration. Animals were then replaced in the home cage, where they were maintained for the five-minute interval between trials and this sequence was repeated three thrice for each animal.

Aversive stimulation and learning phase: passive-avoidance acquisition test. Each animal was forced into the smaller compartment and the sliding door between the two compartments was closed following the last exploration trial. Then, 3 strong electric foot pulses of 50 Hertz, 1.5 milliamps, 1.0 second in duration were administered at five-second intervals, and the animal was returned to their home cage.

Memory retention task. The memory retention task was done twenty-four hours after the previously described acquisition test. For this test, the animals were maintained in the center of the large compartment and each animal was permitted to explore the compartments for three minutes after which they were returned to their home cages. This sequence was repeated three times with an interval between trials of five minutes. Time in the large compartment, time in the small compartment and number of crossings from large to small compartment were recorded as measures of exploration.

2.7 Data analysis

Analysis of variance (ANOVA) with Bonferroni's post-hoc test was performed to estimate the statistical significance of differences between groups (GraphPad Prism, version 5). Across the groups, correlations between the most relevant morphometric and behavioral measurements were evaluated by Pearson's product moment correlation coefficient (r). Neurogenesis parameters were compared for similar experiments performed under conditions of PEI, aerobic (swimming) exercise and another form of environmental enrichment [1–3]. Statistical significances were guaranteed at $P \leq 0.05$.

3. Results

3.1 Morphometric measurements in hippocampus, amygdala and motor cortex

Figure 3 shows the effects of the PEI, with and without KA lesioning, on the CA3 area of hippocampus by light microscopy. The PEI was associated with

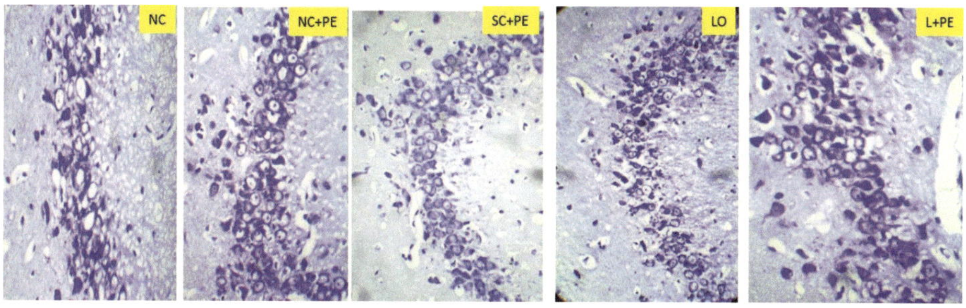

Figure 3.
Effects of a pyramid exploration environmental intervention on neurons in area CA3 of hippocampus. Photomicrographs showing the surviving neurons in groups of 4 month-old male Wistar rats exposed to the following conditions: Normal control (NC), normal control followed by pyramid exploration, PE (NC + PE), sham-operated control followed by environmental enrichment (SC + PE), kainic acid-induced lesioning and seizures (LO) followed by immediate, 1-d post-lesion exposure to the PE (L + PE). Magnification 40x.

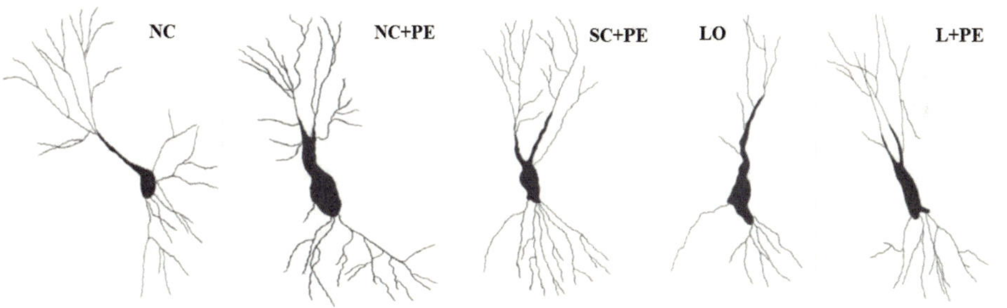

Figure 4.
Effects of a pyramid exploration environmental intervention on dendritic branching depicted by camera lucida. Effects of pyramid exploration (PE) on the dendritic branch points and intersections of the surviving neurons in hippocampal area CA3 depicted by light microscopic camera lucida tracings subjects are groups of 4 month-old male Wistar rats exposed to the following conditions: Normal control (NC), normal control followed by PE, (NC + PE), sham-operated control followed by PE (SC + PE), kainic acid-induced lesioning and seizures (LO) followed by PE (L + PE).

significant increases in the numbers of surviving neurons in the normal and sham-operated control groups and after KA lesioning in the experimental group (data not shown). The PEI also produced significant increases in the numbers of surviving neurons in hippocampal area CA1, dentate gyrus, basolateral amygdala and motor cortex in the controls and in the KA-lesioned animals (data not shown).

Figure 4 depicts the effects of the PEI on the dendritic branching of the surviving neurons in hippocampal area CA3 by light microscopic camera lucida tracings.

Figure 5 shows the morphometric measurements of the effects of the PEI on the counts of branch points and intersections in hippocampal area CA3. These data demonstrate that exposure to the PEI produced significant increases in the branch points and intersections both in the presence and in the absence of KA lesioning. Similar increases were found in dentate gyrus, amygdala and motor cortex and in animals subjected to delayed exposure to the PEI after a delay of 60 d, postictal.

3.2 Behavioral measurements

The PEI was associated with significant increases in the percent bias, percentage of correct responses and the number of alternations on the T-maze learning task.

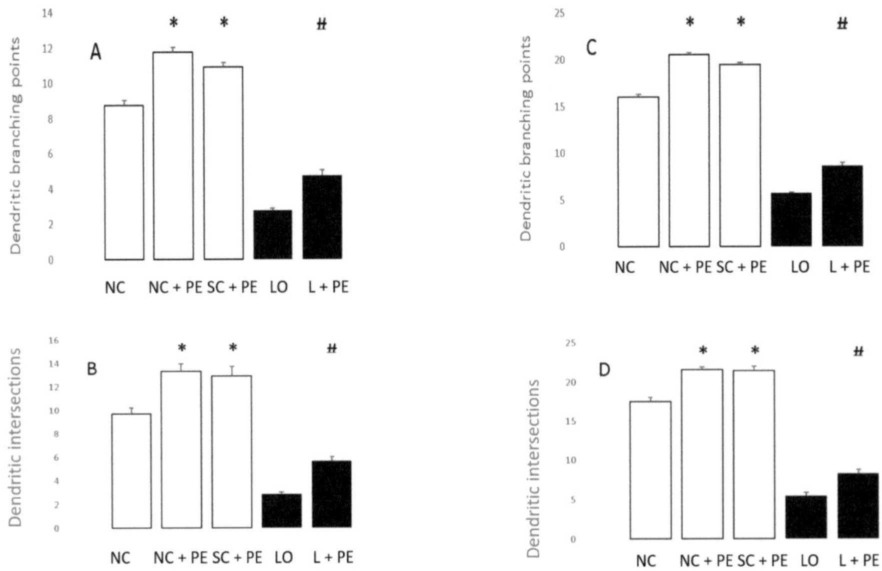

Figure 5.
*Effects of a pyramid exploration environmental intervention on dendritic branch points and intersections in hippocampus. Morphometric cell counts of the surviving neurons in hippocampal area CA3 for groups of 4 month-old male Wistar rats exposed to the following conditions: Normal control (NC), normal control followed by pyramid exploration PE (NC + PE), sham-operated control followed by PE (SC + PE), kainic acid esioning and seizures (LO) followed by PE (L + PE). Panels A and C: Effects of the PE intervention initiated 1-d following grouping in the controls, 1-d postsurgical in the sham-operated controls and 1-d postictal in the kainate-lesioned rats. Panels B and D: Effects of the PE intervention initiated 60-d following grouping in the normal controls, 60-d postsurgical in the sham-operated controls and 60-d postictal in the kainate-lesioned rats. Intergroup differences significant at *$P < 0.05$, #$P < 0.01$.*

Percentage of correct responses for the animals subjected to the PEI for 30 d starting at the first postictal day was positively correlated with the number of surviving neurons in all the brain areas studied, across the five study groups ($r = 0.92$-0.97, $P < 0.001$). Percentage of correct responses for these animals was also positively correlated with the number of apical and basal dendritic branch points and intersections in the same brain areas, across the five study groups ($r = 0.88$-0.94, $P < 0.01$).

Figure 6 presents the effects of the PEI on the exploration and retention phases of passive-avoidance testing. The PEI was associated with significant decrements in the time spent within a small compartment where an aversive stimulus was previously administered and in the number of crossings. The same pattern of behavioral responses was observed in animals subjected to the PEI for 30 d immediately, starting 1-d postictal, as well as, after a 60-d delay postictal. Similar to the morphometric and T-maze data, these changes were observed in the animals subjected to the PEI. Time spent in the small compartment avoiding the aversive stimulus was negatively correlated with the number of surviving neurons in all the brain areas studied, across the five study groups ($r = -0.93$ to -0.99, $P < 0.001$). Time spent in the small compartment was also negatively correlated with the number of apical and basal dendritic branch points and intersections in the same brain areas, across the five study groups ($r = -0.88$ to -0.95, $P < 0.01$).

Table 1 summarizes comparisons of the effects of the pyramid exploration intervention (PEI), environmental enrichment in the absence of pyramid exploration (EE) and aerobic (swimming) exercise (EX) on the numbers of surviving neurons in hippocampal area CA3. There were no significant differences in neurogenesis between these three interventions ($P > 0.1$). Similar results were found for the dendritic branch points and intersections in area CA3 (data not shown).

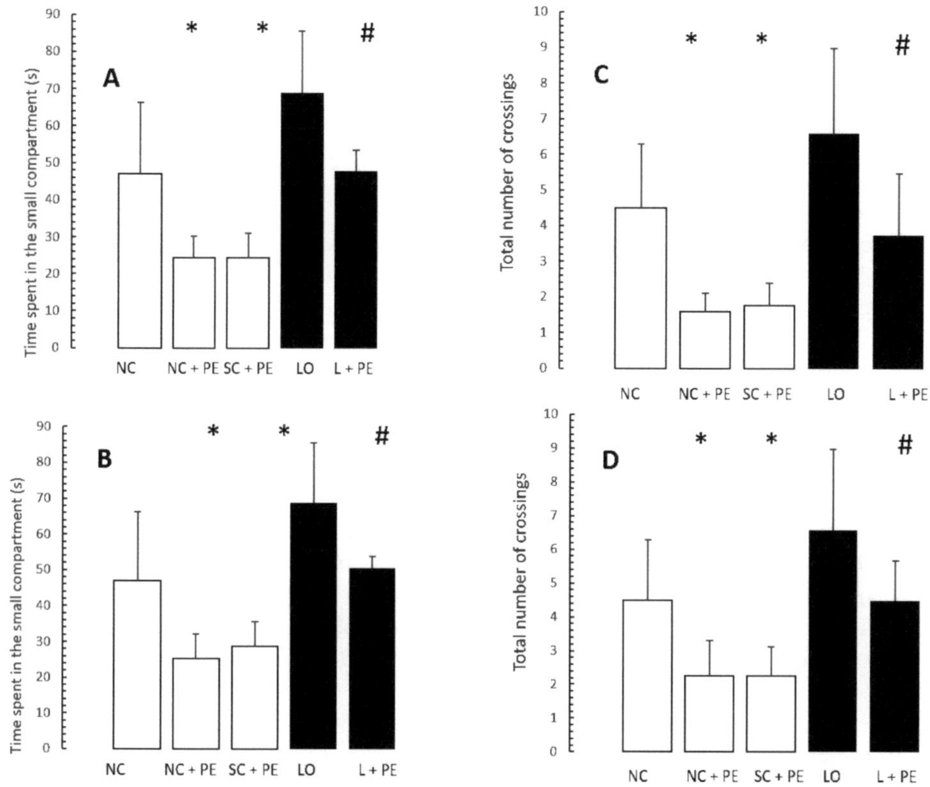

Figure 6.
Effects of a pyramid exploration environmental intervention on a memory passive-avoidance task. Bars compare means ± standard deviations of time spent in a small compartment where there was previous exposure to an aversive stimulus, expressed in s/trial) and total number of crossings in groups of 4 month-old male Wistar rats exposed to the following conditions: Normal control (NC), normal control plus pyramid exploration, PE (NC + PE) and sham-operated control plus PE (SC + PE), kainic acid lesioning and seizures (LO) followed by PE (L + PE). Panels A and B: Effects of the PE intervention initiated 1-d following grouping in the normal controls, 1-d postsurgical in the sham-operated controls and 1-d postictal in the kainate-lesioned rats. Panels C and D: Effects of the PE intervention initiated 60-d following grouping in the normal controls, 60-d postsurgical in the sham-operated controls and 60-d postictal in the kainate-lesioned rats. Intergroup differences significant at $^{*}P < 0.05$, $^{\#}P < 0.01$.

PEI	**104.3 ± 4.457**	**EE**	**108.8 ± 3.601**	**EX**	**105.7 ± 4.412**
SC	103.3 ± 8.359	SC	104.3 ± 4.457	SC	98.83 ± 7.055
KA	60.33 ± 1.966	KA	68.50 ± 3.146	KA	64.83 ± 4.491

PEI = pyramid exploration intervention; EE = environmental enrichment; EX = aerobic swimming exercise; SC = sham control; KA = kainic acid lesion.
Data expressed in means ± standard deviations.
PEI vs. EE vs. EX were not significantly different, P > 0.1.

Table 1.
Number of surviving neurons in hippocampal area CA3.

4. Discussion

The main findings of this study are that morphometrically-measured rat brain neurogenesis and performance-measured learning and memory behavioral tasks are augmented by a pyramidal exploration intervention (PEI). The PEI permitted rats to explore a wooden pyramid for 3 h/d. The PEI was associated with increments in the numbers of surviving neurons, apical and basal dendritic branch points and intersections at hippocampal areas CA1 and CA3, amygdala and motor cortex suggestive of increased neurogenesis and improved learning and memory under control and postictal conditions. This evidence of increased neurogenesis is bolstered by highly significant correlations, across the five study groups. We found significant positive correlations between the animals' percentage of correct responses on a T-maze (learning) task, the numbers of surviving neurons and the numbers of dendritic branch points (r = 0.88-0.94). We found similar significant, but negative, correlations between the time the animals spent in a small compartment avoiding an aversive stimulus (memory task) and the numbers of surviving neurons, dendritic branch points and intersections (r = −0.88 to −0.99). These findings demonstrate that, whether a control or an experimental animal, rats with more neurons and more dendritic intersections (synapses) in the four brain areas studied had greater learning of a T-maze strategy, as well as, greater memory for avoiding an aversive stimulus.

We have previously shown increases in rat brain neurogenesis and improvements in performance on the same learning and memory tasks as employed in the present study associated with an environmental enrichment intervention involving exploration of a wooden square structure containing novel objects in novel configurations for 3 h/d [3]. We designed the present study to expand the previous studies to a different type of environmental intervention, the exploration of a pyramid-shaped wooden house for 3 h/d. We used a pyramid-shaped structure to emulate prior studies demonstrating that housing in pyramid while exposed to restraint stress counteracts the parameters of oxidative stress associated with the animal restraint [5]. Oxidative stress causes accumulation of superoxide and other free radicals—highly reactive oxygen and nitrogen species such as superoxide and hydroxyl radical anions, nitric oxide, nitrogen dioxide and peroxynitrite [15]. These highly reactive oxygen and nitrogen species (ROS/RNS) do not accumulate under normal conditions because they are neutralized/scavenged by antioxidant enzymes such as superoxide dismutase, catalase and glutathione reductase synthesized by, and stored in, each normal healthy cell [16]. Oxidative stress occurs when the balance between production and neutralizing/scavenging favors accumulation of ROS/RNS [17]. Such accumulation of ROS/RNS causes peroxidation of lipids in the cell's plasma and organelle membranes [16]. ROS/RNS-dependent enzymes are known to function normally under conditions of very low, physiological levels of ROS/RNS [17].

The aforementioned pyramid exposure appears to protect against the restraint stress-induced atrophy of the hippocampus [5]. Oxidative stress is shown to be a pathophysiologic feature of KA-induced seizures [18]. The PEI in the present study is, like the aforementioned pyramid study involving stress restraint, associated with physiologically-significant effects, evidenced by significant correlations between morphometric and behavioral measurements across the five study groups. Pyramid exposure is also shown to increase the amplitude of electroencephalographically-measured alpha waves [19], and positive mood responses associated with meditation [20, 21]. Electroencephalography and monitoring of emotional functions were beyond the scope of the present study. However, hippocampus is an important source of emotional responsiveness and theta waves [22]. Theta and alpha waves propagate together in the neocortex when cognitive tasks are performed [23]. It is, therefore, plausible that the increases in neurogenesis and improvements in behavior observed in the present study are likely to have been reflected in brain waves and emotional responses.

KA-induced seizures are also a stimulus for neurogenesis, associated with increased numbers of neural progenitor (stem) cells within the subgranular zone of hippocampus, amygdala sensorimotor cortex [24] but motor cortex neurogenesis has not been extensively studied. It was beyond the scope of the present study to identify neural stem cells and to measure the immediate effect of the KA-induced seizures but we assume that our morphometric counts of surviving neurons, dendritic branch points and intersections after a 30-d period is a fair reflection of the seizure-induced neuronal death followed by neural stem cell proliferation known to occur in the KA rat model of TLE.

5. Conclusion

The results of this study demonstrate that regular exposure of rats to a wooden, pyramidal-shaped environment for their exploration 3 h/d increases neurogenesis learning and memory, under normal control conditions, after a (sham) surgical intervention and following KA-induced seizures. These findings should be interpreted cautiously because previous studies from our laboratory have shown that the same benefits accrue from an environmental enrichment by exposing animals to exploration of a rectangular wooden cage with novel objects in novel configurations for 3 h/d and aerobic (swimming) exercise [1–3]. It is, therefore, likely that pyramid effects are nonspecific and are the result of exposing animals to any novel environment. We, therefore, conclude that pyramid exposure is probably not different than other modes of environmental enrichment for augmenting brain neurogenesis and improving learning and memory functions. Future studies should determine whether exposure to novel environments are effective as complementary or alternative treatments for the wide variety of neurological diseases wherein full recovery of learning and memory functions may be limited by ineffective neurogenesis.

Acknowledgements

This work was funded by a grant from Manipal University.

Conflict of interest statement

The authors report no conflicts-of-interest.

Data availability

The data supporting this research is available upon request to the corresponding author.

Author details

Vasavi R. Gorantla[1*], Sabyasachi Maity[2] and Richard M. Millis[3]

1 Department of Anatomy, St. George's University School of Medicine, Grenada, West Indies

2 Department of Physiology, St. George's University School of Medicine, Grenada, West Indies

3 Department of Pathophysiology, American University of Antigua College of Medicine, Antigua and Barbuda, West Indies

*Address all correspondence to: vgorantl@sgu.edu

References

[1] Gorantla VR, Sirigiri A, Volkova YA, Millis RM. Effects of Swimming Exercise on Limbic and Motor Cortex Neurogenesis in the Kainate-Lesion Model of Temporal Lobe Epilepsy. Cardiovasc Psychiatry Neurol. 2016;2016:3915767. doi: 10.1155/2016/3915767. Epub 2016 May 22. PMID: 27313873; PMCID: PMC4893441.

[2] Gorantla VR, Pemminati S, Bond V, Meyers DG, Millis RM. Effects of Swimming Exercise on Learning and Memory in the Kainate-Lesion Model of Temporal Lobe Epilepsy. J Clin Diagn Res. 2016 Nov;10(11):CF01-CF05. doi: 10.7860/JCDR/2016/22100.8835. Epub 2016 Nov 1. PMID: 28050361; PMCID: PMC5198314.

[3] Gorantla VR, Thomas SE, Millis RM. Environmental Enrichment and Brain Neuroplasticity in the Kainate Rat Model of Temporal Lobe Epilepsy. J Epilepsy Res. 2019 Jun 30;9(1):51-64. doi: 10.14581/jer.19006. PMID: 31482057; PMCID: PMC6706649.

[4] Méndez-Armenta M, Nava-Ruíz C, Juárez-Rebollar D, Rodríguez-Martínez E, Gómez PY. Oxidative stress associated with neuronal apoptosis in experimental models of epilepsy. Oxid Med Cell Longev. 2014;2014:293689. doi: 10.1155/2014/293689. Epub 2014 Dec 29. PMID: 25614776; PMCID: PMC4295154.

[5] Bhat MS, Rao G, Murthy KD, Bhat PG. Housing in pyramid counteracts neuroendocrine and oxidative stress caused by chronic restraint in rats. Evid Based Complement Alternat Med. 2007 Mar;4(1):35-42. doi: 10.1093/ecam/nel049. Epub 2006 Jul 26. PMID: 17342239; PMCID: PMC1810373.

[6] Bradley R. Nikola Tesla, a man of his time. Physics Today, https://doi.org/10.1063/PT.3.4432 **73**, 3, 51 (2020)

[7] Balezin, Mikhail & Baryshnikova, Kseniia & Kapitanova, Polina & Evlyukhin, Andrey. (2018). Electromagnetic properties of the Great Pyramid: First multipole resonances and energy concentration. Journal of Applied Physics. 124. 034903. 10.1063/1.5026556.

[8] Kumar S, Johnson TW, Wood CK, Qu T, Wittenberg NJ, Otto LM, Shaver J, Long NJ, Victora RH, Edel JB, Oh SH. Template-Stripped Multifunctional Wedge and Pyramid Arrays for Magnetic Nanofocusing and Optical Sensing. ACS Appl Mater Interfaces. 2016 Apr 13;8(14):9319-26. doi: 10.1021/acsami.5b12157. Epub 2016 Feb 29. PMID: 26837912; PMCID: PMC4832397.

[9] Herculano-Houzel S. The human brain in numbers: a linearly scaled-up primate brain. Front Hum Neurosci. 2009 Nov 9;3:31. doi: 10.3389/neuro.09.031.2009. PMID: 19915731; PMCID: PMC2776484.

[10] Tudor M, Tudor L, Tudor KI. Hans Berger (1873-1941)--povijest elektroencefalografije [Hans Berger (1873-1941)--the history of electroencephalography]. Acta Med Croatica. 2005;59(4):307-13. Croatian. PMID: 16334737.

[11] Nunez PL, Srinivasan R, Fields RD. EEG functional connectivity, axon delays and white matter disease. Clin Neurophysiol. 2015 Jan;126(1):110-20. doi: 10.1016/j.clinph.2014.04.003. Epub 2014 Apr 13. PMID: 24815984; PMCID: PMC5018992.

[12] Paxinos G, Watson C. *The Rat Brain in Stereotaxic Coordinates*, Academic Press, 7th edition. 2013.

[13] Shankaranarayana BS, Raju TR. The Golgi techniques for staining neurons. In: Raju TR, et al (ed). *Brain and behavior*. Bangalore, India:

National Institute of Mental Health and Neurosciences. 2004:108-11.

[14] Sholl DA. Dendritic organization in the neurons of the visual and motor cortices of the cat. J Anat. 1953 Oct;87(4):387-406. PMID: 13117757; PMCID: PMC1244622.

[15] Phaniendra A, Jestadi DB, Periyasamy L. Free radicals: properties, sources, targets, and their implication in various diseases. Indian J Clin Biochem. 2015 Jan;30(1):11-26. doi: 10.1007/s12291-014-0446-0. Epub 2014 Jul 15. PMID: 25646037; PMCID: PMC4310837.

[16] Di Meo S, Reed TT, Venditti P, Victor VM. Role of ROS and RNS Sources in Physiological and Pathological Conditions. Oxid Med Cell Longev. 2016;2016:1245049. doi: 10.1155/2016/1245049. Epub 2016 Jul 12. PMID: 27478531; PMCID: PMC4960346.

[17] Ayala A, Muñoz MF, Argüelles S. Lipid peroxidation: production, metabolism, and signaling mechanisms of malondialdehyde and 4-hydroxy-2-nonenal. Oxid Med Cell Longev. 2014;2014:360438. doi: 10.1155/2014/360438. Epub 2014 May 8. PMID: 24999379; PMCID: PMC4066722.

[18] Shin EJ, Jeong JH, Chung YH, Kim WK, Ko KH, Bach JH, Hong JS, Yoneda Y, Kim HC. Role of oxidative stress in epileptic seizures. Neurochem Int. 2011 Aug;59(2):122-37. doi: 10.1016/j.neuint.2011.03.025. Epub 2011 Jun 13. PMID: 21672578; PMCID: PMC3606551.

[19] Stark NH. What can a pyramid do? In: The First Practical Pyramid Book, KS: Sheed Andrews and McMeel Inc., Kansas City, 1977, 29.

[20] Schul B, Pettit E. The pyramid and altered states of consciousness. In: The Secret Power of Pyramids, New York: Fawcett Gold Medal, 1975, 61-177.

[21] Toth M, Nielsen G. Transform yourself with pyramid energy. In: Pyramid Power, Vermont, USA, Inner Traditions India, 1985, 124-38.

[22] Tyng CM, Amin HU, Saad MNM, Malik AS. The Influences of Emotion on Learning and Memory. Front Psychol. 2017 Aug 24;8:1454. doi: 10.3389/fpsyg.2017.01454. PMID: 28883804; PMCID: PMC5573739.

[23] Alamia A, VanRullen R. Alpha oscillations and traveling waves: Signatures of predictive coding? PLoS Biol. 2019 Oct 3;17(10):e3000487. doi: 10.1371/journal.pbio.3000487. PMID: 31581198; PMCID: PMC6776260.

[24] Vessal M, Darian-Smith C. Adult neurogenesis occurs in primate sensorimotor cortex following cervical dorsal rhizotomy. Version 2. J Neurosci. 2010 Jun 23;30(25):8613-23. doi: 10.1523/JNEUROSCI.5272-09.2010. PMID: 20573907; PMCID: PMC2897730.

Chapter 15

Current Status and Potential Challenges of Cell-Based Therapy for Treating Status Epilepticus and Chronic Epilepsy

Huifang Zhao and Zhiyuan Li

Abstract

Epilepsy is the fourth most common neurological condition characterized by recurrent unprovoked seizures. Chronic and recurrent seizures may give rise to cell necrosis, astrocyte activation, neuron death, reactive oxygen species (ROS) production, and mitochondria dysfunction. Recent studies have shown that cell-based therapy is a promising treatment option for epilepsy. Various stem cell types were used for treatment of epilepsy in basic and experimental researches. It is especially vital to gauge the efficacy of distinct donor cell types, such as the embryonic stem cells and induced pluripotent stem cells (iPSCs), mesenchymal stem cells (MSCs), hippocampal precursor cells, γ-aminobutyric acid-ergic progenitors, neural stem cells. The goal of this chapter is to evaluate the progress made hitherto in this area and to discuss the prospect for cell-based therapy for epilepsy.

Keywords: epilepsy, seizures, mesenchymal stem cells, neural stem cell transplantation

1. Introduction

Epilepsy is a neurological disorder, characterized by recurrent (two or more) epileptic seizures resulting from excessive and abnormal cortical neural activity. There are tens of millions people experiencing epilepsy [1]. Causes of epilepsy are complex, such as a toxic ingestion, serious head injury, stroke, tumor, complications of other brain diseases and genetic mutation. Epilepsy may occur after some brain infections such as meningitis, herpes simplex encephalitis, pork tapeworm (cysticercosis), cerebral malaria, toxoplasmosis, and toxocariasis. Genetics is believed to be involved in the majority of cases, either directly or indirectly. Around 0.095% of all deaths are on account of status epilepticus or seizure [2]. Approximately 30% of epileptic patients have temporal lobe epilepsy(TLE) which causes neuronal cell death, aberrant mossy fiber sprouting (MFS) [3], hippocampal damage [4] and cognitive deteriorations [5]. The past 30 years have seen the introduction of over fifteen kinds of third-generation antiepileptic drugs (AEDs) that provide more options for different types of seizures [6]. However, approximately 30% of patients continue to have process of epilepsies [7, 8]. For drug-resistant epilepsy, AEDs are unable to prevent or reverse the process of disease. The treatment was not effective [9]. Furthermore, the patients that respond to AEDs typically experience adverse systemic side effects, underscoring the urgent need to develop new therapies that target epileptic foci rather than more systemic interventions.

Based on the high incidence of this disease and the limited treatment options available, it makes sense to explore and analyze the new treatment strategies to inhibit or prevent epileptic-related neuronal changes. Due to the potential for providing neuroprotection, diminishing inflammation and curbing epileptogenesis of Mesenchymal stem cells, the development of chronic epilepsy typified by spontaneous seizures and learning and memory impairments may be restrained. In this chapter, the efficacy of MSCs to restrain neurodegeneration, inflammation, and epileptogenesis were discussed [10]. Neural stem cells and neural progenitors (NSC/NPCs) have broad application prospect in neuro-restorative therapy due to their survival of intracerebral grafting, remarkable capacity for self-renewal, release a multitude of neurotrophic factors, plasticity, and ability to integrate into host brain circuitry [11]. This paper reviewed different cell sources and strategies of using MSC and progenitor cells to treat epilepsy by establishing new neurons that incorporate into host brain circuits.

2. Mesenchymal stem cells and epilepsy

2.1 Properties of mesenchymal stem cells

MSCs were discovered in bone marrow in 1966 for the first time [12]. The therapeutic potential of bone marrow mesenchymal stem cell (BMSC) transplantation has recently been investigated in various pathological conditions of the central nervous system (CNS) [13–16]. Subsequently, MSCs were widely and gradually isolated from various tissues, including adipose, tooth root, umbilical cord, muscle [17–19]. For more scientific comparison and contrast of research results, the minimal criteria for MSCs was defined by the International Society for Cellular Therapy (ISCT) including plastic adherent growth, express CD105, CD73 and CD90, and lack expression of CD45, CD34, CD14 or CD11b, CD79 or CD19 and HLA-DR surface molecules [20]. MSC were able to differentiate into adipocytes, cardiomyocytes, chondrocytes, osteocytes, and myoblasts, both in vitro and in vivo. Early studies showed that MSC can differentiate into CNS glia and neurons and express neural cell markers in vivo. In addition, these cells are readily available as donor cells because MSCs can be obtained freshly from human umbilical cord, bone marrow and cord blood. MSCs or MSC-like cells can also be amplified from fresh and frozen samples of several other tissues.

2.2 MSC-based therapy for epilepsy

Some evidence shows that MSC secretes a large number of cytokines and growth factors through a paracrine mechanism to stimulate endogenous protection and recovery responses [21, 22]. In addition, mesenchymal stem cells express gene-encoded proteins, which are involved in a variety of biological activities, including immunity, angiogenesis, and neuronal functions [23]. After an experimental stroke in rats, intravenous injection of human mesenchymal stem cells can enhance the production of neurotrophins and reduce the death of ischemic tissue [24]. Direct implantation of human mesenchymal stem cells into the hippocampus of mice can induce the proliferation, migration, differentiation and neurogenesis of endogenous neural stem cells [25]. Mesenchymal stem cells have neuroprotective properties by enhancing the antioxidant effect of cells in nerve cells in vitro. At the same time, they also show immunomodulatory effects in vitro, including inhibiting the maturation of dendritic cells and the proliferation of T cells and B cells [26]. Mesenchymal stem cells have the ability to transdifferentiate into nerve cells and have the properties of immune regulation and neuroprotection. Thus, mesenchymal stem cells are involved in many physiological and pathological processes, including cell homeostasis, aging, tissue damage, and inflammatory diseases.

A number of approaches have been tested using cell therapy in epilepsy models (**Table 1**). The pilocarpine model of rat epilepsy is the most common model in the study, because it is similar to the characteristics of human epilepsy. After the injection of pilocarpine, the animal has cholinergic effects, seizures and subsequent chronic epilepsy symptom. 3×10^6 rat autologous BMSCs in 500 μl PBS were injected intravenously to adult male Sprague–Dawley rats 24 and 36 hours after the first seizure. The results of the behavioral test revealed that the number of seizures in the treatment group was significantly reduced. The histopathology of untreated rat tissue showed cell death and neurophagy. The digital density of neurons in each area was significantly higher in the treated group than in the untreated group [27].

Gianina Teribele Venturin et al. found that bone marrow mononuclear cells (BMMCs) transplantation to chronic epileptic rats via tail vein injection decreased the frequency of spontaneous recurrent seizures (SRS), prevented the learning and memory deterioration [28]. In that work, 1×10^7 cells were administered 22 days after Status epilepticus (SE). Here, they showed for the first time that BMMCs reduced the frequency but not the duration of SRS. To evaluate whether BMMCs can reverse the cognitive deficits, the Morris water maze was used to test spatial memory. A 60-s probe test confirmed that lithium–pilocarpine impairs the acquisition of spatial memory and that BMMCs reverse this effect. In other words, Transplantation of BMMCs improved the learning and long-term spatial memory impairments after cell transplantation. This is a pioneering study providing behavioral evidence supporting cell-based therapy for chronic epilepsy. Further research is needed to clarify the mechanism by which transplanted cells exert their effects.

Another study in a mouse model examined the effects of intravenous route of EGFP transgenic mice or male Wistar rats BM-derived MSCs [29]. Transplantation of BMCs prevents spontaneous seizures in pilocarpine-treated rats. They also examined the electrophysiological properties of rat brain sections from the different experimental groups. In saline-epileptic animals, the field excitatory postsynaptic potentials (fEPSPs) by stimulation of Schaffer's vein was reduced 10 days after SE compared with the non-epileptic rats in the control group; however, an incremental increase in fEPSPs amplitude was observed in the BMC-epileptic animals. Qualitative analysis of Nissl-stained neurons showed histological lesions in the epileptic rats including neuron shrunken, pycnotic nuclei and severe reduction in the neuronal density. The digital density of neurons in each area was significantly higher in the treated group than in the untreated group. After transplantation, cells were localized in the cortex and/or hippocampus, perirhinal cortex and basomedial amygdale. In addition, no tissue damage or tumor formation was found in animals transplanted with BMSCs, and no systemic complications or increased morbidity occurred in epileptic animals with intravenous BMSCs.

Several studies have also examined the bystander effects of the mesenchymal stem cells that modulate the host environment. Daejong Jeon et al. demonstrate that a cytosolic extract of human ASCs (ASCs-E) mitigated the activity of seizure spikes following diazepam treatment and inhibited SRS in mice [30]. The evidence indicates that ASCs-E can effectively regulate the pathogenesis in epilepsy models and improved behavioral performance. They also suggest a stem cell–based, noninvasive therapy for the treatment of epilepsy. Further investigation of the capability of MSCs for anticonvulsant potential showed matching results.

References	Model	Type of MSC	Number of MSC	Route of administration	Period after SE	Outcome measures examined	Major findings
[29]	SE injecting pilocarpine	BMCs from EGFP transgenic mice	1×10^6 cells	Intravenous route via the tail vein	15-21 days 110-117 days	Electrophysiological immunofluorescence volume estimation neuronal density	Reduced seizures in the chronic phase Protective effects on LTP Decreased neurodegeneration Engrafting of some BM-MNCs into the hippocampus and cortex
[30]	SE injecting pilocarpine	Human ASCs	1×10^6 cells	Intraperitoneally administrated to C57BL/6 mice	7 days	Blood-brain barrier (BBB) leakage EEG Behavioral tasks	Earlier attenuation of seizure spike activities; reduction of BBB leakage, and inhibition of the development of epilepsy. Human ASCs-E treatment (for 7 days) during the chronic epileptic stage suppressed SRS and reduced abnormal epileptic behavioral phenotypes.
[32]	Pentylenetetrazole (PTZ)-induced epileptogenesis	MSCs	1×10^6 cells	Intravenous injection	Two weeks	Determination of GABA level by HPLC; immunohistochemistry; determination of oxidant and antioxidant markers; assessment of cognitive function and motor coordination	Enhanced the motor coordination; increased ambulation frequency; they enhanced the GABA neurotransmitter levels;
[37]	Pilocarpine-induced SE	Human umbilical mesenchymal stem cells	1×10^5cells	Intra-hippocampal transplantation	Two to four weeks	Simultaneous video and electroencephalographic recordings	The number of SRMS was significantly decreased; reduced pyramidal neuron loss

DOI: http://dx.doi.org/10.5772/intechopen.93811

References	Model	Type of MSC	Number of MSC	Route of administration	Period after SE	Outcome measures examined	Major findings
[38]	Pilocarpine-induced SE	BMSCs	1×10^5 cells	Injected either intravenously (IV) or in hippocampus bilaterally (1C)	15 days	Determination of reduced glutathione content, lipid peroxidation, paraoxonase activity, IL-1β and TNF-α; histopathological investigation; immunohistochemical assay	Ameliorated the pilocarpine-induced neurochemical and histological changes, retained amino acid neurotransmitters to the normal level, downregulated the immunoreactivity to insulin growth factor-1 receptor, synaptophysin, and caspase-3 and reduced oxidative insult and inflammatory markers.

Table 1.
Stem cell transplantation studies in epilepsy models.

The results of Filip et al. [31] clearly demonstrated that gabapentin enhances GABA-ergic neurotransmission and reduced the severity of epilepsy caused by PTZ kindling. Their results showed that the injection of mesenchymal stem cells enhanced the level of GABA inhibitory neurotransmitter and had a greater reduction in the severity of epilepsy [32]. In addition, research results showed that MSCs can not only improve the severity of seizures and oxidative stress damage, but also improve pentylenetetrazol (PTZ)-induced motor incoordination and cognitive impairment. These functions may benefit from the ability of mesenchymal stem cells to migrate and return to damaged areas, and self-renewal and differentiation potential for neuronal death during epilepsy [33, 34]. In this study, they also found that the expression of microglia and neuronal markers were increased after injections of MSCs, which can be clearly seen from the immunohistochemical expression of the glial cell marker S100β protein. Previous studies have reported that mesenchymal stem cells can differentiate into glial cell-like cells in phenotype and function, and can be used as a suitable glial cell substitute for nerve repair and regeneration in clinical applications [35]. In addition, transplanted cells can provide a large amount of neurotrophic factors including brain-derived neurotrophic factor, nerve growth factor, and neurotrophic factor-3 [36]. In conclusion, MSCs could be a promising therapeutic option in the management of chronic epilepsy.

Indeed, a follow-up study using a mouse model of status epilepticus demonstrated that transplantation of human umbilical mesenchymal stem cells (HUMSCs) into bilateral hippocampi ameliorated seizure activity [37]. They examined the effects of intra-hippocampal transplantation of HUMSCs on pilocarpine-treated rats. The results of video and electroencephalography (EEG) recordings from two to four week after PBS injection or HUMSC implantation showed that pilocarpine-induced SE in terms of onset, incidence, and duration were attenuated. In addition, other pathological changes after pilocarpine-induced SE such as brain edema, hippocampal cytoarchitecture, and integrity of the hippocampal pyramidal neurons were evaluated. Magnetic resonance imaging [MRI] was performed on each rat at one week before SE and one, eight, 15, 22, and 29 days afterward. The edema in the lateral ventricles, piriform cortex, and hippocampus at eight days was similar to that at one day after HUMSCs transplantation. Then, histo-morphologically on Nissl stained coronal sections was performed to examine possible changes in the cytoarchitecture. The dorsal hippocampus was significantly enlarged in the SE + HUMSC group than those in the SE group, suggesting the neuroprotective potential of transplanted HUMSCs. In general, intra-hippocampal transplantation of HUMSCs can prevent tissue damage and neuronal loss, provide supplemental neuronal protection and stimulate neurogenesis, and suppress the spontaneous recurrent seizures in a pilocarpine TLE model.

Another study examined the effects of implantation of Bone marrow derived mesenchymal stem cells either through intravenously (IV) or in hippocampus bilaterally (IC). BMSCs treatment reduced the hippocampal excitatory amino acid neurotransmitters, downregulated inflammatory cytokines (TNF-α, IL-1β), ameliorated histological changes, and reduced oxidative insult and inflammatory markers [38]. After 22 days of Pilocarpine induction of status epilepticus [SE], intrahippocampal injection of BMSCs was performed. Hippocampal GABA content is lower in SE epileptic animals than the sham control group. BMSCs transplantation through both routes significantly elevated hippocampal GABA content as compared to SE rats. In addition, the frequency of epileptic seizures in video surveillance analysis showed a significant reduction in the number of animals injected with MSC compared with the carrier group.

One study reported that BMSCs transplantation reduced hippocampal excitatory amino acid neurotransmitters and inhibited BDNF-mediated excitatory toxicity by either I.V. or I.C. pathways, similar to inhibition of synaptophysin immune response. The observed improvements extended to neurotransmitter balance, in which inhibitory tension was increased and excitatory metastases were observed in rats with epilepsy restored to normal balance. Bone marrow mesenchymal stem cell therapy improved the neurochemical and histological changes induced by triclosan, retained amino acid neurotransmitters to normal levels, down-regulated immune responses to insulin growth factor 1 receptors, synaptophysin, and caspase-3, and reduced detection of oxidative damage and inflammatory markers in epileptic models.

The number of GAD67+ GABAergic inhibitory neurons was significantly decreased in the CA1 and DH regions in the vehicle group at 2 months after SE inducing by the lithium-pilocarpine [39]. Furthermore, both Manganese-enhanced magnetic resonance imaging (MEMRI) and Timm (zinc) staining showed that the abnormal mossy fiber sprouting of the hippocampus in the MSC group was lower. Therefore, their results showed that intravenous infusion of bone marrow mesenchymal stem cells reduced the occurrence of epilepsy by inhibiting abnormal MFS in the SE rat model. Moreover, previous research has focused on reducing the loss of inhibitory neurons as a therapeutic mechanism for infused mesenchymal stem cells. Injection of mesenchymal stem cells inhibited the onset of epilepsy after SE and retained cognitive function. Injected GFP+ MSCs accumulated in the hippocampus and were related to the preservation of GAD67+ and NeuN+ hippocampal neurons.

3. Neural stem/progenitor cell and epilepsy

3.1 Potential of NSC/NPC for epilepsy

Epilepsy affects 1%-2% of the population worldwide [40]. Approximately 40% of epilepsy patients have temporal lobe epilepsy (TLE). Up to 35% of patients with TLE continue to have chronic seizures due to resistant to antiepileptic drugs [41, 42]. TLE is characterized by complex partial seizures hippocampal sclerosis, inhibitive gamma aminobutyric acid-ergic (GABAergic) interneuron loss, gliosis in hippocampal [43]. The main pathological changes of human temporal lobe epilepsy are hippocampal sclerosis and mossy fiber sprouting (MFS). Hippocampal sclerosis is mainly manifested in morphology as hippocampal atrophy and induration, and in histology, it is mainly manifested as necrosis of selective CA3 pyramidal neurons and secondary glial fibrosis. Mossy fibers (MF) are the axons of granular cells in the dentate gyrus, which normally project to the dendrites of pyramidal neurons in the CA3 and CA4 regions. MFS means that the postsynaptic site of MF is vacant and the target area of its normal projection disappears, resulting in budding to the inner molecular layer after the death of pyramidal neurons in these areas [44]. At the molecular level, the imbalance of excitatory and inhibitory neurotransmitters may be the main factor of seizures.

Although surgical removal of the hippocampus decreased seizure activity, this choice is bound to cognitive impairment [45], loss of viable tissue during resection [46], hemiplegia, hemianopia, and memory impairment. Bilateral resection is not suitable for patients with bilateral hippocampal sclerosis. Therefore, exploring through neural stem cells transplantation for the repair and reconstruction of hippocampal function has important clinical significance. Hence, the development of alternative therapies that have the potential for both reversing the epileptogenic circuitry and suppressing chronic epileptic seizures is extremely valuable.

Neural stem cells exist in the nervous system. After transplantation into the damaged central nervous system, they may differentiate into nerve neurons, astrocytes and oligodendrocytes by asymmetric division. Release of chemokines after partial tissue injury attracts neural stem cells to the site of injury. Neural stem cells also secrete a variety of neurotrophic factors to promote the repair of damaged cells.

Neural stem cells contribute to strengthen synaptic connections and create new neural circuits. It is proved that the directional differentiation of neural stem cells makes the repair and replacement of dead nerve cells possible. In order to reduce the sequelae of nerve injury, delay or inhibit the further development of the disease, and achieve better recovery effect, it is very necessary to repair and activate necrotic nerve cells fundamentally.

Neural stem cells have the capacity of self-renewal and express various growth factors. Multipotent NSCs can be obtained from multiple sources such as embryonic stem cells (ESCs), induced pluripotent stem cells (iPSCs), fetal, postnatal and adult brain tissues [47, 48]. NSCs can survive well intracerebral grafting, migrate into regions of the brain displaying neuron loss, increase concentration of proinflammatory cytokines, positively influence the survival of host cells and tissues, replace significant numbers of lost interneurons, promote functional recovery and maintain normal network function [49, 50].

3.2 Efficacy of neural stem/progenitor cell grafts in rat model

Astrocytes have the capable of secreting beneficial neurotrophic factors that promote neuroprotection, reduce frequencies of SRMS [51] and enhance neurogenesis. It provides an attractive approach for stimulation neurogenesis endogenous NSCs in the dentate subgranular zone [52, 53]. NSC transplantation can suppress neuroinflammation. Therefore, neural stem cells become potential donor cells for the treatment of brain injury or neurodegenerative diseases. Transplantation of NSCs in hippocampal injury rat is efficacious for thwarting mood and memory dysfunction and abnormal neurogenesis [54]. Studies have shown that in animal models with TLE seizures, the number of hippocampal GABA-ergic interneurons decreased [55, 56]. Status epilepticus [SE] typically progresses into temporal lobe epilepsy [TLE].

Several studies have examined the efficacy of NSCs for controlling seizures when administered in SE model (**Table 2**). A study reported that the transplant intravenously of beta galactosidase-encoded human NSCs could prevent spontaneous recurrent seizure formation in adult rats with pilocarpine-induced status epilepticus [57]. Ruschenschmidt et al. [58] have demonstrated that embryonic stem cell-derived neurons displayed intrinsic and synaptic properties characteristic of neurons when transplanted into the hippocampus of chronic epileptic animals. Transplantation techniques using bilaterally placed grafts of striatal precursors in the acute phase of the disease reduced the frequency of spontaneous recurrent motor seizures (SRMS) on a long-term basis in the chronic epilepsy period [59]. Adult neural stem cells had anti-epileptic effect in rats with status epilepticus (SE) induced by kainic acid. NSC transplantation increased the number of neuropeptide Y (NPY) and glutamic decarboxylase 67 (GAD67) positive interneurons, and inhibited the moss fiber germination to the inner molecular layer [60, 61].

Hong Shen et al. [62] demonstrated that Hippocampal stem cells (HSCs) derived from the postnatal hippocampus have the potential of promoting repairs in the epileptic brain. In this study, Hippocampal stem cells were transplanted into the right hippocampus in rats with kainite acid [KA]-induced epilepsy. At 1, 4, 8, and 24 weeks posttransplantation, Timm's stain, Nissl staining, electroencephalogram were performed. The results showed that sharp waves were reduced, Aberrant MFS induced by KA-lesion was suppressed by HSC grafts, and the loss of CA3 pyramidal

References	Model	Type of NSC	Number of NSC	Route of administration	Period after SE	Outcome measures examined	Major findings
[51]	Kainic acid-induced status epilepticus (SE)	NSCs embryonic medial ganglionic eminence (MGE)	8×10^4	Graft into hippocampi of adult rats	Two months	Measurement of postgrafting SRMS; Analyses of learning and memory function	Reduced frequencies of SRMS, duration of individual SRMS and the total time spent in seizures
[57]	Status epilepticus induced by pilocarpine	H7 hESC differentiated into MGE cells	5×10^4	Hippocampus	2 weeks	Behavioral analysis; immunohistochemistry; transmission electron; microscopy (TEM); electrophysiology; neurolucida tracing	Grafted neurons were capable of suppressing seizures and ameliorating behavioral abnormalities such as cognitive deficits, aggressiveness and hyperactivity.
[59]	Kainite acid (KA)-induced epilepsy	Striatal precursors	1×10^5	Hippocampus	9–12 months	Calbindin; immunostaining; neuropeptide Y; immunostaining; Nissl staining analyses of spontaneous recurrent motor seizures	Grafting considerably preserved hippocampal Calbindin but had no effects on aberrant mossy fiber sprouting, reduced the frequency of SRMS on a long-term basis
[62]	Kainite acid (KA)-induced epilepsy	Hippocampal stem cells (HSC)	5×10^5	Transplant HSCs into the right hippocampus	24 weeks	EEG recording; Timm's staining; Nissl staining	Reduced frequency restore the loss of CA3 pyramidal neurons; aberrant MFS was notably suppressed
[63]	Maximum electroconvulsive shock (MES)	GABAergic precursor	5×10^4	Neocortex bilaterally	Sixty days	Immunohistochemistry; MES test	Altered the course of MES acute seizures, increasing seizure threshold, and/or blocked the generalized convulsive activity

References	Model	Type of NSC	Number of NSC	Route of administration	Period after SE	Outcome measures examined	Major findings
[64]	Status epilepticus induced by pilocarpine	Human neural stem/progenitor cells	4×10^5	CA3 region of the right hippocampus	2 weeks	Evaluation of NSPC grafts on kindled seizures and SRMS; Morris water maze; Timm staining	Reduced behavioral seizure duration, after discharge duration on electroencephalograms, and seizure stage in the kindling model, as well as the frequency and the duration of spontaneous recurrent motor seizures
[65]	Status epilepticus induced by Li-pilocarpine	NPCs derived from the medial ganglionic eminence and ventral mesencephalon	STN (8×10^4 or 1.5×10^5 NPCs) or SNr (8×10^4 or 5×10^4 NPCs)	Graft into subthalamic nucleus (STN) or substantia nigra pars reticulata (SNr)	4 months	Immunohistological; effect of intrasubthalamic; cell grafting on seizure thresholds.	Average clonic seizure threshold increased above pre-grafting

Table 2.
Stem cell transplantation studies in epilepsy models.

neurons was partially restored. Given these results, HSC grafts have the therapeutic potentials for the treatment of epilepsy. Further investigation of the capability of NSCs for providing neuroprotection using a maximum electroconvulsive shock (MES) mode showed matching results [63]. Transplantation of medial ganglionic eminence (MGE) cells altered the course of MES acute onset, increased the onset threshold, and increased GABA interneuron selectivity compensates for excitatory activity, thereby reducing susceptibility to epileptic seizures.

Over the past decades, embryonic stem cells, neural stem cells, or neural precursors have been tested in rat models of epilepsy: Li-pilocarpine-induced status epilepticus, kainic acid-induced status epilepticus or kindling-based TLE models. Haejin Lee et al. investigated whether transplantation of human fetal brain-derived NSPC grafts into the hippocampus in both kindling and pilocarpine induced TLE models could improve the epileptic phenotypes [64]. In the study, huNSPCs for transplantation were derived from a cadaver at 13 weeks of gestation. In vitro, huNSPCs can differentiate into three types of nerve cells in vitro: neurons, oligodendrocytes, and astrocytes. Differentiation of human NSPCs was analyzed at 8 weeks posttransplantation in epileptic rats. Confocal microscopic images revealed that grafted cells differentiated into oligodendrocytes, astrocytes and TUJ1+ neurons in kindled rats. In the pilocarpine model, TUJ1+ neurons, GFAP+ astrocytes, and OLIG2+ oligodendrocyte progenitors were observed in confocal microscopy images. In the kindled rats, EEG examination, behavioral seizure duration, and seizure stage were substantial decreased. Nevertheless, the anticonvulsant effect is not persistent and gradually disappeared after 7 weeks. The frequency and severity of spontaneous recurrent motor seizures (SRMS) were significantly reduced at 2 and 3 months after grafting in epileptic rats. Furthermore, the average total time spent in SRMS was significant decreased at 2 and 3 months after grafting. Timm staining show that aberrant sprouting of mossy fibers was not significantly different between the two groups. Water maze testing and probe test were performed at 9 weeks after grafting. The ability of spatial learning and memory function in kindled rats showed no significant difference. Another study examined the effects of transplantation of NPCs from three different donor species [65]. Clonic seizure thresholds were analyzed by statistical evaluation. Average clonic seizure threshold increased above pre-grafting control were observed during this time-point investigation after grafting.

3.3 GABA-ergic progenitors/neuron and epilepsy

Interneurons are a type of nerve cells that can release neurotransmitters such as GABA. They mainly exist in brain areas such as the cerebral cortex and hippocampus [66]. Interneurons account for about 25% to 30% of the total number of brain neurons [67] and play an important role in the regulation of brain functions. Gamma-amino butyric acid (GABA) intermediate neurons refer to nerve cells with GABA as the main transmitter, accounting for about 20% of total neurons in cerebral cortex [68]. GABA intermediate neurons form extensive synaptic connections with pyramidal cells and play an important role in regulating the activity of pyramidal cells and maintaining the excitatory/inhibitory balance of cerebral cortical circuits [69, 70]. In the cerebral cortex, different types of neurons form complex circuits and work together to process and store information in a timely manner. They also interact with glutamate pyramidal cell input in specific ways and support the temporal dynamics of synapses, network oscillations, selection of cell combinations, and realization of brain states. This cellular diversity gives the ability to perform complex biological processes. The relatively uniform pyramidal cells are supported by a rich variety of GABAergic interneurons, which provide general inhibition and also regulate pyramidal cell activity over time. The type of GABAergic interneuron is not unique to the CA1 region. Similar neurons are also present in the hippocampus and most other areas of the foreign cortex [71]. In addition, these GABAergic inter-neurons can also be found in the cortex of mice, rats, cats, monkeys and humans. Examination of epileptic tissue removed from TLE patients revealed a loss of interneurons that release inhibitory neurotransmitter GABA [72, 73]. GABA-mediated inhibition has been repeatedly demonstrated to be weakened in TLE animal models [74] (**Table 3**).

Several studies have tested the effects of neurons. Neural transplantation of GABA-producing cells into subthalamic nucleus (STN) aims to correct imbalance between excitatory and inhibitory neurotransmission. Grafting of GABA-producing cells into the STN suppressed seizure activity. The STN can be considered a target region [75]. hPSC-derived maturing GABAergic interneurons suppressed seizures and ameliorated behavioral abnormalities such as cognitive deficits, aggressiveness, and hyperactivity. In addition, substantial numbers of the GABA-ergic interneurons and GDNF-secreting cells mediate seizure suppression. Neural cell grafting has shown considerable efficiency for inducing the reactivation of the host hippocampal GABA-ergic interneurons and diminishing the aberrant mossy fiber sprouting in the dentate gyrus. Furthermore, the synaptic integration of graft-derived GABA-ergic interneurons effects host brain activity at both cellular and network levels.

4. Challenges and potential

Currently, MSC-based therapy and Neural stem cell and neurons grafting for epilepsy has become an increasing focus of research. Stem cells can be targeted to focal areas of epileptogenesis and tailored to affect only the dysfunctional constituents of the epileptic circuit. Stem cells could theoretically be used in areas of eloquent cortex and could be more widely inserted into a region of epileptogenesis based on clinical response. Neural stem cells can engraft into the injured brain areas, positively influence the survival of host cells and tissues, and promote functional recovery. Afterward, function of these cells for suppressing seizures and improving cognitive function in chronic epilepsy were determined.

Stem cell therapy for epilepsy mainly involves the replacement of damaged neurons with stem cell differentiation, secretion of protective factors and anti-inflammatory factors to prevent clinical deterioration. Mesenchymal stem cells have great potential in cell therapy because they are easy to obtain, easy to amplify, and can be autologous transplanted with little immune rejection. There is ample evidence that mesenchymal stem cells can differentiate into neuronal destinies and secrete a range of anti-inflammatory, protective cytokines. In addition, bone marrow mesenchymal stem cells have been shown to point to damaged areas, meaning they could be used as vehicles for therapeutic drugs. In fact, various beneficial effects have been reported after transplantation of human bone marrow mesenchymal stem cells into rodent models of epilepsy, such as neurotrophic factor-mediated protection, enhanced neurogenesis, inflammation regulation, and removal of abnormal protein aggregates.

At present, the application of NSCs to repair central nervous system damage mainly takes two ways, namely exogenous transplantation replacement therapy and endogenous activation complementary therapy. Therefore, the function of NSCs to treat neurological diseases is of great significance, and certain progress has been examined in experimental research on the treatment of temporal lobe epilepsy. NSCs have the capacity of self-renewing, highly migratory, low immunogenic, and differentiate into different types of nerve cells. In theory, it overcomes many of the above shortcomings of embryonic tissue and is attractive for the treatment of nervous system diseases.

References	Model	Type of NSC/ Neuron	Number of Neuron	Route of administration	Period after SE (days)	Outcome measures examined	Major findings
[74]	Intravenous pentylenetetrazol e (PTZ) rat	GABAergic cell line hGAD-overexpressing cell line	8×10^4	Grafting into substantia nigra pars reticulata and subthalamic nucleus	10/11 days, 3-5 weeks	Histological analysis thionine (Nissl) and bisbenzimide staining	Anticonvulsant effects can be induced by bilateral transplantation of GABAergic M213-20 cells and hGAD-overexpressing cells into the STN; anticonvulsant effect; more long-lasting than transplantation of the same cell line into the SNr of amygdala-kindled rats
[75]	Pilocarpine intraperitoneally, status epilepticus (SE)	Human MGE Cells	5×10^4	Hippocampus	7 days, 2 weeks	EEG recording; Y maze novel object recognition test; locomotion test handling test; immunohistochemistry	PSC-derived human mGINs migrate extensively within the epileptic hippocampus, integrate into host circuitry and reduce seizure activity and other behavioral abnormalities
[76]	Pilocarpine-induced status epilepticus in mice	Mouse ES cell-derived neural progenitors (ESNPs)	1×10^5	Hilus of the dentate gyrus	2–3 months	Graft differentiation, mossy fiber sprouting, cellular morphology, and electrophysiological	New cells functionally integrate into epileptic hippocampal circuitry; ESNP-derived neurons formed dense axonal arborizations in the inner molecular layer and throughout the hilus

Table 3.
Stem cell transplantation studies in epilepsy models.

A number of experimental studies have shown that cell transplantation can reduce the attack frequency of TLE, inhibit the pathological process of epilepsy, and repair the damaged nerve structure. However, several key problems still need to be solved before cell transplantation therapy for epilepsy can move from preclinical research to clinical research. This means that grafted cells should meet the following requirements.

(1) The activity of transplanted cells should be guaranteed normal physiological activities. They can establish functional synaptic connections with the host and carry out functional integration to meet the requirements of repairing damaged neural pathways; (2) the transplanted cells have a strong ability to migrate from the transplanted area to the appropriate cell layer; and (3) the transplanted cells should have normal differentiation and proliferation ability.

In view of the therapeutic effect of different cell types, application of combined strategies may be considered. This may include transplanting MSC and nerve cells (hippocampus or MGE progenitors or NSCs) into the hippocampus: (1) systemic administration of hippocampal neurogenesis enhancers such as small molecules, antidepressants, antioxidants, or neurotrophic factors; (2) MSC and Neural stem cells engineered to release neurogenic enhancers and adenosine. Enhancing the overall rate of transplantation-derived GABA-ergic intermediate neuron and GDNF derived cells has enormous potential to significantly reduce the neurogenic regional recovery of the hippocampus in the pre-clinical models of chronic frame [77, 78].

5. Conclusions

To sum up, it is of great significance to explore the way of cell transplantation, find a treatment method that can replace the lost neurons, repair the damaged nervous system, increase the secretion of inhibitory neurotransmitter, and effectively control the occurrence and development of epilepsy. At the same time, the method can overcome the shortcomings of drug treatment and surgical treatment, fundamentally cure epilepsy. MSC and Progenitors/Stem cell derived from multiple sources can reduce epileptogenesis and improved cognitive function with grafting performed to epileptic brain regions. This has been demonstrated in animal prototypes of chronic TLE, kindling, SE and absence seizures, and in mutant mice displaying SRS. These abundant studies have laid a solid foundation for the early application of cell transplantation therapy in clinical practice.

Acknowledgements

We would like to thank Lang He for suggestion.

Conflict of interest

The authors declare that they have no competing interests.

Nomenclature

ROS	reactive oxygen species
BBB	damage of blood–brain barrier
iPSCs	induced pluripotent stem cells

MSCs	mesenchymal stem cells
TLE	temporal lobe epilepsy
MFS	mossy fiber sprouting
AEDs	antiepileptic drugs
NSC	neural stem cells
NPC	neural progenitors
BMSC	bone marrow mesenchymal stem cell
CNS	central nervous system
ISCT	International Society for Cellular Therapy
BMMCs	bone marrow mononuclear cells
SRS	spontaneous recurrent seizures
SE	status epilepticus
fEPSPs	excitatory postsynaptic potentials
ASCs-E	extract of human ASCs
PTZ	pentylenetetrazol
HUMSCs	human umbilical mesenchymal stem cells
EEG	electroencephalography
MRI	magnetic resonance imaging
IV	intravenously
IC	hippocampus bilaterally
MEMRI	manganese-enhanced magnetic resonance imaging
MF	mossy fibers
ESCs	embryonic stem cells
SRMS	spontaneous recurrent motor seizures
NPY	neuropeptide Y
GAD67	glutamic decarboxylase 67
KA	kainite acid
HSCs	hippocampal stem cells
MES	maximum electroconvulsive shock
MGE	medial ganglionic eminence
huNSPCs	human neural stem/progenitor cells
TUJ1	β-tubulin III
STN	subthalamic nucleus

Author details

Huifang Zhao and Zhiyuan Li*
CAS Key Laboratory of Regenerative Biology, Guangdong Provincial Key Laboratory of Stem Cell and Regenerative Medicine, Guangzhou Institutes of Biomedicine and Health, Chinese Academy of Sciences, Guangzhou, China

*Address all correspondence to: li_zhiyuan@gibh.ac.cn

References

[1] Global, regional, and national incidence, prevalence, and years lived with disability for 301 acute and chronic diseases and injuries in 188 countries, 1990-2013: a systematic analysis for the Global Burden of Disease Study 2013. Lancet. 2015; 386 (9995):743-800. DOI: 10.1016/S0140-6736(15)60692-4

[2] Maria Thom, Maura Boldrini, Elizabeth Bundock, Mary N. Sheppard, Orrin Devinsky. The past, present and future challenges in epilepsy related and sudden deaths and biobanking. Neuropathol Appl Neurobiol. 2018; 44(1): 32-55. DOI: 10.1111/nan.12453

[3] F.E. Dudek, T.P. Sutula. Epileptogenesis in the dentate gyrus: a critical perspective Prog. Brain Res. 2007; 163:755-773. DOI /10.1016/S0079-6123(07)63041-6

[4] A. Finegersh, C. Avedissian, S. Shamim, I. Dustin, P.M. Thompson, W.H. Theodore. Bilateral hippocampal atrophy in temporal lobe epilepsy: effect of depressive symptoms and febrile seizures. Epilepsia. 2011 Apr; 52(4): 689-697. DOI: 10.1111/j.1528-1167.2010.02928.x

[5] J. Detour, H. Schroeder, D. Desor, A. Nehlig. A 5-month period of epilepsy impairs spatial memory, decreases anxiety, but spares object recognition in the lithium-pilocarpine model in adult rats. Epilepsia. 2005;46: 499-508. DOI/10.1111/j.0013-9580.2005.38704.x

[6] Löscher W, Klitgaard H, Twyman RE, Schmidt D. New avenues for anti-epileptic drug discovery and development. Nat Rev Drug Discov. 2013; 12:757-776. DOI: 10.1038/nrd4126

[7] Temkin, N. R. Preventing and treating posttraumatic seizures: the human experience. Epilepsia. 2009; 50 (Suppl. 2), 10-13. 8. DOI: 10.1038/nrd4126

[8] Schmidt, D. Is antiepileptogenesis a realistic goal in clinical trials? Concerns and new horizons. Epilept Disord. 2012; 14, 105-113. DOI:10.1684/epd.2012.0512

[9] Löscher, W, Schmidt, D. Modern antiepileptic drug development has failed to deliver: ways out of the current dilemma. Epilepsia. 2011; 52, 657-678. DOI: /10.1111/j.1528-1167.2011.03024.x

[10] Satish Agadi, Ashok K Shetty. Concise Review: Prospects of Bone Marrow Mononuclear Cells and Mesenchymal Stem Cells for Treating Status Epilepticus and Chronic Epilepsy. STEM CELLS. 2015;33:2093-2103. doi: 10.1002/stem.2029. Epub 2015 May 13.

[11] Steven N. Roper, Dennis A. Steindler. Stem cells as a potential therapy for epilepsy. Exp Neurol. 2013; 244: 59-66. DOI:10.1016/j.expneurol.2012.01.004

[12] Friedenstein AJ, Piatetzky S II, Petrakova K V Petrakova. Osteogenesis in transplants of bone marrow cells. J Embryol Exp Morphol. 1966;16:381-90. DOI: 10.1002/jcp.1040740209

[13] Azizi SA, Stokes D, Augelli BJ et al. Engraftment and migration of human bone marrow stromal cells implanted in the brains of albino rats similarities to astrocyte grafts. Proc Natl Acad Sci U S A 1998;95:3908-3913. DOI: 10.1073/pnas.95.7.3908

[14] Jiang Y, Jahagirdar BN, Reinhardt RL et al. Pluripotency of mesenchymal stem cells derived from adult marrow. Nature. 2002;418:41-49. DOI: 10.1038/nature00870

[15] Sanchez-Ramos J, Song S, Cardozo-Pelaez F et al. Adult bone marrow stromal cells differentiate into neural cells in vitro. Exp Neurol. 2000; 164:247-256. DOI:10.1006/exnr.2000.7389.

[16] A Voulgari-Kokota 1, R Fairless, M Karamita, V Kyrargyri, V Tseveleki. Mesenchymal stem cells protect CNS neurons against glutamate excitotoxicity by inhibiting glutamate receptor expression and function. Exp Neurol.2012;236:161-70. DOI: 10.1016/j.expneurol.2012.04.011

[17] Ferrari G, Cusella-De Angelis G, Coletta M, Paolucci E, Stornaiuolo A et al. Muscle regeneration by bone marrow-derived myogenic progenitors. Science. 1998;279: 1528-1530. DOI: 10.1126/science.279.5356.1528

[18] De Ugarte DA, Morizono K, Elbarbary A, Alfonso Z, Zuk PA, Zhu M et al. Comparison of multi-lineage cells from human adipose tissue and bone marrow. Cells Tissues Organs. 2003; 174: 101-109. doi: 10.1159/000071150

[19] Rogers I, Casper RF. Umbilical cord blood stem cells. Best Pract Res Clin Obstet Gynaecol. 2004;18:893-908. DOI: 10.1016/j.bpobgyn.2004.06.004

[20] Dominici M, Le Blanc K, Mueller I, et al. Minimal criteria for defining multipotent mesenchymal stromal cells. The International Society for Cellular Therapy position statement. Cytotherapy. 2006;12:315-7. DOI: 10.1080/14653240600855905

[21] Phinney, D.G., Prockop, D.J. Concise review: mesenchymal stem/multipotent stromal cells: the state of transdifferentiation and modes of tissue repair—current views. Stem Cells. 2007; 25, 2896-2902. DOI: 10.1634/stemcells.2007-0637

[22] Uccelli, A., Moretta, L., Pistoia, V., Mesenchymal stem cells in health and disease. Nat Rev Immunol. 2008;8, 726-736. DOI: 10.1038/nri2395.

[23] Phinney, D.G., Hill, K., Michelson, C., DuTreil, M., Hughes, C., Humphries, S., Wilkinson, R., Baddoo, M., Bayly, E. Biological activities encoded by the murine mesenchymal stem cell transcriptome provide a basis for their developmental potential and broad therapeutic efficacy. Stem Cells. 2006; 24, 186-198. DOI: 10.1634/stemcells.2004-0236

[24] Li, Y., Chen, J., Chen, X.G., Wang, L., Gautam, S.C., Xu, Y.X., Katakowski, M., Zhang, L.J., Lu, M., Janakiraman, N., Chopp, M. Human marrow stromal cell therapy for stroke in rat: neurotrophins and functional recovery. Neurology. 2002; 59, 514-523. doi:10.1212/wnl.59.4.514.

[25] Munoz, J.R., Stoutenger, B.R., Robinson, A.P., Spees, J.L., Prockop, D.J. Human stem/progenitor cells from bone marrow promote neurogenesis of endogenous neural stem cells in the hippocampus of mice. Proc Natl Acad Sci U S A. 2005; 102, 18171-18176.DOI: 10.1073/pnas.0508945102

[26] Lanza, C., Morando, S., Voci, A., Canesi, L., Principato, M.C., Serpero, L.D., Mancardi, G., Uccelli, A., Vergani, L. Neuroprotective mesenchymal stem cells are endowed with a potent antioxidant effect in vivo. J. Neurochem. 2009; 110, 1674-1684. DOI: 10.1111/j.1471-4159.2009.06268.x

[27] Alireza Abdanipour, Taki Tiraihi, Javad Mirnajafi-Zadeh. Improvement of the pilocarpine epilepsy model in rat using bone marrow stromal cell therapy. Neurological Research. 2011;33(6):625-32.DOI: 10.1179/1743132810Y.0000000018

[28] Gianina Teribele Venturin, Samuel Greggio, Daniel Rodrigo Marinowic, et al. Bone marrow mononuclear cells reduce seizure frequency and improve cognitive outcome in chronic epileptic rats. Life Sciences. Life Sci. 2011;15;89(7-8):229-34. DOI: 10.1016/j.lfs.2011.06.006

[29] Costa-Ferro ZS, Vitola AS, Pedroso MF et al. Prevention of seizures

and reorganization of hippocampal functions by transplantation of bone marrow cells in the acute phase of experimental epilepsy. Seizure. 2010; 19:84-92. DOI: 10.1016/j.seizure.2009.12.003

[30] Daejong Jeon, Kon Chu, Soon-Tae Lee, Keun-Hwa Jung et al. A cell-free extract from human adipose stem cells protects mice against epilepsy. Epilepsia. 2011;52(9):1617-26.DOI: 10.1111/j.1528-1167.2011.03182.x.

[31] Filip M, Frankowska M, Gołda A, Zaniewska M, Vetulani J, Przegaliński E: Various GABAmimetic drugs differently affect cocaine evoked hyperlocomotion and sensitization. Eur J Pharmacol. 2006; 541:163-170. DOI: 10.1016/j.ejphar.2006.05.011

[32] Amira S Mohammed, Mohammed M Ewais, Mona K Tawfik, Soha S Essawy. Effects of Intravenous Human Umbilical Cord Blood Mesenchymal Stem Cell Therapy versus Gabapentin in Pentylenetetrazole-Induced Chronic Epilepsy in Rats. Pharmacology. 2014;94(1-2):41-50. DOI: 10.1159/000365219

[33] Leal MM, Costa-Ferro ZS, Souza BS et al. Earl transplantation of bone marrow mononuclear cells promotes neuroprotection and modulation of inflammation after status epilepticus in mice by paracrine mechanisms. Neurochem Res. 2014;39:259-268. DOI: 10.1007/s11064-013-1217-7

[34] Yasuhara T, Hara K, Maki M, Xu L, Yu G, Ali M, Masuda T, Yu S, Bae E, Hayashi T, MatsukawaN,KanekoY,Kuzmin-NicholsN, Ellovitch S, Cruz E, Klasko S, Sanberg C, Sanberg P, Borlongan C. Mannitol facilitates neurotrophic factor up-regulation and behavioural recovery in neonatal hypoxic-ischaemic rats with human umbilical cord blood grafts. J Cell Mol Med. 2010;14:914-921. DOI: 10.1111/j.1582-4934.2008.00671.x

[35] Sadan O, Shemesh N, Barzilay R, Bahat Stromza M, Melamed E, Cohen Y. Migration of neurotrophic factors-secreting mesenchymal stem cells toward a quinolinic acid lesion as viewed by magnetic resonance imaging. Stem Cells. 2008;26:2542-2551. DOI: 10.1634/stemcells.2008-0240

[36] Ziegler L, Grigoryan S, Yang I, Thakor N, Goldstein R. Efficient generation of Schwann cells from human embryonic stem cell-derived neurospheres. Stem Cell Rev. 2011;7: 394-403. DOI: 10.1007/s12015-010-9198-2.

[37] Xenograft of human umbilical mesenchymal stem cells from Wharton's jelly as a potential therapy for rat pilocarpine-induced epilepsy. Brain Behav Immun.2016; 54:45-58. DOI: 10.1016/j.bbi.2015.12.021

[38] Neveen A Salem, Marwa El-Shamarka, Yasser Khadrawy, Shaimaa El-Shebiney. New prospects of mesenchymal stem cells for ameliorating temporal lobe epilepsy. Inflammopharmacology. 2018;26(4):963-972. DOI: 10.1007/s10787-018-0456-2

[39] Shinobu Fukumura, Masanori Sasaki, Yuko Kataoka-Sasaki, Shinichi Oka, Masahito Nakazaki. Intravenous infusion of mesenchymal stem cells reduces epileptogenesis in a rat model of status epilepticus. Epilepsy Res. 2018 ;141:56-63. DOI: 10.1016/j.eplepsyres.2018.02.008

[40] Strine TW, Kobau R, Chapman DP, et al. Psychological distress, comorbidities, and health behaviors among U.S. adults with seizures: results from the 2002 National Health Interview Survey. Epilepsia. 2005;46:1133-1139. DOI: 10.1111/j.1528-1167.2005.01605.x

[41] Engel J Jr. Intractable epilepsy: Definition and neurobiology.

Epilepsia. 2001;42 Suppl 6:3. DOI: 10.1046/j.1528-1157.2001.0420s6003.x

[42] Litt, B., Esteller, R., Echauz, J., et al. Epileptic seizures may begin hours in advance of clinical onset: A report of five patients. Neuron. 2001; 30(1), 51-64. DOI: 10.1016/s0896-6273(01)00262-8

[43] Dudek, FE, & Sutula, TP. Epileptogenesis in the dentate gyrus: A critical perspective. Prog Brain Res. 2007;163:755-73. DOI: 10.1016/S0079-6123(07)63041-6

[44] Shibley H, Smith BN. Pilocarpine-induced status epilepticus results in mossy fiber sprouting and spontaneous seizures in C57BL/6 and CD-1 mice. Epilepsy Res. 2002; 49(2):109-20. DOI: 10.1016/s0920-1211(02)00012-8

[45] Helmstaedter C. Temporal lobe resection--does the prospect of seizure freedom outweigh the cognitive risks?. Nat Clin Pract Neurol. 2008;4(2):66-7. DOI: 10.1038/ncpneuro0657

[46] Shamim S, Wiggs E, Heiss J, et al. Temporal lobectomy: resection volume, neuropsychological effects, and seizure outcome. Epilepsy Behav. 2009;16:311-314. DOI: 10.1016/j.yebeh.2009.07.040

[47] Xu T, Zhang M, Laurent T, Xie M, Ding S. Concise review: chemical approaches for modulating lineage-specific stem cells and progenitors. Stem Cells Transl Med. 2013; 2:355-361. DOI: 10.5966/sctm.2012-0172

[48] Shetty AK. Hippocampal injury-induced cognitive and mood dysfunction, altered neurogenesis, and epilepsy: Can early neural stem cell grafting intervention provide protection? Epilepsy & Behav. 2014; 38:117-124. DOI: 10.1016/j.yebeh.2013.12.001

[49] Ryu JK, Cho T, Wang YT, McLarnon JG. Neural progenitor cells attenuate inflammatory reactivity and neuronal loss in an animal model of inflamed AD brain. J Neuroinflammation. 2009; 6:39. DOI: 10.1186/1742-2094-6-39

[50] Blurton-Jones M, Kitazawa M, Martinez-Coria H, Castello NA, Müller FJ, Loring JF, et al. Neural stem cells improve cognition via BDNF in a transgenic model of Alzheimer disease. Proc Natl Acad Sci USA. 2009; 106:13594-13599. DOI: 10.1073/pnas.0901402106

[51] Waldau B, Hattiangady B, Kuruba R, et al. Medial ganglionic eminence-derived neural stem cell grafts ease spontaneous seizures and restore GDNF expression in a rat model of chronic temporal lobe epilepsy. Stem Cells. 2010; 28:1153-1164. DOI: 10.1002/stem.446

[52] Teng YD, Benn SC, Kalkanis SN, Shefner JM, Onario RC, Cheng B, et al. Multimodal actions of neural stem cells in a mouse model of ALS: a meta-analysis. Sci Transl Med. 2012; 4:165ra164. DOI: 10.1126/scitranslmed.3004579

[53] de Lanerolle NC, Kim JH, Robbins RJ, et al. Hippocampal interneuron loss and plasticity in human temporal lobe epilepsy. Brain Res. 1989;495:387-395. DOI:10.1016/0006-8993(89)90234-5.

[54] Shetty AK, Turner DA. Fetal hippocampal grafts containing CA3 cells restore host hippocampal glutamate decarboxylase-positive interneuron numbers in a rat model of temporal lobe epilepsy. J Neurosci. 2000;20:8788-8801. DOI: 10.1523/JNEUROSCI.20-23-08788.2000

[55] Hattiangady B, Shetty AK. Neural stem cell grafting counteracts hippocampal injury-induced impairments in mood, memory and neurogenesis. Stem Cell Transl

Med. 2012; 1:696-708. DOI: 10.5966/sctm.2012-0050

[56] Henderson KW, Gupta J, Tagliatela S, Litvina E, Zheng X, Van Zandt MA, Woods N, Grund E, Lin D, Royston S, Yanagawa Y, Aaron GB, Naegele JR. Long-term seizure suppression and optogenetic analyses of synaptic connectivity in epileptic mice with hippocampal grafts of GABAergic interneurons. J Neurosci. 2014; 34:13492-13504. doi: 10.1523/JNEUROSCI.0005-14.2014.

[57] Cunningham M, Cho JH, Leung A, Savvidis G, Ahn S, Moon M, Lee PK, Han JJ, Azimi N, Kim KS, Bolshakov VY, Chung S. hPSC-derived maturing GABAergic interneurons ameliorate seizures and abnormal behavior in epileptic mice. Cell Stem Cell. 2014; 15:559-573. DOI: 10.1016/j.stem.2014.10.006

[58] Chu K, Kim M, Jung KH, Jeon D, Lee ST, Kim J, et al. Human neural stem cell transplantation reduces spontaneous recurrent seizures following pilocarpine induced status epilepticus in adult rats. Brain Res 2004;1023(2):213-21. DOI: 10.1016/j.brainres.2004.07.045

[59] Hattiangady B, Rao MS, Shetty AK. Grafting of striatal precursor cells into hippocampus shortly after status epilepticus restrains chronic temporal lobe epilepsy. Exp Neurol. 2008;212(2):468-81. DOI: 10.1016/j.expneurol.2008.04.040

[60] Jing M, Shingo T, Yasuhara T, Kondo A, Morimoto T, Wang F, et al. The combined therapy of intrahippocampal transplantation of adult neural stem cells and intraventricular erythropoietin-infusion ameliorates spontaneous recurrent seizures by suppression of abnormal mossy fiber sprouting. Brain Res. 2009;1295:203-17. DOI: 10.1016/j.brainres.2009.07.079

[61] Ruschenschmidt C, Koch PG, Brustle O, Beck H. Functional properties of ES cell-derived neurons engrafted into the hippocampus of adult normal and chronically epileptic rats. Epilepsia. 2005;46(Suppl. 5):174-83. DOI: 10.1111/j.1528-1167.2005.01028.x

[62] Shen H, Liu L, Huo Z, Lin Z. Hippocampal stem cell grafting-mediated recovery of injured hippocampus in the rat model of temporal lobe epilepsy. Int J Neurosci. 2010;120 (10):647-54. DOI: 10.3109/00207454.2010.509526

[63] Maria E Calcagnotto, Lorena P Ruiz, Miriam M Blanco, Jair G Santos-Junior, Maria F Valente, Camila Patti et al. Effect of neuronal precursor cells derived from medial ganglionic eminence in an acute epileptic seizure model. Epilepsia. 2010 ;51 Suppl 3:71-5 DOI: 10.1111/j.1528-1167.2010.02614.x

[64] Haejin Lee, Seokhwan Yun, Il-Sun Kim, Il-Shin Lee, Jeong Eun Shin, Soo Chul Park, Won-Joo Kim, Kook In Park. Human Fetal Brain-Derived Neural Stem/Progenitor Cells Grafted into the Adult Epileptic Brain Restrain Seizures in Rat Models of Temporal Lobe Epilepsy. PLoS One. 2014 Aug 8;9(8):e104092.DOI: 10.1371/journal.pone.0104092.

[65] Bianca Backofen-Wehrhahn, Laura Gey, Sonja Bröer. Anticonvulsant effects after grafting of rat, porcine, and human mesencephalic neural progenitor cells into the rat subthalamic nucleus. Exp Neurol. 2018 ;310:70-83. DOI: 10.1016/j.expneurol.2018.09.004

[66] Lodato S, Arlotta P. Generating neuronal diversity in the mammalian cerebral cortex. Annu Rev Cell Dev Biol. 2015;31,699-720. DOI: 10.1146/annurev-cellbio-100814-125353

[67] Ascoli GA, Alonso-Nanclares L, Anderson SA, Barrionuevo G, Benavides-Piccione R, Burkhalter A,

Buzsaki G, Cauli B, Defelipe J, Fairen A, et al. Petilla terminology: Nomenclature of features of GABAergic interneurons of the cerebral cortex. Nat Rev Neurosci. 2008;9: 557-568. DOI: 10.1038/nrn2402

[68] Freund TF, Buzsa´ki G. 1996. Interneurons of the hippocampus. Hippocampus 6: 347-470. DOI: 10.1002/(SICI)1098-1063(1996)6:4<347::AID-HIPO1>3.0.CO;2-I

[69] Lewis DA, Curley AA, Glausier JR, Volk DW. Cortical parvalbumin interneurons and cognitive dysfunction in schizophrenia. Trends Neurosci. 2012; 35, 57-67. DOI: 10.1016/j.tins.2011.10.004

[70] Klausberger T, Somogyi P. Neuronal diversity and temporal dynamics: the unity of hippocampal circuit operations. Science. 2008; 321:53-57. DOI: 10.1126/science.1149381

[71] Lund JS, Lewis DA. J. Comp. Local circuit neurons of developing and mature macaque prefrontal cortex: Golgi and immunocytochemical characteristics. Neurol. 1993; 328(2):282-312.DOI: 10.1002/cne.903280209

[72] Marco P, Sola RG, Pulido P, Alijarde MT, Sanchez A, Ramon y Cajal S, DeFelipe J. Inhibitory neurons in the human epileptogenic temporal neocortex. An immunocytochemical study. Brain. 1996; 119(Pt 4):1327-1347. DOI: 10.1093/brain/119.4.1327

[73] Spreafico R, Battaglia G, Arcelli P, Andermann F, Dubeau F, Palmini A, Olivier A, Villemure JG, Tampieri D, Avanzini G, et al. Cortical dysplasia: an immunocytochemical study of three patients. Neurology. 1998; 50:27-36. DOI: 10.1212/wnl.50.1.27

[74] Annelie Handreck, Bianca Backofen-Wehrhahn, Sonja Bröer, Wolfgang Löscher, Manuela Gernert Anticonvulsant Effects by Bilateral and Unilateral Transplantation of GABA-Producing Cells Into the Subthalamic Nucleus in an Acute Seizure Model. Cell Transplant. 2014; 23(1):111-32. DOI: 10.3727/096368912X658944

[75] Miles Cunningham, Jun-Hyeong Cho, Amanda Leung, George Savvidis, Sandra Ahn. hPSC-Derived Maturing GABAergic Interneurons Ameliorate Seizures and Abnormal Behavior in Epileptic Mice. Cell Stem Cell. 2014; 15(5):559-73. DOI: 10.1016/j.stem.2014.10.006

[76] Shetty AK, Turner DA. Fetal hippocampal CA3 cell transplants restore host hippocampal GAD-positive interneuron numbers in a rat model of TLE. J Neurosci. 2000;20:8788-8801.DOI: 10.1523/JNEUROSCI.20-23-08788.2000

[77] Hattiangady B, Rao MS, Shetty AK. Chronic temporal lobe epilepsy is associated with severely diminished dentate neurogenesis in the adult hippocampus. Neurobiol Dis. 2004;17:473-490. DOI: 10.1016/j.nbd.2004.08.008

[78] Hattiangady B, Shetty AK. Decreased neuronal differentiation of newly generated cells underlies reduced hippocampal neurogenesis in chronic temporal lobe epilepsy. Hippocampus. 2010;20:97-112. DOI: 10.1002/hipo.20594